The Doctor of Nursing Practice Scholarly Project
A Framework for Success

SECOND EDITION

EDITED BY

Katherine Moran, DNP, RN, CDE, FAADE
McAuley School of Nursing
University of Detroit Mercy
My Self-Management Team, Inc.
Detroit, Michigan

Rosanne Burson, DNP, ACNS-BC, CDE, FAADE
McAuley School of Nursing
University of Detroit Mercy
My Self-Management Team, Inc.
Detroit, Michigan

Dianne Conrad, DNP, RN, FNP-BC, CDE, FNAP
Kirkhof College of Nursing
Grand Valley State University
Grand Rapids, Michigan
Cadillac Family Physicians, PC
Cadillac, Michigan

D0962457

JONES & BARTL
LEARNING

World Headquarters
Jones & Bartlett Learning
5 Wall Street
Burlington, MA 01803
978-443-5000
info@jblearning.com
www.jblearning.com

Jones & Bartlett Learning books and products are available through most bookstores and online booksellers.
To contact Jones & Bartlett Learning directly, call 800-832-0034, fax 978-443-8000, or visit our website,
www.jblearning.com.

Substantial discounts on bulk quantities of Jones & Bartlett Learning publications are available to corporations, professional associations, and other qualified organizations. For details and specific discount information, contact the special sales department at Jones & Bartlett Learning via the above contact information or send an email to specialsales@jblearning.com.

Production Credits
VP, Executive Publisher: David D. Cella
Executive Editor: Amanda Martin
Associate Acquisitions Editor: Rebecca Myrick
Editorial Assistant: Lauren Vaughn
Senior Production Editor: Amanda Clerkin
Senior Marketing Manager: Jennifer Scherzay
Project Fulfillment Manager: Wendy Kilborn

Composition: S4Carlisle Publishing Services
Cover Design: Kristin E. Parker
Rights & Media Specialist: Wes DeShano
Media Development Editor: Troy Liston
Cover Image: © totally out/Shutterstock
Printing and Binding: Edwards Brothers Malloy
Cover Printing: Edwards Brothers Malloy

Library of Congress Cataloging-in-Publication Data
Names: Moran, Katherine J., 1959- , editor. | Burson, Rosanne, 1957- , editor. | Conrad, Dianne, 1956- , editor.
Title: The doctor of nursing practice scholarly project : a framework for success / edited by Katherine Moran,
  Rosanne Burson, Dianne Conrad.
Description: Second edition. | Burlington, Massachusetts : Jones & Bartlett Learning, [2017] | Includes bibliographical
  references and index.
Identifiers: LCCN 2015045331 | ISBN 9781284079685
Subjects: | MESH: Advanced Practice Nursing--education--United States. | Education, Nursing,
  Graduate--United States. | Nursing Research--education--United States. | Program Development--United States.
Classification: LCC RT75 | NLM WY 18.5 | DDC 610.73071/1--dc23 LC
record available at http://lccn.loc.gov/2015045331

6048

Printed in the United States of America
20 19 18 17   10 9 8 7 6 5 4 3

Dedication

Katherine Moran

In dedication to my family . . . my husband Dave for always believing in me; my parents, James and Margaret Porrett, for their valuable life lessons; my son David, daughter-in-law Amy, daughter Nicole and son-in-law Steven for continuing to inspire me; my sisters Lori and Lisa for their unwavering support; and my grandchildren Caleb, Ana, Ayla, Ella, and Connor for the *absolute joy* that they have brought to my life . . . I am blessed.

Rosanne Burson

This book is dedicated to my husband Steve, who has supported every endeavor along the way. Thank you for being an exemplary partner for every facet of our life and a wonderful role model for our children, Lisa and Schuyler. Special thanks to my parents, Bev and Don, for always encouraging and believing in me.

Dianne Conrad

I dedicate this book to my husband and lifelong partner, Alan J. Conrad, MD. He has always valued higher education and has encouraged me, as well as our sons, Paul and Mark, to prepare for our respective professions. He has made it possible and walked alongside me as I pursued each nursing degree from diploma to DNP. He is my mentor and collaborator in exemplifying the art and science of excellence in providing primary health care.

I also dedicate this book to my parents, Daniel and Carol Koval, who provided the foundation of instilling the values of hard work, dedication, and perseverance, as well as encouragement throughout my lifetime.

Contents

Acknowledgments   xi

Contributors   xiii

Foreword   xv

Preface   xix

Purpose   xxi

Section I   **The Doctor of Nursing Practice Degree   1**

Chapter 1   **Setting the Stage for the Doctor of Nursing Practice
                    Scholarly Project   3**
                    Katherine Moran
                        Taking the Journey   4
                        The Purpose of the Scholarly Project   6
                        Chapters at a Glance   8
                        Summary   13

Chapter 2   **The Journey to the Doctor of Nursing Practice Degree   15**
                    Donna Behler McArthur
                        Evolution of the DNP Degree   16
                        Acceleration of Movement to the DNP Degree   21
                        Challenges Moving Forward   22
                        Assessing Rigor   25
                        Opportunities for the Future   28
                        Making an Impact   30

Chapter 3   **Defining the Doctor of Nursing Practice:
                    Current Trends   35**
                    Dianne Conrad and Karen Kesten
                        Defining the Practice Doctorate in Nursing   36

Comparison of the DNP and PhD in Nursing   40
Current Trends in Doctoral Education   43
Reports Affecting DNP Education   44
Summary of Trends   54
Summary   55

Chapter 4   **Scholarship in Practice   59**
Rosanne Burson
What Is Scholarship?   60
History of Scholarship and Nursing Practice   61
Scholarship Evolution   62
Types of Scholarship   65
Practice Scholarship and Nursing Theory   67
What Is the Purpose of the DNP Project?   72
What Is the Potential Impact of the DNP Project?   76
What Qualifies as a DNP Project?   77
Current Views of the DNP Project   77
Scholarship Beyond the DNP Project   78
Recommendations   79

Section II   **The Scholarly Project   87**

Chapter 5   **The Phenomenon of Interest   89**
Katherine Moran and Rosanne Burson
The Expertise of Nursing Practice   90
Identifying the Phenomenon of Interest   92
Identification of a Problem/Concern   95
Using Nursing Theory to Explore
    a Phenomenon   97
Looking at a Phenomenon Through
    a Different Lens   100
Keeping Your Options Open   110

Chapter 6   **Developing the Scholarly Project   117**
Katherine Moran
Developing the DNP Project   118
Defining the Project Type   137

Chapter 7   **Interprofessional and Intraprofessional Collaboration
in the Scholarly Project   151**
Dianne Conrad
Gathering Resources for the DNP Project   152
Definitions   153

Components of Collaboration in the DNP Project:
Who, What, Where, When, and How 154
What Type of Information Is Needed? 160
Where and When Does Collaboration Take Place? 162
How to Accomplish a Successful Scholarly Project
Using Collaboration 163
Summary 167

Chapter 8   **The DNP Project Team 171**
Marisa L. Wilson, Shannon Reedy Idzik, and Dianne Conrad
Thesis, Dissertation, and the DNP Project 172
Choosing the DNP Project Faculty Mentor and Project
Team Members 174
Roles and Expectations of Project Team Members 176
Defining the Timeline for the DNP Project 177
Enhancing Team Productivity 178
Alternative Approaches to a Traditional Committee
for Project Supervision 181
Crediting the Project Team 184
Summary 184

Chapter 9   **Creating and Developing the Project Plan 189**
Rosanne Burson and Katherine Moran
Creation of Innovation 191
The DNP Project Plan 192
Appendix A 206
Appendix B 207
Appendix C 208
Collaborating with Content Experts 209
Institutional Review Board Approval 209
Submitting for Grant Support 212
Preparing for Implementation of the DNP Project 213

Chapter 10   **Driving the Practicum to Impact
the Scholarly Project 223**
Rosanne Burson
Practicum Purpose 224
Identifying the Setting 225
Matching Student Competency with Project Needs 227
Site Agreements 230
Practicum Hours 230
Choosing a Mentor 231
Developing Objectives for the Practicum 238

Practicum Deliverables   240
Presenting the Practicum Plan   242
Implementing the Practicum   243
Practicum Evaluation—Were the Objectives Met?   244
Setting the Stage for the DNP Project   244
Closing Out the Practicum   244

Chapter 11   The Proposal   247
Katherine Moran
Professional Writing   248
Writing the Proposal   251
Components of the Proposal   253
Project Design   260
Citing References   267
Appendices   267
Writing Tips   268

Chapter 12   The Scholarly Project Toolbox   287
Katherine Moran, Rosanne Burson, and Dianne Conrad
Utilizing the Toolbox   288
Summary   307

Chapter 13   Project Implementation   329
Katherine Moran and Rosanne Burson
The Implementation Process   330
What Constitutes Project Success?   332
Factors to Consider During Project Implementation   333

Section III   Doctor of Nursing Practice Outcomes   345

**Chapter 14   Aligning Design, Method, and Evaluation
with the Clinical Question   347**
Patricia Rouen
It Starts with Design   348
Diversity in DNP Projects   356
Driven by Design: Data Collection Methods   357
Resources for Data Collection:
    Registries and Surveys   362
It Takes a Team: Data Collection   363
Data Management   364
Data Entry   365
Data Analysis   366
Telling the Story   368

Chapter 15   **Disseminating the Results   375**
             Rosanne Burson
                 What Are the Deliverables?   376
                 Public Presentations   377
                 Portfolios   381
                 Written Manuscript   382
                 Tips for Successful Journal Submission   382

Chapter 16   **The Rest of the Story—Evaluating the Doctor
             of Nursing Practice   397**
             Dianne Conrad and David G. Campbell-O'Dell
                 The DNP: Continuous Quality Improvement of the
                     Degree, DNP Graduate Practice, and the Impact
                     on Outcomes   399
                 Structure—DNP Education   399
                 Process—Healthcare Delivery by the DNP   410
                 Outcomes—The Impact of the DNP-Prepared Nurse
                     on Patients, Systems, Populations, and Policy   412
                 The Impact of the DNP Graduate in Practice   418
                 Summary   422

             Index   425

Acknowledgments

Our heartfelt thanks go out to the DNP faculty at Madonna University who were there when we started our DNP journey. Your vision, encouragement, and continued support provided us with a wonderful foundation for which we are most grateful. We extend our gratitude to Amanda J. Martin, Jones & Bartlett Learning Executive Editor, for recognizing the value of this project; Rebecca Myrick, Associate Acquisitions Editor, Nursing; Lauren Vaughn, Editorial Assistant, Nursing; and Amanda Clerkin, Senior Production Editor for guidance in completing this project. Finally, we thank Lisa Merriman for enriching our book with her artistic contribution and Evelyn Clingerman, PhD, CNE, RN, FNAP for support and contributions to our scholarship team.

Contributors

Rosanne Burson, DNP, ACNS-BC, CDE, FAADE
DNP Program Coordinator
McAuley School of Nursing
University of Detroit Mercy
My Self-Management Team, Inc.
Detroit, Michigan

Evelyn Clingerman, PhD, CNE, RN, FNAP
Executive Director
The Bonnie Wesorick Center for Health Care Transformation
Kirkhof College of Nursing
Grand Valley State University
Grand Rapids, Michigan

Dianne Conrad, DNP, RN, FNP-BC, CDE, FNAP
Kirkhof College of Nursing
Grand Valley State University
Grand Rapids, Michigan
Cadillac Family Physicians, PC
Cadillac, Michigan

Shannon Reedy Idzik, DNP, CRNP, FAANP
Associate Professor
Associate Dean, Doctor of Nursing Practice Program
University of Maryland School of Nursing
Baltimore, Maryland

Karen Kesten, DNP, APRN, CCRN, PCCN, CCNS, CNE
Director of Educational Innovations
American Association of Colleges of Nursing
Washington, DC

Donna Behler McArthur, PhD, FNP-BC, FAANP
Clinical Professor, University of Arizona, College of Nursing
Clinical Professor, Department of Neurology, College of Medicine
Tucson, Arizona

Katherine Moran, DNP, RN, CDE, FAADE
Assistant Professor
McAuley School of Nursing
College of Health Professions
University of Detroit Mercy
My Self-Management Team, Inc.
Detroit, Michigan

David G. Campbell-O'Dell, DNP, ARNP, FNP-BC
Doctors of Nursing Practice, Inc.
Key West, Florida

Patricia Rouen, PhD, FNP-BC
Associate Professor
McAuley School of Nursing
College of Health Professions
University of Detroit Mercy
Detroit, Michigan

Melissa Willmarth-Stec, DNP, APRN, CNM, FACNM
Associate Professor of Clinical
    Nursing, Director, DNP Program
University of Cincinnati College of
    Nursing
Cincinnati, Ohio

Marisa L. Wilson, DNSc, MHSc, RN-BC, CPHIMS
Associate Professor
University of Alabama at Birmingham
Birmingham, Alabama

Foreword

Lisa Chism, DNP, GNP, BC, NCMP, FAANP

In 1999, the Institute of Medicine (IOM) published a report, *To Err Is Human: Building a Safer Health System.* This report summarized the errors made in health care and estimated the cost of these errors to be between $17 billion and $29 billion per year in hospitals nationwide (Kohn, Corrigan, & Donaldson, 1999). This publication was the catalyst for a substantial shift in the education and preparation of healthcare providers that has dramatically shaped the future direction of nursing education.

In response to this report, the publication *Crossing the Quality Chasm: A New Health System for the 21st Century* was released by the IOM in 2001. This publication focused on how the health system may be reinvented to foster innovation and improve the delivery of care. To assist in achieving this goal, *Health Professions Education: A Bridge to Quality* was published in 2003 (Greiner & Knebel, 2003). This report was instrumental in shaping the recommendations for educating *all* healthcare professionals. Further, *Health Professions Education: A Bridge to Quality* summarized for educators and accreditation, licensing, and certification organizations specific competencies that all healthcare students and professionals should develop and maintain:

- Delivering patient-centered care
- Working as part of interdisciplinary teams
- Practicing evidence-based medicine
- Focusing on quality improvement
- Using information technology (Greiner & Knebel, 2003)

In addition, a report released by the IOM in 2010, *The Future of Nursing: Leading Change, Advancing Health,* recommended that:

- Nurses should practice to the full extent of their education and training.
- Nurses should achieve higher levels of education and training through an improved education system that promotes seamless academic progression.
- Nurses should be full partners, with physicians and other healthcare professionals, in redesigning health care in the United States.
- Effective workforce planning and policy making require better data collection and information infrastructure (IOM, 2010).

To achieve the recommendations of the IOM, it was also recommended that the number of doctorally prepared nurses (practice and research-focused) be doubled by the year 2020 (IOM, 2010).

Nursing responded to the recommendations set forth by the IOM. Dialogue began in 2002 among nursing leaders, healthcare organization leaders, and stakeholders that focused on nursing's response to the immediate needs of healthcare and nursing education. In 2004, the American Association of Colleges of Nursing (AACN) exhibited true innovation and assigned a task force to develop a new practice doctorate in nursing. This task force resulted in the development and approval of the *Position Statement on the Practice Doctorate in Nursing* (AACN, 2004). This position statement formalized the doctor of nursing practice (DNP) degree as the highest level of preparation for nursing practice, as well as a transition to doctoral-level preparation from traditional master's-level preparation for advanced nursing practice. The year 2015 was also set as the target date to complete this transition.

As a result of the recommendations of this task force, AACN published *The Essentials of Doctoral Education for Advanced Nursing Practice* (AACN, 2006). These essentials are reflective of the IOM's recommended competencies for all healthcare students and professionals and are the curriculum standards for the DNP degree.

Through the innovation and leadership exhibited by the AACN, the DNP degree finally took shape. The DNP degree, focusing *on practice,* was developed and instituted a dramatic transition in nursing education. This transition continues as more DNP degree programs are developed and more students enroll.

The Essentials of Doctoral Education for Advanced Nursing Practice (AACN, 2006) have shaped the curriculum standards of DNP programs and are consistent with the recommendations of the IOM. Within the curriculum standards, a scholarly project is required of all graduates of DNP programs, and this is perhaps the most daunting requirement for many students. Traditionally, there has been a lack of clarity as to what a scholarly project for a DNP program should include. Consistent themes of DNP project requirements include rigor, the translation of research into practice, and the application of knowledge. The AACN (2006) summarized that "the final DNP project produce a tangible and deliverable academic product that is derived from the practice immersion experience and is reviewed and evaluated by an academic committee" (p. 20). Further, the AACN relates that the final DNP project "documents outcomes of the student's educational experiences, provides a measurable medium for evaluating the immersion experience, and summarizes the student's growth in knowledge and expertise . . . (and) serves as a foundation for future scholarly practice" (AACN, 2006, p. 20).

However, as stated in the preface of this book, there truly is a paucity of information available on the specifics of the DNP project. Therefore, this very timely publication has filled a void regarding all aspects of the DNP project. Students from all DNP programs have benefited from this clear, concise, and inclusive text.

This comprehensive guide not only provides a context for the DNP project but also takes the reader on a journey that begins with selecting a phenomenon of interest, the development of a project plan, and finally the culmination and evaluation of the scholarly project. This unique and innovative text thoughtfully describes a *process* designed to help the DNP student succeed in completing a meaningful DNP project. A unique feature of this text is the lived experiences of DNP graduates included in each chapter, which have been updated in this edition. These exemplars provide valuable insights regarding how the scholarly project serves as DNP students' foundation for continued scholarship and contributions to nursing and health care.

The second edition of this valuable resource is also updated to include new reports that demonstrate trends in DNP education, curriculum, and the DNP project. New content in this edition also addresses the importance of completing an organizational assessment regarding the scholarly project within the context of the organization. This added dimension will enhance project implementation, organizational change, and sustainability. To further elucidate the importance of a DNP project's implementation, a section describing implementation science was also added. In addition, "Tips" on scholarly writing were included as a guide to assist DNP students with the challenges of writing on a graduate level. Written and edited by DNP graduates, this updated text is a wonderful resource and exemplar of how DNP graduates are shaping health care and nursing education. The commitment and dedication to transform and improve health care is clearly evidenced by the valuable contributions of DNP graduates in all practice arenas.

REFERENCES

American Association of Colleges of Nursing. (2004). *Position statement on the practice doctorate in nursing.* Retrieved from http://www.aacn.nche.edu/publications/position/DNPpositionstatement.pdf

American Association of Colleges of Nursing. (2006). *The essentials of doctoral education for advanced nursing practice.* Retrieved from http://www.aacn.nche.edu/publications/position/DNPEssentials.pdf

Greiner, A. C., & Knebel, E. (Eds.). (2003). *Health professions education: A bridge to quality.* Washington, DC: National Academies Press.

Institute of Medicine. (2001). *Crossing the quality chasm: A new health system for the 21st century.* Washington, DC: National Academies Press.

Institute of Medicine. (2010). *The future of nursing: Leading change, advancing health.* Retrieved from http://www.iom.edu/Reports/2010/The-Future-of-Nursing-Leading-Change-Advancing-Health/Report-Brief-Education.aspx

Kohn, L. T., Corrigan, J. M., & Donaldson, M. S. (Eds.). (1999). *To err is human: Building a safer health system.* Committee on Quality of Health Care in America, Institute of Medicine. Washington, DC: National Academy Press.

Preface

Healthcare reform has been on the minds of many individuals across the United States since the introduction of the Patient Protection and Affordable Care Act in March 2010. As decisions are made about implementing reform, it is important to thoughtfully consider how we as a nation will meet the healthcare needs of the people. Regardless of the outcome, it is clear that the availability of highly educated nurses to care for individuals is imperative to the health of our nation.

The Institute of Medicine (IOM) and the Robert Wood Johnson Foundation (RWJF) have recognized the need to strengthen the largest component of the healthcare workforce—nurses—to become partners and leaders in improving the delivery of care and the healthcare system as a whole (IOM, 2010, p. ix). Both the IOM and RWJF agree that accessible, high-quality care cannot be achieved without exceptional nursing care/leadership and, as such, have partnered in creating the RWJF Initiative on the Future of Nursing to explore challenges central to the future of the nursing profession (IOM, 2010, p. ix). Two specific recommendations coming from this report that are relevant involve (1) ensuring nurses achieve higher levels of education and training and (2) ensuring nurses become full partners with physicians and other healthcare professionals in redesigning health care.

In 2004, the American Association of Colleges of Nursing recognized the need to develop nurses as healthcare leaders and subsequently released a position statement advocating that by 2015 a doctor of nursing practice (DNP) degree be required for advanced practice nurses. Since that time, schools of nursing across the nation have introduced this terminal degree into their respective programs (American Association of Colleges of Nursing, 2011).

One universal requirement for any DNP candidate, regardless of the institution attended, is the successful completion of a DNP project that uses evidence-based practice (EBP) for improved delivery of care, patient outcomes, and clinical systems management (AACN, 2004). The requirements for the DNP project are similar to the dissertation requirement for the PhD candidate insofar as both require rigorous scholarly work. The difference is in the focus; for the PhD candidate, the focus is generally on knowledge generation and discovery, whereas the focus for the DNP student is to apply this knowledge in some meaningful way to ultimately serve the needs of society. As mentioned in Chapter 4, Scholarship in Practice, both types of scholars contribute to knowledge generation and are interdependent to fully impact health.

Unfortunately, there is a paucity of comprehensive resources available to guide students in completing the DNP project. Therefore, there is a need for a book that not only explores the journey the student embarks on when completing scholarly work but also a book that provides a framework for success. For these reasons, this book was designed and written by advanced practice nurses who have an earned DNP degree especially for nurses working toward that end.

Some of the unique features of this book include clearly identified learning objectives at the beginning of each chapter, multiple examples to help illustrate key points, as well as significant features that are highlighted for easy reference. Where applicable, chapters conclude with key messages and an action plan to help the student through the DNP project development and implementation process.

The authors are proud to include work from DNP scholars across the country that is highlighted in various chapters throughout the book. There is also a chapter dedicated specifically to tools and templates that the DNP student may find useful when embarking on the project process. The authors include an example of a published project manuscript in the appendix after Chapter 15 to encourage students to disseminate their work for the good of nursing and the health of our nation. Ultimately, this book is a demonstration of intraprofessional collaboration of DNP-prepared nurses with PhD and doctor of nursing science (DNSc) colleagues as contributing authors, to produce a resource for enhancing the nursing profession.

REFERENCES

American Association of Colleges of Nursing. (2004). *Position statement on the practice doctorate in nursing.* Retrieved from http://www.aacn.nche.edu/publications/position/DNPpositionstatement.pdf

American Association of Colleges of Nursing. (2011). *Fact sheet: The doctor of nursing practice.* Retrieved from http://www.aacn.nche.edu/media-relations/fact-sheets/dnp

Institute of Medicine. (2010). *The future of nursing: Leading change, advancing health.* Washington, DC: The National Academies Press.

Purpose

The purpose of this book is to provide a road map for DNP students to use on their journey from project conception through completion and dissemination. The goal is to introduce a *process* that will enable DNP students to work through their project in a more effective, efficient manner and will assist in resolving the current variability of scholarly projects within DNP programs around the country. This book is not intended to be prescriptive. Rather, it was developed from a broad, inclusive perspective to address the varying needs of DNP students across the country. The authors hope that it will be useful for practical application and that it gives a framework for the scholarly work process.

This book will also serve as an aid to assist faculty who are mentoring, counseling, or coaching students on the process of completing DNP scholarly work. Finally, this resource will assist preceptors and mentors of DNP students in health organizations as many DNP projects are completed within these systems.

The Doctor of Nursing Practice Degree

CHAPTER 1

Setting the Stage for the Doctor of Nursing Practice Scholarly Project

Katherine Moran

CHAPTER OVERVIEW

The purpose of this chapter is to help the student recognize the value of doctoral education and the practice doctorate and understand the significance of the doctor of nursing practice (DNP) project. This will be accomplished by introducing the student to concepts that will be discussed throughout this textbook and by highlighting a framework that students can use to complete the scholarly project, which reflects attainment of the DNP *Essentials*.

CHAPTER OBJECTIVES

After completing the chapter, the learner will be able to:
1. Describe the DNP scholar
2. Conceptualize the evolutionary nature of the scholarly project
3. Discern the purpose of the DNP project

TAKING THE JOURNEY

It is well known that the healthcare needs of our nation are becoming more complex, the cost of health care is increasing, and the quality of health care is being questioned. Many Americans are concerned about how these issues will be resolved. Recognizing these challenges, two reports were released from the Institute of Medicine, *Crossing the Quality Chasm* and the *Future of Nursing*, making an urgent call for fundamental change in healthcare delivery.

In many ways, the DNP degree was designed to help meet these and other challenges within health care. The DNP possesses *advanced competencies* for increasingly complex clinical, faculty, and leadership roles; enhanced *knowledge* to improve nursing practice and patient outcomes; and enhanced *leadership* skills to strengthen practice and healthcare delivery; in addition, the DNP gives nursing parity with other health professions, most of which have a doctorate as the credential required for practice (American Association of Colleges of Nursing [AACN], 2004). In essence, DNP-prepared nurses have been called to lead and manage collaborative efforts with other healthcare practitioners to improve health care.

> The decision to enter a DNP program marks the beginning of what will become a *transformative experience* for many students.

It should be no surprise, then, that the decision to enter a DNP program marks the beginning of what will become a *transformative experience* for many students. The program is both challenging and rewarding. Through the process of personal development, one begins to recognize the need to view the world through multiple lenses, to continue the quest for new nursing knowledge, to apply that knowledge in a practice setting in a meaningful way, and to collaborate with other healthcare practitioners to meet the ever increasing and complex healthcare needs of the nation. It is a journey where the student travels conceptually from one place in his or her clinical practice to a new place in practice. The insight gleaned through the process gives the student a new frame of reference to continue to build a more comprehensive understanding of nursing praxis, which will ultimately benefit nursing as a profession and society as a whole.

It is important to recognize that the DNP degree is in a state of evolution and that *all DNP-prepared nurses need to influence the outcome*. The practice doctorate must demonstrate through knowledge synthesis, skill refinement, and the completion of the DNP project that they are prepared for doctoral nursing practice. DNP-prepared nurses will need to continue to make a concerted effort to demonstrate those nursing-specific improved healthcare outcomes that establish the value of the practice doctorate and elevate the science-based *practice* of the nursing profession. Only then will society begin to see the impact of practice scholarship and, therefore, the associated benefit of the practice doctorate.

Soon after the student begins the doctoral program, he or she will begin the work on the final program deliverable: the DNP project. Each doctoral-level course provides an opportunity for the student to gain new knowledge that will help him or her complete the project. Through this journey, the student may refine original project ideas, or the student may end up going in an entirely new direction. Be assured that this is part of the process. In the end, the scholarly project will be a carefully selected project that not only meets program requirements but also fulfills the student's professional goals, the organization's goals (where the project is implemented), and contributes to the overall goals of the DNP-prepared nurse as a healthcare professional: to *positively influence health care now and in the future.*

After graduating from a DNP program and completing a scholarly project as a final deliverable to prepare us as practice scholars, the authors want to share their experience and personal insights regarding the topic of the DNP project. Our hopes are to help future DNP students on their journey, to be a guide on the side that lends a helping hand when needed. The goal of this textbook is to give the student a frame of reference when embarking on the DNP project. However, because there are virtually limitless DNP project ideas being developed, it is impossible to speak to the needs of each of these specifically. Therefore, this textbook was designed to include the potential requirements for the most comprehensive project even though some DNP projects may not require such detail. This is not meant to suggest that all projects should mirror the examples provided; rather, this text is intended to be a reference or a framework that allows the student to choose items that will help inform his or her project and challenges the student to consider new perspectives that foster creativity and the development of innovative ideas. At the same time, it is our hope that doctoral nursing educators, team members, and other healthcare professionals interfacing with DNP students find this textbook helpful when guiding the DNP student through the scholarly project process.

Developing the DNP project is not a linear process; it is created through a series of explorations that result in a comprehensive, well-thought-out project plan. As such, the student should recognize that

> Developing the DNP project is not a linear process; it is created through a series of explorations that result in a comprehensive, well-thought-out project plan.

although the topics in this textbook are presented in a stepwise framework to help him or her through the process, some of the work may occur simultaneously because of the evolutionary nature of the project.

Many different DNP programs are available across the United States. All of the programs meet the needs of the community they serve; however, they may accomplish this via different methods. As a result, *program structures will vary*; some may include a formal DNP project team while others may use a completely different approach. For example, some universities may use a model that requires only one faculty advisor who guides the DNP student through the process, while others may use a dyad approach that includes one faculty member from the university and one representative from the community. The same is true regarding the final program deliverable requirements. In an attempt to better understand the characteristics of these programs, the authors have collaborated with many individuals either providing DNP education in programs throughout the United States or informing DNP education, such as the American Association of Colleges of Nursing (AACN), to better understand the needs of DNP students, faculty, and others working with students to complete the DNP project. We have learned that DNP education and the recommended requirements of DNP projects and teams are continuing to evolve (see Chapter 3, Defining the Doctor of Nursing Practice: Current Trends). Recognizing this, the authors sought to meet the various scholarly requirement needs of these programs by providing a wide variety of options and perspectives for the student to consider and reference where applicable. While there are many examples, templates, and other formats provided as tools for the journey, the intent is to give the student options, not be directive.

THE PURPOSE OF THE SCHOLARLY PROJECT

A debate has been ongoing for many years regarding what one should consider as *scholarship*, especially in academe. Many learned individuals have weighed in on this debate over the years, including Ernest L. Boyer, a well-known educator who at one point served as the United States Commissioner on Education. In 1990, Boyer, then president of the Carnegie Foundation for Advancement of Teaching, suggested that for "America's colleges and universities to remain vital a new vision of scholarship is required" (Boyer, 1990, p. 13). It is clear that the scholarship debate began long before the DNP degree; however, since the introduction of this degree, the discussion has shifted to include *practice scholarship*.

In an effort to contribute to the richness of this dialogue, a discussion regarding the evolving scholarship of practice is provided in Chapter 4, Scholarship in Practice.

> A *scholar* is a learned person, who is specialized in an area of knowledge; one who has gained mastery in a particular discipline ("Scholar," 2015).

For the purposes of introduction to the DNP project, though, it is important to recognize, from a very literal sense, that the term *scholar* is defined as a learned person, who is specialized in an area of knowledge; one who has gained mastery in a particular discipline ("Scholar," 2015). Taking this definition and applying it to the DNP project helps one recognize that this project provides the student with a vehicle through which he or she can demonstrate advanced knowledge in a particular area. This is in alignment with AACN, which believes that the final DNP project should demonstrate "synthesis of the student's work" and that it should lay the groundwork for future scholarship (2006, p. 20). Certainly, the project should demonstrate the student's achievement of the eight DNP *Essentials of Doctoral Education* for advanced nursing practice, as outlined by the AACN. A detailed discussion regarding these competencies and current trends in DNP education is provided in Chapter 3.

It should be clear that the DNP project is many things: a required program deliverable, the demonstration of doctoral competencies, and a means to achieve professional goals as well as the goals of the organization where the project is implemented; in addition, it is hoped that the project is only the beginning of many future scholarly contributions by the DNP-prepared nurse that lead to improvement in health care and add to nursing knowledge. Therefore, the DNP project plays a very important role in doctoral education; it affords the DNP student an opportunity to *launch into scholarly practice*.

> The DNP project plays a very important role in doctoral education; it affords the DNP student an opportunity to launch into scholarly practice.

The DNP-prepared nurse will have many opportunities to transcend current barriers and positively impact health care in the United States as we know it today—to build a bridge between research and practice, as well as between theory and practice. These are indeed exciting times!

In many ways, the creation of this textbook is an example of DNP scholarly work. The authors collaborated with thought leaders in the field, demonstrating the skills attained in Essential VI: *interprofessional collaboration for improving patient and population health outcomes*. Then, using the skills garnered in DNP Essential III: *clinical scholarship and analytical methods for evidence-based practice*, the authors reviewed the current literature and resources available for students on this topic. The authors also collaborated with other practice experts across the United States, considered their personal experiences as DNP graduates, and determined that a resource designated specifically for the completion of the DNP project would be a useful resource for DNP students, DNP faculty, and members of healthcare organizations.

In essence, the authors formed a *scholarship team* and worked together to meet the perceived needs of DNP students in programs throughout the country to provide the final deliverable, which correlates with DNP Essential VIII: *advanced nursing practice*.

CHAPTERS AT A GLANCE

The reader will note that each chapter begins with an image of Greek Ionic style columns that symbolize the cumulative doctoral work and overall achievement of the DNP student. The columns represent the eight DNP Essentials and corresponding knowledge and skills that are developed or strengthened by completing a practice doctorate program. Finally, the *capstone* that rests on the top of the structure represents the highest point of achievement, when the student successfully completes the final doctoral project.

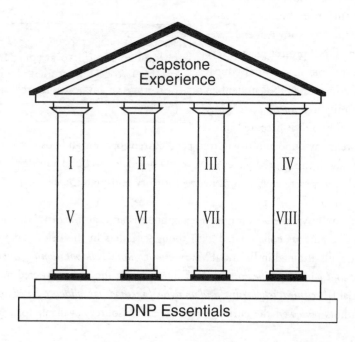

The DNP Essentials are referenced in each chapter where they apply to the chapter discussion. As mentioned in the preface, the student will also note that significant points of the discussion are highlighted in *boxes* throughout the chapter, and *key messages* are reiterated at the end of each chapter. To facilitate learning and to help move the student along in the development of the DNP project, each chapter begins with learning objectives and concludes with an action plan and *helpful resources* (where applicable).

Section I: The Doctor of Nursing Practice Degree

Every good framework begins with a solid foundation. To that end, the focus of the first section of this textbook is providing an overview of the DNP degree that includes the history leading to the degree, the purpose of the degree, and the current trends, as well as defining the purpose of the DNP project and the current view of potential projects. The student is reminded that both the practice- and research-based doctorate will need to collaborate to impact nursing and health care and that the collaboration between the two doctoral levels of preparation will determine the future of nursing and its impact on health care.

The goal of this section is to help the student develop an understanding of scholarship as it relates to the practice doctorate, to conceptualize the types of projects that can be and are being considered by DNP students in programs across the United States, to examine potential topics of interest in relation to the appropriate level of scholarship, and recognize the ultimate significance of the DNP project—*to validate the effectiveness of the DNP-prepared nurse.*

Section II: The Scholarly Project

Section II is devoted to guiding the reader through the DNP project process. The complex nature of nursing practice is discussed, as well as how practice provides many opportunities to explore nursing phenomena. The student is introduced to a variety of strategies to help him or her select a phenomenon of interest and to explore the topic comprehensively. The value of identifying a project that will lead to an improvement in clinical practice is stressed. Further, the DNP student is introduced to elements of a scholarly project that need to be considered early in the development phase, including conducting a literature search, writing a literature review to support the value and/or the need to study the phenomenon of interest, performing a needs assessment, formulating a problem statement, defining the project goal and project scope, and developing a project framework.

Nationally, nurses are being called to actively collaborate within interprofessional teams to improve quality, cost-effective, and efficient care and improve outcomes (Institute of Medicine, 2003). Therefore, another focus of this section is to help the student understand that (1) the DNP project provides him or her with an opportunity to attain and refine the competencies needed for collaborative team participation and leadership; (2) the DNP student will need additional resources to assist in assessing, planning, implementing, and evaluating the DNP project; and (3) this is best achieved through collaboration.

The student is guided through these and other processes that influence the development and implementation of the DNP project by the faculty mentor and/or project team. Therefore, the composition and roles of the project team, including the faculty mentor and other members, are reviewed. This information is important because project team dynamics, including making the most of team meetings and resources to form a cohesive and collegial team that will work together, is vital to the student's success in completing the DNP project.

Another important component of project development is the project plan. A broad overview of points to consider when preparing for project implementation is provided, such as taking into consideration the client and personnel, monitoring requirements, problem solving/troubleshooting demands, the need to communicate with key stakeholders, and the characteristics and skill set of effective leaders. Samples of a variety of tools are provided for the student to use throughout the scholarly project development and implementation cycle to help ensure a successful outcome. Further, the value of the practicum is stressed in this section to help the student recognize (1) how the experience will support the development of DNP competencies and professional scholarly growth and (2) the potential to use the practicum in preparation for implementation of the DNP project. The project plan provided as an example is fairly detailed to capture the elements needed in a complex or comprehensive project. However, the student is reminded that *all the elements presented may not be applicable to every potential project.*

Finally, this section concludes with a discussion regarding how the DNP project proposal represents the student's intellectual ability, knowledge in the subject area, and contributions to nursing. To help the student with the proposal writing process, information is provided to (1) help the student recognize early in the process when he or she may need some additional writing support, (2) introduce the student to the components included in a sample project proposal, and (3) provide a reference for writing the DNP project proposal.

Section III: Doctor of Nursing Practice Outcomes

The last section of this textbook, Section III, concludes by reaffirming the importance of the DNP project and the need to disseminate the results. A review of the various approaches used to obtain data and the methods used to work with the data received is provided. Various formats for disseminating the results are reviewed, such as public presentation, a defense of the project, a written manuscript for the university, and a manuscript submission to a scholarly journal. To this point, valuable insight is offered from several journal editors who share their advice on how to successfully submit a manuscript for publication. The importance of communicating and disseminating the results of the DNP project is stressed not only because it may be a required program deliverable but also because of the knowledge translation that occurs; benefiting both nursing as a profession and, even more broadly, the health of our nation. The student is reminded that the scholarly project is a product of DNP education that reflects the attainment of knowledge and skills that launches the DNP graduate into scholarly practice. The point is made, however, that it is important to recognize the need to evaluate the outcomes of this doctoral degree in nursing for effectiveness in accomplishing the goals of improving the nursing profession and health care and meeting societal needs. Recognizing that this will be an important focus for the DNP, an evaluation strategy is proposed using a framework based on the Donabedian model, the gold standard for defining quality management.

Finally, in many of the chapters, there is an excerpt from the perspective of the DNP student regarding the topic of discussion in the specific chapter. For instance, in Chapter 5, The Phenomenon of Interest, the student shares her experience of narrowing the topic related to her clinical expertise, the societal need, data from the organization, and the evidence in the literature.

These examples are included to showcase aspects of the DNP project, to show the potential for the DNP scholarly project as a program deliverable, to provide evidence of healthcare transformation, and to illustrate the impact of the practice doctorate in nursing. Although it is evident that these projects certainly contribute to the health of individual populations, as a whole, they demonstrate that doctorally prepared nurses provide more than protection, promotion, and optimization of health and abilities; these nurses facilitate healing and wellness through human connection. DNP-prepared nurses are *demonstrating* their value to society through practice scholarship that improves healthcare outcomes. As a result of these efforts, society is beginning to see the impact of practice scholarship and the associated benefit of the practice doctorate.

The first excerpt, provided by Dr. Deonne Brown Benedict, focuses on her work as a nurse practitioner entrepreneur and the impact that a single nurse practitioner can make in meeting the needs of the community.

Nurse Practitioner Entrepreneurship
Deonne Brown Benedict, DNP, ARNP, FNP-BC

My DNP project was a three-pronged undertaking. It evaluated consumer perspectives on nurse practitioners (NPs), interviewed NP entrepreneurs to determine success factors for NP clinic ownership, and studied NP business knowledge. I also evaluated a variety of other local factors for clinic start-up. With these data, I was able to determine many of the components that lead to a successful clinic venture. After completing my DNP degree, I studied several potential clinic models, including free clinics and the "ideal medical practice model." These efforts culminated in the development of a unique hybrid model for my practice, allowing me to meet the needs of both insured clients and uninsured clients who may not be able to afford typical care. This clinic model does not require outside grant support but is able to serve the needs of insured, uninsured, and Medicaid clients, many of whom were previously not receiving adequate care. It also allows for longer visits, valuable time for establishing rapport, educating clients, and living out the philosophy and ideals of NPs.

In 2009, I opened a nurse-owned and managed clinic based on this low-overhead, high-tech, and high-touch model. The clinic paid off its start-up costs in several months and has provided me with a wonderful opportunity to serve my community while maintaining a rewarding job with a reasonable income. I no longer see 20–30 patients a day, but rather spend an hour with new patients and 30 minutes in follow-ups for chronic conditions. Patients love the "concierge" type care they receive (really just great NP care), and the paperless office and secure electronic communications make my job easier. I have used the knowledge I gained in the process to consult with NPs across the country with tips for getting their own practices started and have published and spoken to university NP students and NP groups in support of nurse entrepreneurship.

SUMMARY

The journey to the DNP degree may still be via a winding and rugged road; however, given the potential for DNP graduates to improve healthcare outcomes and to positively impact the nursing profession, these authors hope that more and more of our nursing colleagues recognize the value of doctoral education and join us on the journey. For the current DNP student, our hopes are that this textbook will provide a broad view of the scholarly project and shed light on the DNP project journey.

Finally, where healthcare reform is concerned, it is evident that the Institute of Medicine has recognized nurses as valuable players in this process. Therefore, it is time for nurses, especially DNP-prepared nurses, to see health care as something we shape—DNPs are called to lead and manage collaborative efforts with other healthcare practitioners to improve health care.

Do not go where the path may lead, go instead where there is no path and leave a trail.
                                                              —Ralph Waldo Emerson

Key Messages

- The decision to enter a DNP program marks the beginning of what will become a transformative experience for many students.
- Developing the scholarly project is not a linear process; it is created through a series of explorations that result in a comprehensive, well-thought-out project plan.
- The DNP project is a required program deliverable that demonstrates achievement of doctoral competencies and advanced knowledge in a particular area.
- The DNP project is a means to achieve professional goals and marks the beginning of many future scholarly contributions.

Action Plan—Next Steps

1. Consider the value of the DNP scholarly project.
2. Open the mind to a variety of potential project topics.
3. Take advantage of learning opportunities.
4. Enjoy the journey!

REFERENCES

American Association of Colleges of Nursing. (2004). *AACN position statement on the practice doctorate in nursing.* Retrieved from http://www.aacn.nche.edu/publications/position/DNPpositionstatement.pdf

American Association of Colleges of Nursing. (2006). *The essentials for doctoral education for advanced nursing practice.* Washington, DC: Author.

Boyer, E. (1990). *Scholarship reconsidered: Priorities of the professoriate.* The Carnegie Foundation for the Advancement of Teaching. New York, NY: John Wiley & Sons.

Institute of Medicine. (2003). *Health professions education: A bridge to quality.* Retrieved from http://www.nap.edu/openbook.php?record_id=10681&page=45

Scholar. (2015). *The Free Dictionary.* Retrieved from http://www.thefreedictionary.com/scholar

CHAPTER 2

The Journey to the Doctor of Nursing Practice Degree

Donna Behler McArthur

CHAPTER OVERVIEW

The doctor of nursing practice (DNP) degree represents the highest level of formal education for advanced nursing practice. This chapter describes the evolution of the DNP degree within the context of burgeoning knowledge, changes in healthcare delivery, escalating demands of chronic illness care, diverse patient populations, and globalization. Propelling forces from the Institute of Medicine (IOM) and the American Association of Colleges of Nursing (AACN) are described to include early adopters and national initiatives. Likewise, criticisms of the timing of DNP programs related to nurse practitioner (NP) capacity in the face of healthcare reform are related. While schools of nursing have made progress in transitioning to the DNP degree by 2015, facilitators and barriers related to this transition have been identified in a study conducted by the RAND Corporation, commissioned by the AACN board of directors (Auerbach et al., 2014). Challenges moving forward related to program variability, project designs, and assessing program rigor are recognized. A hallmark of the practice doctorate is a program of study that develops the practice expertise within the specialty as well as core knowledge regarding quality improvement initiatives.

EVOLUTION OF THE DNP DEGREE

Background for Change

Fueled by the rapid expansion of knowledge underpinning practice, complexity of patient care, national concerns about the quality of health care and patient safety, and shortages of nursing personnel and faculty, a higher level of education for advanced nursing practice leaders was realized prior to the turn of the 21st century. Several reports from the IOM underscored the need for an appropriately trained workforce to meet the challenges of the 21st

> Reports from the IOM underscored the need for an appropriately trained workforce to meet the challenges of the 21st century.

century: *To Err Is Human: Building a Safer Health System* (1999), *Crossing the Quality Chasm* (2001), and *Health Professions Education: A Bridge to Quality* (2003a). Core competencies for healthcare professionals were noted: (1) provide patient-centered care, (2) work in interdisciplinary teams, (3) employ evidence-based practice, (4) apply quality improvement, and (5) utilize informatics (IOM, 2003a). Given the dynamic nature of the science and evidence base in health care, innovative educational approaches were needed to teach advanced nursing practice students how to manage knowledge, use effective tools to support clinical decision making, and apply methodological rules to evaluate the evidence. I am sharing my perspective of the journey toward the DNP degree through the lens of a family nurse practitioner (FNP), educator, and former Director of two DNP programs—University of Arizona College of Nursing and Vanderbilt University School of Nursing (VUSN).

Advanced nursing practice is broadly defined by the AACN (2004) to include the administration of nursing and healthcare organizations and the development and implementation of health policy. Often referred to as "indirect" care,

> Advanced nursing practice includes the administration of nursing and healthcare organizations and the development and implementation of health policy (AACN, 2004).

this definition broadens the applicability of the DNP degree beyond advanced practice registered nurses (NPs, certified registered nurse anesthetists, clinical nurse specialists, and certified nurse midwives) to include master's-prepared nurse administrators, informatics nurse specialists, and health policy experts. Nursing education has not been included as a stand-alone advanced nursing practice specialty. Reflecting on the definition of advanced nursing practice, the IOM (2003b) called for nurse executives and managers to have educational preparation to ensure readiness to participate in executive leadership within healthcare organizations.

Early Adopters

The concept of a practice (or clinical) doctorate has been unfolding for over three decades (AACN, 2004). Case Western Reserve University is generally credited with beginning the first doctor of nursing (ND) program as an entry-level nursing degree in 1979. Graduates were prepared as generalist nurses with expanded skills and knowledge. In 1990, the ND program was changed from an entry-level program to a post-master's clinical doctorate (http://fpb.case.edu/DNP/history.shtm).

As of June 2015, there were 264 established DNP programs accepting students, with another 60 in the planning stages, representing 48 states and the District of Columbia (AACN, 2015a) (see **Figure 2-1**). Over 18,350 students attended these programs in 2014 with 3,065 having graduated (AACN, 2015b).

These numbers are striking considering that in 2003, there were four programs with active ND programs (Case Western Reserve University, Rush University, University of Colorado, University of South Carolina), one DNP program (University of Kentucky), and one doctor of nursing science (DNSc) program (University of Tennessee-Memphis). Several other schools were planning programs, most notably Columbia University (doctor of nursing practice [DrNP]) (Marion et al., 2003).

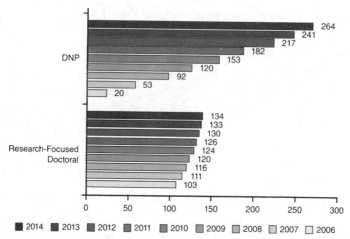

FIGURE 2-1 Represents doctoral nursing program growth from 2006–2014.

Although the ND and DrNP degrees share many of the components of the current DNP degree, confusion surrounded different designations. Hence, the determination was made by AACN to use one degree, the DNP.

National Initiatives

The NONPF Practice Doctorate Task Force was established in 2001 to explore issues surrounding the shift in academic preparation for NPs. Although research supports that advanced practice registered nurses (APRNs) provide safe, high-quality care in all specialties and practice sites (Brooten et al., 2010; Cragin & Kennedy, 2006; Mundinger et al., 2000; Newhouse et al., 2011; Pine, Holt, & Lou, 2003), APRNs are among the few healthcare professionals educated and then licensed as independent practitioners at the master's degree level rather than the doctoral degree level (others include pharmacists, medical doctors, dentists, psychologists, and audiologists). A seminal article supporting the development of the practice doctorate and its commitment to provide leadership in this initiative was authored by members of the NONPF task force (Marion et al., 2003). Encouraging nursing to adopt a shared vision to

> APRNs are among the few healthcare professionals educated and then licensed as independent practitioners at the master's degree level rather than the doctoral level.

move the practice doctorate forward, these nurse leaders reiterated the challenges for advanced nursing practice in the face of the need for expert clinical teachers, shifts in information technology, demographic changes, disparities in healthcare delivery and access, and stakeholder expectations. The practice doctorate, focusing on direct care of patient populations and leadership, would respond to the following: evaluating the evidence base for care, delivering the care, setting healthcare policy, and leading and managing clinical care units and healthcare systems.

The AACN board of directors took the lead in transforming APRN education and created an 11-member task force on the practice doctorate in nursing, with Dr. Betty Lenz, then dean of the School of Nursing at Ohio State University, as the chairperson. The charge put to the task force was to clarify the purpose of the professional clinical doctorate, especially core content and core competencies; describe trends over time in clinical doctoral education; assess the need for clinically focused doctoral programs; identify preferred goals, titles, outcomes, and resources; discuss the elements of a unified approach versus a diverse approach; determine the potential implications for advanced practice nursing; make recommendations regarding related issues and resources; and describe potential for various tracks or role options (AACN, 2006b). The work of the task force included performing comprehensive reviews of existing practice doctorates across disciplines, collaborating with NONPF, interviewing key informants (e.g., deans, program directors, graduates) at the eight current programs in the United States, and conducting open discussions at the AACN doctoral education conferences and master's education conferences. Task force findings addressed each charge, to include the major recommendation: that is, the DNP is the terminal degree for advanced nursing practice preparation. Additional findings included that practice-focused doctoral programs should be accredited by a nursing accreditation body, with the DNP degree being associated with practice-focused doctoral education. As daunting as it sounded to master's-prepared APRNs, the task force recommended a transition period to provide a mechanism for master's-prepared nurses to pursue the degree.

> The DNP is the terminal degree for advanced nursing practice preparation (AACN, 2004).

The preceding findings begged the question, "Why now?" Findings supporting the move to the DNP degree included a better match of program requirements and credits. Indeed, since the evolution of NP programs, for example, the credits have increased to mirror those in many PhD programs. Likewise, task force members recognized that enhanced knowledge and leadership skills were needed to strengthen practice and healthcare delivery. Other supportive statements included the need for faculty, parity with other professions, and an improved image of nursing.

The AACN position statement, created by the task force, was reviewed by an eight-member external reaction panel and approved by the AACN membership in October 2004 (AACN, 2004). AACN member institutions represented at the meeting voted to move the current level of advanced nursing practice from the master's degree to the doctoral degree by 2015. Thereafter, a flurry of activity commenced within schools and colleges of nursing regarding the targeted implementation date. The Task Force on the Practice Doctorate in Nursing recommended the development of a document addressing educational standards, indicators of quality for practice doctoral programs, and core content/competencies. The DNP Essentials Task Force was created to develop this document. *The Essentials of Doctoral Education for Advanced Nursing Practice* document, which provided a framework to guide program development and accreditation, was disseminated in 2006. In addition, the DNP Roadmap Task Force was created and charged with developing an implementation plan that provided a roadmap for achieving the goals of the AACN position statement by 2015 (http://www.aacn .nche.edu/dnp/roadmapreport.pdf). AACN member institutions represented at the meeting voted to move the current level of advanced nursing practice from the master's degree to the doctoral degree by 2015.

From 2004 to 2006, the original AACN Task Force on the Practice Doctorate and subsequent task forces related to the *Essentials* and the *Roadmap* documents conducted forums and invitational meetings to collect input on the DNP degree from education and practice stakeholders. Internet surveys of schools were conducted, and regional conferences in cooperation with the Essentials Task Force were held in five locations, to include a national stakeholder conference in Washington, DC, with 65 leaders from 44 professional organizations. Major resources were developed, which have been updated and remain in popular use today by faculty, administrators, potential students, DNP students, and healthcare consumers; the most notable is the DNP Tool Kit and a Frequently Asked Questions reference (http://www.aacn.nche.edu/DNP/dnpfaq.htm).

Several schools described the development of their DNP programs to provide exemplars; one of these programs was at the University of Washington. Magyary, Whitney, and Brown (2006) described the development of practice inquiry and collaborative research endeavors with the DNP graduate as the science partner. They described practice inquiry as the "ongoing, systematic, investigation of questions about nursing therapeutics and clinical phenomena with the intent to appraise and translate all forms of best evidence to practice, and to evaluate the translational impact on the quality of health care and health outcomes" (p. 143).

ACCELERATION OF MOVEMENT TO THE DNP DEGREE

The notion of a practice doctorate (DNP degree) as the terminal degree for the education of APRNs has not been universally accepted by all disciplines, including nursing. Discord among some medical organizations was no surprise; however, the rapid rollout of the DNP degree created angst among nursing academicians and practitioners. Challenges were presented to accrediting, certifying, and licensing bodies. Graduate nursing programs had to realign curricula with the AACN recommendations while recognizing faculty preparation, student applicant pools, and resource allocation. Discussions ensued within major nursing organizations (e.g., the American Academy of Nurse Practitioners, the National Organization of Nurse Anesthetists, and the American College of Nurse-Midwives).

Compelling arguments against the DNP degree as the appropriate terminal degree in nursing at this time have been made (Cronenwett et al., 2011; Dracup, Cronenwett, Meleis, & Benner, 2005). History, timing, substance, and marginalization shaped the overall discussions. Different types of doctorates have been offered, including the doctor of nursing science (DNS or DNSc), the doctor of science in nursing (DSN), the doctor of education (EdD), and the doctor of nursing (ND). Often the degrees were offered and administered by the school of nursing rather than the graduate school of the university. When the schools could definitively support that they had a critical mass of doctorally prepared faculty and a rigorous research program, they submitted an application to change the program to a PhD degree, thus decreasing marginalization (Meleis & Dracup, 2005). Institutional issues remain today surrounding options to house the DNP degree within the respective school of nursing. Dracup et al. (2005) questioned the widening of the chasm between nurse scientists and clinicians with the creation of an additional doctoral track and recommended continued dialogue within and outside the profession before the adoption of the DNP degree. Indeed, discussions have ensued, and DNP programs continue to proliferate.

Economic challenges facing the United States since the AACN 2004 position paper was disseminated have had a major impact on the ability of some schools to develop new programs and to recruit students, perhaps lessening the overall quality of the programs (Cronenwett et al., 2011). Embracing the 2015 target for the DNP degree to be the terminal degree for APNs, many schools of nursing immediately transitioned their program to the DNP degree without the option of a master's degree exit point—hence, additional years of education prior to certification and practice coupled with student financial burdens. From a workforce perspective, questions have been raised regarding the capacity of APRNs, particularly NPs, to meet the healthcare needs of the millions of Americans expected to gain health insurance through healthcare reform initiatives (Buerhaus, 2010).

The majority of schools with advanced APRN programs offer or are planning to offer a DNP degree at the post-baccalaureate and/or post-master's level (AACN, 2014). That said, the AACN board of directors acknowledged issues surrounding the transition to the practice doctorate by 2015 and in 2013 commissioned the RAND Corporation to conduct a study in order to understand schools' program curriculum to prepare APRNs with rationale. In addition, barriers and facilitators to schools' adoption of the DNP degree were identified. A mixed methodology was used with the researchers conducting a national survey of 400 schools of nursing offering APRN programs. Qualitative interviews were conducted with 29 deans/directors. The level of support for the BSN-DNP degree among the participants interviewed ranged from enthusiastic to moderate to opposing (Auerbach et al., 2014). See Chapter 3 for more on the Rand Report recommendations for DNP education.

> . . . the number of students enrolling in DNP programs and the continued impact within work environments speak to the evolving success of DNP programs.

Dialogue has continued related to workforce concerns and economic challenges. That said, the number of students enrolling in DNP programs and the continued impact within specific work environments speak to the evolving success of many DNP programs.

CHALLENGES MOVING FORWARD

Program Variability

With the rapid rollout and proliferation of programs throughout the United States, variability is inevitable. First, the institutional infrastructure and support are major considerations. New programs typically must be approved by multiple layers of university approving bodies (e.g., the individual school, the faculty senate, and the board of regents). For universities that offer research and professional doctorate degrees, the addition of a new practice doctorate may be facilitated. In these cases, the DNP degree may fall under the graduate school instead of within the school or college of nursing. The graduate school will require quality standards across all doctoral degrees, often requiring comprehensive written and oral exams. Explicating the difference between a DNP project and a dissertation while supporting the notion of the DNP graduate as a practice scholar invites critical dialogue and stakeholder education. For some programs, the DNP degree represented the first doctoral degree within the institution, which speaks to potential difficulty in building a critical mass of scholars within the larger community as well as getting stakeholder buy-in.

Variability is evident not only across programs but also within programs. For example, in response to the AACN recommendations, many BSN entry-level NP programs with a master's degree exit were converted into BSN-DNP programs. Other programs offered a master's degree exit as part of the BSN-DNP sequence, enabling graduates to complete the specialty certification exam and begin practicing as advanced practice nurses. Still other programs continued with the BSN-MSN programs while adding the post-master's DNP option. According to the RAND Report, the movement toward offering the BSN-DNP option and closing master's-level APRN programs is expected to accelerate (Auerbach et al., 2014).

Issues have surfaced regarding the scholarly project of BSN-DNP students, who are new to advanced practice nursing roles, compared with expert practitioners, who enter as post-master's DNP students (Roberts & McArthur, 2015). The core DNP courses are identical; the requirements for a scholarly project and a designated number of practice hours in which to integrate DNP coursework and develop the project are consistent. However, students may represent distinct differences in their levels of practice expertise and potential to identify a meaningful inquiry from practice. In addition, BSN entry-level DNP students most likely will require additional semesters of clinical supervision and closer oversight of their projects.

What's in a Name? The DNP Project

Variability as to the types of projects merits discussion. Reiterating the AACN's description of the *Final DNP Project* (AACN, 2004), the project is to demonstrate the synthesis of the student's work and lays the groundwork for future scholarship, to include mastery of specialty content. In contrast to the dissertation as the deliverable in a research-focused doctoral program, the final

DNP project has been called a capstone project, clinical dissertation, system change project, portfolio, translational research project, and practice inquiry, among other titles. Early examples of project types included the development of a practice portfolio (Committee on DrNP Competencies, 2003), practice change initiative, pilot study, program evaluation, quality improvement project, evaluation of a new practice model, consulting project, or integrated critical literature review. Projects have been evolving from the practice portfolio and the integrated literature review to focus more on implementation and evaluation components that impact patients, populations, organizations and the health of the nation. The scope of projects reflects the diversity of advanced nursing practice specialties and population foci, as well as the supporting coursework and faculty mentors. The different pathways to the DNP degree—BSN-MSN-DNP, BSN-DNP, MSN-DNP, and PhD-DNP—create opportunities and challenges for the identification, development, and implementation of a project. Practice partners may be agencies and organizations with an increased number of group projects (Brown & Crabtree, 2013). The challenges for faculty and students are to assess available resources within individual DNP programs and recognize the need for students and faculty to identify strengths and provide guidance to students in identifying meaningful projects that can be implemented within a realistic timeframe. Although further implementation and evaluation of the project may occur post-graduation, the student should have mastered the competencies necessary to identify, plan, implement, and evaluate the project. Titles and abstracts of DNP projects are located on organization websites (Sigma Theta Tau library, Doctors of Nursing Practice Inc., NONPF) as well as individual programs. At this time, there is no central repository of all projects.

Recognizing the variability among program requirements for the DNP final product, the AACN board of directors implemented the DNP Task Force in 2014. A major charge of the task force was to develop a white paper clarifying the purpose of the DNP final scholarly product. In addition to addressing the current state of the products, the task force defines resources needed to support the development of quality products and develop a set of recommendations and exemplars (www.aacn.nche.edu/about-aacn/committees-task-forces). Areas of recommendation include a focus on implementation science, faculty development, empirical evaluation of the impact of the DNP graduate, and the project as a synthesis of learning. See Chapter 3 for the final recommendations of the Implementation of the DNP Task Force (AACN, 2015c).

ASSESSING RIGOR

The concept of rigor is difficult to define and is very context specific. For example, the competencies to be achieved through a practice doctorate are different from those achieved through a research doctorate. Hence, the criteria used to assess quality should be unique to the specific program. The quality indicators designated for research-focused doctoral programs in nursing are applicable to doctoral programs leading to a PhD or DNS degree, not the DNP degree (AACN, 2006b). The respective doctorates impact health care in different yet complementary ways. Both should be congruent with the organizational mission and goals, reflecting their unique contributions. The purpose of the research-focused doctoral program in nursing is to develop nurse scientists. The expected outcomes and curricular elements of PhD programs in nursing are divided into three key roles, each with inherent competencies: (1) develop the science, (2) be a steward of the discipline, and (3) educate the next generation (AACN, 2010). Many of the expected outcomes and core curricular elements mirror those of the *Essentials* document but are specifically related to conducting original research instead of conducting quality improvement initiatives or implementing practice changes; for example, theoretical and scientific underpinnings and practice knowledge that informs nursing science are included.

The quality of practice-focused doctoral programs is measured in several dimensions by multiple stakeholders. Unlike the research-focused doctorates, the ongoing reviews and quality assessment are not carried out by the graduate schools (AACN, 2004). The purpose of the practice-based doctorate is to "prepare nurse specialists at the highest level of advanced practice" (AACN, 2006a, p. 53). Characteristics of DNP programs, faculty, and graduates are defined by AACN (2006b) in the document *The Essentials of Doctoral Education for Advanced Nursing Practice*. The AACN *Position Statement on the Practice Doctorate in Nursing* (2004) states that "practice-focused doctoral programs need to be accredited by a nursing accrediting agency recognized by the U.S. Secretary of Education" (p. 14).

Although most DNP faculty and students are familiar with the AACN documents, the National League for Nursing (NLN) also has developed outcomes and competencies across practical/vocational through doctorate programs in nursing. The overarching outcomes are: competencies in human flourishing, nursing judgment, professional identity, and spirit of inquiry (NLN, 2010).

> ... doctoral education in nursing is designed to prepare nurses for the highest level of leadership in practice and scientific inquiry.

In summary, doctoral education in nursing is designed to prepare nurses for the highest level of leadership in practice and scientific inquiry. Although the goals and competencies for the two doctorates differ, there is overlap, and partnerships exist within the context of practice.

Formative and Summative Evaluations

Formative evaluations are completed at various times within an educational program with the intention of obtaining student and faculty input regarding overall program goals, which inform curriculum and program development. Summative evaluations occur at the completion of the program of study and are related largely to the performance of graduates. Graff, Russell, and Stegbauer (2007) described the formative and summative evaluation data provided by students and graduates from the University of Tennessee Health Science Center College of Nursing practice doctorate program. Their findings provide a resource for educators and students alike. Three student cohorts participated in a series of focus groups ($n = 35$) facilitated by qualitative researchers to obtain data about the implementation and effects of the new DNP program. Questions posed to the groups focused on perceptions of how their roles may change as a result of the program and how the courses they were taking contributed to any role change development. Students noted the evolutionary process with changes in function and relationships. Students described how they approached problems differently and how their clinical practices were changed (p. 175). Surveys of students on exit ($n = 57$) and one year post-graduation ($n = 31$) evaluated the accomplishment of program outcomes. The findings supported the conclusion that the program was successful in helping them meet the expected outcomes.

At VUSN, formative and summative evaluation metrics similar to those of Graff et al. (2007) are in place to include the addition of an anonymous survey disseminated after each on-campus intensive experience, which occurs the beginning of each semester. Beuscher and Cook (2014) conducted a formative program evaluation through a qualitative study with VUSN's first DNP student cohort that addressed the topics of challenges, facilitating aspects of the program, and perceived value of the program. Their findings suggested student challenges related to time management, being the first cohort, and dealing with new teaching technology, and issues related to teaching faculty. Facilitators within the program included a community of peers, supportive faculty, and program flexibility. Last, the perceived value of the program included building a toolkit of knowledge, professional credibility, and empowerment. The importance of embracing students' perspectives in program evaluations speaks to a student-centric community and can impact future program development, innovation, and marketing.

Kaplan and Brown (2009) describe the formation of formative and summative evaluations of the University of Washington DNP Program recognizing the need to transcend standard curriculum evaluation. The evaluation plan addresses program effectiveness as well as the experience of transition as described by students and faculty. Data collection includes surveys, interviews, and review of student files. Evaluation components include program benchmarks, student perspectives, faculty and preceptor perspectives, curriculum evaluation, collaboration, and end-of-program and post-program evaluation.

The majority of DNP programs have the infrastructure (committee, faculty/administration) responsible for program evaluation of the DNP degree program. They often work with student and academic services to assess student competency at the end of the program and at designated intervals post-graduation. Data are reviewed with findings used to inform curricular changes.

Recommendations from the RAND report include the need for outcomes studies to assess the impact of the DNP graduates related to patient care and the dissemination to stakeholders (e.g., employers) as to the added value of the DNP-prepared APRN (Auerbach et al., 2014).

Accreditation of DNP Programs

Program accreditation by a nursing or nursing-related accreditation organization recognized by the U.S. Department of Education (USDE) and/or the Council for Higher Education Accreditation (CHEA) is required. The two bodies within nursing that accredit DNP programs are the Commission on Collegiate Nursing Education (CCNE) and the National League for Nursing Accrediting Commission (NLNAC). Both organizations accredit BSN and MSN programs as well. CCNE was the first organization to evaluate and accredit DNP programs beginning during the 2008–2009 academic year. The majority of DNP programs seek accreditation upon enrollment of the first cohort. Institutions offering the DNP degree must provide the accrediting body specific program information prior to scheduling an on-site visit and developing a comprehensive document addressing specific criteria. For example, the DNP program must be developed in accordance with *The Essentials of Doctoral Education for Advanced Nursing Practice* (AACN, 2006b). In BSN-DNP programs preparing NPs, the revised *Criteria for Evaluation of Nurse Practitioner Programs* (National Task Force, 2008) must be incorporated.

Standards addressed for the accreditation process require evidence to support identified outcomes (http://www.nlnac.org/manuals/SC2008_doctorate.htm). Standards include mission and administrative capacity, faculty and staff, students, curriculum, resources, and outcomes. Programs engaged in distance education may require additional criteria. Reflecting on the previous section, formative and summative evaluations with student input directly impact several standards, particularly outcomes.

OPPORTUNITIES FOR THE FUTURE

The Affordable Care Act (ACA) has the potential to increase health care to over 32 million Americans, coupled with leveling healthcare costs. These changes call for innovative models of care, which speaks to the *Future of Nursing* report (IOM, 2010) calling for healthcare providers to be permitted to practice to the fullest extent of their knowledge and competence. There is variation in aspects of practices in large part because of state-based regulatory barriers (Fairman, Rowe, Hassmiller, & Shalala, 2011). Standardization in terms of scope of practice for nurses is indicated within the context of economic forces, demographics, and the gap between supply and demand, particularly primary care.

Consensus Model for APRN Regulation

As mentioned, the change in educational requirements for APRN practice continues to impact certification and regulation for many specialties. Stakeholders continue to recognize that we are in a time of transition and have many venues to communicate shared initiatives, the major one being the Consensus Model for APRN Regulation: Licensure, Accreditation, Certification & Education (APRN Consensus Work Group & the National Council of State Boards of Nursing, 2008). Further reinforcing the IOM (2010) endorsement of graduate education for nursing and the importance of allowing nurses to practice to the full extent of their education and training, education, accreditation, certification, and licensure of APRNs must be consistent across jurisdictions.

The model for APRN regulation was developed by the APRN Joint Dialogue Group and has been endorsed by 48 professional nursing organizations. The document defines APRN practice, the APRN regulatory model, and specialties and discusses titling, the emergence of new roles and population foci, and strategies for implementation. For example, the BSN-entry DNP student must have the appropriate education to sit for a certification examination to assess national competencies of the APRN core (pathophysiology, pharmacology, and health/physical assessment), role (CNP, CRNA, CNM, CNS), and at least one population area of practice (family, adult/gerontology, neonatal, pediatrics, women's health/gender related, psychiatric mental health). Education, certification, and licensure must be congruent in terms of the role and the population foci. The acronym LACE reflects the communication mechanism of the regulatory organizations representing APRN licensure, accreditation, certification, and education entities.

The DNP Graduate in Academia

The IOM Future of Nursing Committee (IOM, 2010) recommended increasing the proportion of RNs with an earned baccalaureate degree from 50% to 80% by 2020. Unfortunately, nursing schools are turning away thousands of qualified applicants because of budgetary constraints and faculty shortage. Addressing this conundrum, the recommendation was made to double the number of nurses with a doctorate by 2020 to add to the cadre of nurse faculty and researchers. The question remains as to what mix of DNP- and PhD-prepared nurses is needed to address the faculty shortage. Likewise, what is the intraprofessional team composition of DNP- and PhD-prepared nurses needed to solve the problems of 32 million new patients who will need health care as a result of the ACA (Nickitas & Feeg, 2011)?

The DNP graduate is an evolving practice scholar and practice expert and is positioned to assume a faculty position, which assumes a match between the criteria determined by the institution and the qualifications of the applicant. Many post-master's DNP students already have faculty appointments in APRN specialty programs and as preceptors. Informal discussions with other DNP program directors support that the majority of post-master's DNP graduates have academic appointments after graduation. These graduates may teach or co-teach courses and precept students in a contractual basis or through joint appointments. Graduates also may be considered practice faculty with full-time practice appointments. These numbers will continue to increase as the requirements for doctorally prepared practice-active faculty grow.

MAKING AN IMPACT

Clearly there is generation of practice evidence through DNP projects. As alluded to previously, the rigor and diversity among projects vary greatly. There is high heterogeneity in focus and outcomes produced. Likewise, projects are context specific, which means they may not be generalizable to other settings, and the impact may be best measured by case studies at this point. That said, the potential for leadership in improving and sustaining evidence-based practice and practice change through collaboration with agencies/organizations and/or research initiatives is exponential. The impact will be measured through dissemination to key stakeholders, at local, regional, and national meetings, and through publications. Sharing project abstracts with professional organizations permitting Web-based access is another venue for dissemination.

By way of example, I share the evolution of leadership roles of two recent post-master's DNP graduates from VUSN: One graduate has a background in health systems management, and the other is a family nurse practitioner. The project of the first graduate was Preparing the Nurse Manager for Evidence-Based Nursing Practice. The purpose was to design an evidence-based educational program for nurse managers to provide them with the knowledge and skills to support the utilization of evidence-based nursing practice by nurses at the bedside. Based on her clinical and management expertise in pediatrics, coupled with the integration of her DNP project into practice at one institution, she was competitively interviewed and offered a new position as the chief nursing officer of an urban children's hospital in another state.

The second graduate has had a lengthy career as a civilian within a major military organization, largely within primary care. Her DNP project was on chronic nonmalignant pain management and the prevention of prescription drug abuse. Recently, her practice organization created a new NP position in the pain management department, which resulted in a promotion for her as well as increased autonomy and responsibility. The position provided a platform for her to continue her scholarly work. I am certain these two shared experiences resonate with many DNP graduates and faculty.

DNP graduates are improving health care through quality improvement initiatives, evaluation of practice, and policy development. Leadership roles in improving and sustaining evidence-based practice and interprofessional patient-centered outcomes will continue to evolve.

Dr. Jeanne Stein presents her journey of how the DNP degree prepared her to become an expert in the practice field of psychiatric community mental health nursing, as well as an advanced nurse educator of undergraduate and graduate nursing students.

Becoming a DNP: My Story
Jeanne Stein, DNP, MSN, RN, CNS

My professional nursing career started at the age of 19 after graduating from a diploma school of nursing and passing my State Board of Nursing examination. I worked as a staff nurse on a busy medical-surgical unit and a pediatric unit at a small rural hospital. After 2 years, I decided to take a position as an occupational health nurse manager at a large steel company with 1,500 employees. I was involved in performing preventive screenings, practicing health maintenance, and caring for multiple and sometimes life-threatening body injuries. I went on to work at a busy downtown occupational health clinic. At the same time, I decided it was time to go back to school to obtain a bachelor of science in nursing in the evenings. I began to feel a need to add to my mental health nursing knowledge as I cared for people of all ages and walks of life—wanting to care for the "whole person." I felt that I didn't know enough about caring for the person who had anxiety, depression, substance abuse, and other brain disorders. This led me to pursue a master's degree in community mental health nursing with an emphasis on prevention. I began teaching nursing students psychiatric/mental health nursing. Part time, I engaged in nursing practice in the home, hospice, and camp nursing in the summer. At a crossroads in my professional career after considerable years in nursing practice (30 years) and 20 years as a nurse educator and clinical nurse specialist, it was time for me to have another new beginning. Again, I wanted more knowledge and skills.

The DNP degree prepared me to become an expert in my practice field of psychiatric community mental health nursing, as well as enhanced my current role as an advanced nurse educator of undergraduate and graduate nursing students. I was well-prepared to apply my enhanced knowledge and skills in teaching-learning, curriculum and theory development, and program evaluation. I have also been a leader in facilitating program changes in nursing education at my university and in my community. For example, I was instrumental in helping the faculty focus on more critical thinking with student assignments and less arduous paperwork. I designed a student nurse learning outcome tool to assess what were the most helpful assignments in their educational experience each semester. In the community, I participated with a whole interdisciplinary mental health team in becoming a new Mental Health America chapter in my state. Additionally, I developed my own theory-guided model of care, Stein's Theory of Meaning Through Cognitive-Behavioral Process, which I am applying in teaching and my practice.

Key Messages

- The concept of the practice doctorate has evolved over the past 30 years.
- NONPF and AACN combined forces to adopt a shared vision to move the practice doctorate forward.
- National initiatives, to include IOM reports, address the need for nurses with practice doctorates to focus on innovative, evidence-based practice, reflecting application of research findings.
- The *Essentials of Doctoral Education for Advanced Nursing Practice* provides a framework to guide program development and accreditation.
- Challenges in moving forward with DNP programs include program variability, components of scholarly projects, and assessment of rigor.

REFERENCES

American Association of Colleges of Nursing. (2004). *Position statement on the practice doctorate in nursing.* Washington, DC: Author. Retrieved from http://www.aacn.nche.edu/publications/position/DNPpositionstatement.pdf

American Association of Colleges of Nursing. (2006a). *DNP roadmap task force report.* Washington, DC: Author.

American Association of Colleges of Nursing. (2006b). *The essentials of doctoral education for advanced nursing practice.* Washington, DC: Author.

American Association of Colleges of Nursing. (2010). *The research-focused doctoral program in nursing: Pathways to excellence.* Washington, DC: Author.

American Association of Colleges of Nursing. (2014). *Talking points-Rand Study on the DNP by 2015.* Retrieved from http://www.aacn.nche.edu/dnp/talking-points.pdf

American Association of Colleges of Nursing. (2015a). DNP fact sheet. Retrieved from: http://www.aacn.nche.edu/media-relations/fact-sheets/dnp

American Association of Colleges of Nursing (2015b). Custom report on Doctoral Program Enrollments, 1997–2014. Washington, DC: AACN Research and Data Services.

American Association of Colleges of Nursing. (2015c). New white paper on the DNP: Current issues and clarifying recommendations. Retrieved from http://www.aacn .nche.edu/news/articles/2015/dnp-white-paper

APRN Consensus Work Group and the National Council of State Boards of Nursing APRN Advisory Committee. (2008). *Consensus model for APRN regulation: Licensure, accreditation, certification & education.* Retrieved from http://www.ncsbn.org/ Consensus_Model_for_APRN_Regulation July_2008.pdf

Auerbach, D. I., Martsolf, G., Pearson, M. L., Taylor, E. A., Zaydman, M., Muchow, A., . . . Dower, C. (2014). *The DNP by 2015—A study of the institutional, political, and professional issues that facilitate or impede establishing a post-baccalaureate Doctor of Nursing Practice program.* RAND Corporation. Retrieved from www.aacn.nche.edu/DNPstudy

Beuscher, L., & Cook, T. (2014). Aha! moments: Student insights of a new doctor of nursing practice program. *Women's Healthcare,* February 2014, 32–38.

Brooten, D., Youngblut, J., Brown, L., Finkler, S. A., Neff, D. F., & Madigan, E. (2010). A randomized trial of nurse specialist home care for women with high-risk pregnancies: Outcomes and costs. *American Journal of Managed Care, 7*(8), 793–803.

Brown, M. A., & Crabtree, K. (2013). The development of practice scholarship in DNP programs: A paradigm shift. *Journal of Professional Nursing, 29*(6), 330–337.

Buerhaus, P. (2010). Have nurse practitioners reached a tipping point? Interview of a panel of NP thought leaders. *Nursing Economic$, 28*(5), 346–349.

Committee on DrNP Competencies. (2003). *Competencies for a doctor of clinical nursing.* New York, NY: Columbia University School of Nursing.

Cragin, L., & Kennedy, H. P. (2006). Linking obstetric and midwifery practice with optimal outcomes. *Journal of Obstetric, Gynecologic, & Neonatal Nursing, 35*(6), 779–785.

Cronenwett, L., Dracup, K., Grey, M., McCauley, L., Meleis, A., & Salmon, M. (2011). The doctor of nursing practice: A national workforce perspective. *Nursing Outlook, 59,* 9–17.

Dracup, K., Cronenwett, L., Meleis, A., & Benner, P. (2005). Reflections on the doctorate of nursing practice. *Nursing Outlook, 53,* 177–182.

Fairman, J. A., Rowe, J. W., Hassmiller, S., & Shalala, D. E. (2011). Broadening the scope of nursing practice. *New England Journal of Medicine, 364*(3), 193–196.

Graff, J. C., Russell, C. K., & Stegbauer, C. C. (2007). Formative and summative evaluation of a practice doctorate program. *Nurse Educator, 32*(4), 173–177.

Institute of Medicine. (1999). *To err is human: Building a safer health system.* Washington, DC: National Academies Press.

Institute of Medicine. (2001). *Crossing the quality chasm.* Washington, DC: National Academies Press.

Institute of Medicine. (2003a). *Health professions education: A bridge to quality.* Washington, DC: National Academies Press.

Institute of Medicine. (2003b). *Keeping patients safe: Transforming the work environment of nurses.* Washington, DC: National Academies Press.

Institute of Medicine. (2010). *The future of nursing: Leading change, advancing health.* Washington, DC: Author.

Kaplan, L., & Brown, M-A. (2009). Doctor of Nursing Practice program evaluation and beyond: Capturing the profession's transition to the DNP. *Nursing Education Perspectives, 30*(6) (Nov/Dec 2009), 362–366.

Magyary, D., Whitney, J. D., & Brown, M. A. (2006). Advancing practice inquiry: Research foundations of the practice doctorate in nursing. *Nursing Outlook, 54,* 139–151.

Marion, L., Viens, D., O'Sullivan, A., Crabtree, K., Fontana, S., & Price, M. (2003). The practice doctorate in nursing: Future or fringe? *Topics in Advanced Practice Nursing eJournal.* Retrieved from http://www.medscape.com/viewarticle/453247

Meleis, A. I., & Dracup, K. (2005, September 30). The case against the DNP: History, timing, substance, and marginalization. *Online Journal of Issues in Nursing, 10*(3), Manuscript 2. doi:10.3912/OJIN.Vol10No03Man02

Mundinger, M. O., Kane, R. L., Lenz, E. R., Totten, A. M., Tsai, W. Y., Cleary, P. D., . . . Shelanski, M. L. (2000). Primary care outcomes in patients treated by nurse practitioners or physicians: A randomized trial. *Journal of the American Medical Association, 283*, 59–68.

National League for Nursing. (2010). *Outcomes and competencies for graduates of practical/ vocational, diploma, associate degree, baccalaureate, master's, practice doctorate, and research doctorate programs in nursing.* New York, NY: Author.

National Task Force on Quality Nurse Practitioner Education. (2008). *Criteria for evaluation of nurse practitioner programs.* Retrieved from http://www.aacn.nche.edu/ leading-initiatives/education-resources/evalcriteria2008.pdf

Newhouse, R. P., Stanik-Hutt, J., White, K. M., Johantgen, M., Bass, E. B., Zangaro, G., Wilson, R. F., . . . Weiner, J. P. (2011). Advanced practice nurse outcomes 1990–2008: A Systematic review. *Nursing Economic$, 29*(5), 230–250.

Nickitas, D. M., & Feeg, V. (2011). Doubling the number of nurses with a doctorate by 2020: Predicting the right number or getting it right? *Nursing Economic$, 29*(3), 109–110, 125.

Pine, M., Holt, K. D., & Lou, Y. B. (2003). Surgical mortality and type of anesthesia provider. *AANA Journal, 71*(2), 109–116.

Roberts, M. E., & McArthur, D. B. (2015). Chapter 10. The BSN-DNP Path: Opportunities and challenges for DNP students and graduates. In L.A. Chism (Ed.), *The doctor of nursing practice: A guidebook for role development and professional issues* (3rd ed.). Burlington, MA: Jones & Bartlett.

CHAPTER 3

Defining the Doctor of Nursing Practice: Current Trends

Dianne Conrad and Karen Kesten

CHAPTER OVERVIEW

The purpose of this chapter is to define doctoral preparation for nursing and describe nursing practice doctoral education and its role in transforming health care. Current trends in doctor of nursing practice (DNP) education will be explored on how the practice doctorate is evolving to meet the competencies as outlined in *The Essentials for Doctoral Education for Advanced Nursing Practice* (American Association of Colleges of Nursing [AACN], 2006).

CHAPTER OBJECTIVES

After completing the chapter, the learner will be able to:

1. Define "doctor of nursing practice"
2. Describe the state of DNP education
3. Differentiate between the research and practice doctorate degrees
4. Discuss how the practice-based doctorate and the research-based doctorate will collaborate to impact nursing and health care

DEFINING THE PRACTICE DOCTORATE IN NURSING

The time is now for the practice doctorate in nursing. Nursing education has evolved to meet the needs of society in preparing nurses throughout history. The emergence and dramatic growth of DNP programs in the United States reflect this country's demand for highly competent providers to improve the health care of its people.

In 2001, the Institute of Medicine (IOM) outlined aims for healthcare improvement in *Crossing the Quality Chasm: A New Health System for the 21st Century*, which included care that is safe, effective, patient centered, timely, efficient, and equitable. To provide that care, the IOM (2003), in *Health Professions Education: A Bridge to Quality*, called for a change in how healthcare providers are prepared to meet these challenges. Healthcare providers in all professions are to attain the following core competencies:

- Provide patient-centered care
- Work in interdisciplinary teams
- Employ evidence-based practice
- Apply quality improvement
- Utilize informatics

By 2010, the IOM's report *The Future of Nursing: Leading Change, Advancing Health* responded with these key messages:

- Nurses should practice to the full extent of their education and training.
- Nurses should achieve higher levels of education and training through an improved education system that promotes seamless academic progression.
- Nurses should be full partners with physicians and other healthcare professionals in redesigning health care in the United States.
- Effective workforce planning and policy making require better data collection and information infrastructure.

These important documents reflect the changing societal needs for a highly educated workforce prepared to meet the complex challenges of health care in the 21st century and beyond. In response to these challenges, nursing as a profession has developed an educational program at the doctoral level to prepare individuals for advanced nursing practice. The purpose of practice-focused doctoral programs is to *prepare experts in specialized advanced nursing practice,* as defined by the AACN (2006). The programs are to *focus heavily on innovative and evidence-based practice, reflecting the application of credible research findings.*

See **Table 3-1** for a comparison of IOM recommendations on healthcare improvement, the competencies of healthcare professionals, and clinical nursing doctoral preparation *Essentials.*

Table 3-1 Comparison of Institute of Medicine Recommendations on Healthcare Improvement, Competencies of Healthcare Professionals, and Clinical Nursing Doctoral Preparation

Six Aims for Healthcare Improvement (IOM, 2001)	Core Competencies of Healthcare Professionals (IOM, 2003)	The Essentials of Doctoral Education for Advanced Nursing Practice (AACN, 2006)
	DNP Essential VIII *Advanced Nursing Practice*	
Safe: Avoiding injuries to patients from the care that is intended to help them	*Apply quality improvement *Work in interdisciplinary teams	I. Scientific underpinnings for practice II. Organizational and systems leadership for quality improvement and systems thinking VI. Interprofessional collaboration for improving patient and population health outcomes
Effective: Providing services based on scientific knowledge to all who could benefit and refraining from providing services to those not likely to benefit	*Employ evidence-based practice *Utilize informatics	I. Scientific underpinnings for practice II. Organizational and systems leadership for quality improvement and systems thinking III. Clinical scholarship and analytical methods for evidence-based practice IV. Information systems/technology and patient care technology for the improvement and transformation of health care V. Health care policy for advocacy in health care
Patient-centered: Providing care that is respectful of and responsive to individual patient preferences, needs, and values and ensuring that patient values guide all clinical decisions	*Patient-centered care	V. Health care policy for advocacy in health care VII. Clinical prevention and population health for improving the nation's health
Timely: Reducing waits and sometimes harmful delays for both those who receive and those who give care	*Work in interdisciplinary teams *Apply quality improvement *Employ evidence-based practice	II. Organizational and systems leadership for quality improvement and systems thinking VI. Interprofessional collaboration for improving patient and population health outcomes

(Continued)

Table 3-1 Comparison of Institute of Medicine Recommendations on Health-care Improvement, Competencies of Healthcare Professionals, and Clinical Nursing Doctoral Preparation (*Continued*)

Six Aims for Healthcare Improvement (IOM, 2001)	Core Competencies of Healthcare Professionals (IOM, 2003)	The Essentials of Doctoral Education for Advanced Nursing Practice (AACN, 2006)
	DNP Essential VIII *Advanced Nursing Practice*	
Efficient: Avoiding waste, including waste of equipment, supplies, ideas, and energy	˙Work in interdisciplinary teams ˙Utilize informatics ˙Apply quality improvement	I. Scientific underpinnings for practice III. Clinical scholarship and analytical methods for evidence-based practice IV. Information systems/technology and patient care technology for the improvement and transformation of health care V. Healthcare policy for advocacy in health care VI. Interprofessional collaboration for improving patient and population health outcomes
Equitable: Providing care that does not vary in quality because of personal characteristics such as gender, ethnicity, geographic location, and socioeconomic status	˙Patient-centered care ˙Apply quality improvement ˙Utilize informatics	II. Organizational and systems leadership for quality improvement and systems thinking VII. Clinical prevention and population health for improving the nation's health IV. Information systems/technology and patient care technology for the improvement and transformation of health care

Reprinted with permission from American Association of Colleges of Nursing. (2006). The essentials for doctoral education for advanced nursing practice. Washington, DC: Author; Institute of Medicine. (2003). Health professions education: A bridge to quality. Retrieved from http://www.nap.edu/openbook.php?record_id=10681&page=45

The DNP is a *degree*, not a *role*.

The clinical doctorate for nurses, the DNP, is a *degree*, not a *role*. There are many roles in advanced practice nursing. The AACN (2004) defined advanced practice nursing as "any form of nursing intervention that influences healthcare outcomes for individuals or populations, including the direct care of individual patients, management of care for individuals and populations, administration of nursing and healthcare organizations, and the development and implementation of health policy" (p. 2).

Therefore, advanced nursing practice encompasses such roles as nurse practitioner (NP), clinical nurse specialist (CNS), certified nurse-midwife (CNM), nurse anesthetist, nurse administrator, nurse informaticist, and nurse health policy specialist. This list of roles is not inclusive because nursing entrepreneurs continue to pioneer advanced practice roles to meet patient needs in a variety of settings.

There is a special definition of the roles of the advanced practice registered nurse (APRN). In 2008, a report titled *Consensus Model for APRN Regulation: Licensure, Accreditation, Certification & Education* was completed through the work of the APRN Consensus Work Group and the National Council of State Boards of Nursing APRN Advisory Committee (APRN Joint Dialogue Group, 2008). This group defined four specific APRN roles—certified registered nurse anesthetist (CRNA), CNM, CNS, and certified nurse practitioner—for the purpose of standardizing licensure language across the country. However, the group acknowledged that "many nurses with advanced graduate nursing preparation practice in roles and specialties (e.g., informatics, public health, education or administration) that are essential to advance the health of the public but do not focus on direct care to individuals and, therefore, their practice does not require regulatory recognition beyond the Registered Nurse license granted by state boards of nursing. Like the four current APRN roles, practice in these other advanced specialty nursing roles requires specialized knowledge and skills acquired through graduate-level education" (p. 5).

Though the APRN consensus document did not specify the practice doctorate as the education level for these advanced practice roles, graduate-level education was a requirement. Any of these roles benefit from education at the doctoral level to prepare nurses for the challenges of today's healthcare arena. These advanced practice roles are oriented toward providing quality care and improving patient outcomes.

The *Essentials of DNP Education* (AACN, 2006) give these doctorally prepared nurses the tools and competencies they need to carry out their role at the highest level (see **Figure 3-1**).

The AACN (2004) further delineates the benefits of a practice-focused doctorate to:

- develop the needed advanced competencies for increasingly complex practice, faculty, and leadership roles;
- enhance knowledge to improve nursing practice and patient outcomes; and
- enhance leadership skills to strengthen practice and healthcare delivery (p. 4).

Most important, the DNP prepared nurse is able to translate scientific evidence into practice in a timely fashion.

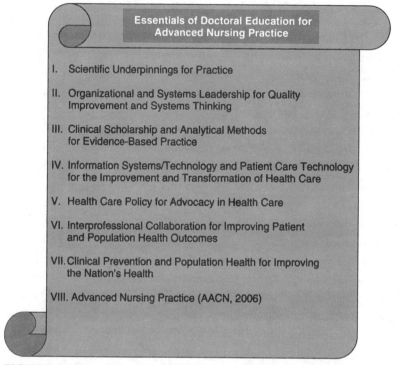

FIGURE 3-1 Essentials of doctoral education for advanced practice nursing.
Data from American Association of Colleges of Nursing. (2006). The essentials for doctoral education for advanced nursing practice. Washington, DC: Author.

COMPARISON OF THE DNP AND PHD IN NURSING

Doctoral preparation in nursing currently has two paths: the research-based doctorate that began in 1934 at New York University and flourished in the 1970s (Chism, 2016), and the current practice doctorate, the DNP, that has been defined and developed by the AACN since 2002. See Chapter 4, Scholarship in Practice, for a discussion of the evolution of the practice doctorate.

The two doctoral programs according to the AACN (2006) are different in their goals and in the competencies of their graduates. The practice doctorate (DNP) and the research doctorates (PhD and Doctor of Nursing Science [DNS]) offer complementary, alternative approaches to attaining the highest level of educational preparation in nursing with rigorous and demanding programs of study. The profession of nursing benefits from scholar leaders who are committed to the advancement of the science and practice of nursing.

A comparison of nursing doctoral programs is outlined in **Table 3-2**.

Table 3-2 Comparison of Doctoral Nursing Programs

	Practice Doctorate DNP	Research Doctorate PhD/DNS
Common Characteristics	• Rigorous and demanding expectations • Scholarly approach to the discipline • Commitment to the advancement of the profession	
Program of Study	Prepares leaders at highest level of nursing practice to improve patient outcomes and translate research into practice	Prepares nurses at the highest level of nursing science to conduct research to advance the science of nursing
Students	• Commitment to practice career • Oriented toward improving outcomes for patient care and population health	• Commitment to research career • Oriented toward developing new nursing knowledge and scientific inquiry
Program Faculty	• Practice or research doctorate in nursing, and expertise in area teaching • Leadership experience in area of role and population practice • High level of expertise in practice congruent with focus of academic program	• Research doctorate in nursing or related field • Leadership experience in area of sustained research funding • High level of expertise in research congruent with focus of academic funding • High level of expertise in research congruent with focus of academic program
Resources	• Mentors and/or preceptors in leadership positions across practice settings • Access to diverse practice settings with appropriate resources for areas of practice • Access to financial aid • Access to information and patient-care technology resources congruent with areas of study	• Mentors and/or preceptors in research settings • Access to research settings with appropriate resources • Access to dissertation support dollars and financial aid • Access to information and research technology resources congruent with program of research

(Continued)

Table 3-2 Comparison of Doctoral Nursing Programs (*Continued*)

	Practice Doctorate DNP	Research Doctorate PhD/DNS
Program Assessment and Evaluation	• Program outcomes: Health-care improvements and contributions via practice, policy change, and practice scholarship • Receives accreditation by nursing accreditor	• Program outcomes: Contributes to healthcare improvements via the development of new knowledge and scholarly products that provide the foundation for the advancement of nursing science • Oversight by the institution's authorized bodies (i.e., graduate school) and regional accreditors

Modified from American Association of Colleges of Nursing. (2014). Key differences between DNP and PhD/DNS programs. Retrieved from: http://www.aacn.nche.edu/dnp/ContrastGrid.pdf

The challenges of healthcare delivery in the 21st century will necessitate the collaboration of interdisciplinary teams (IOM, 2003). Partnering of the research doctorate with the practice doctorate will demonstrate cooperation within nursing that can advance the profession. Lamb (2012) described building collaboration "readiness" with the combination of the PhD in nursing and DNP. She stated that the PhD in nursing brings:

- more minds, more tools, more innovation
- a broader range of theories and more explanatory theoretical models
- an expanded toolkit for research design and methods
- the opportunity for more competitive grants

The DNP brings the following to the team:

- better teamwork, leading to better outcomes
- the contribution of a broader range of evidence
- greater opportunities to accelerate nurse-led and interprofessional practice models

The benefits of interprofessional and intraprofessional collaboration will be discussed further in Chapter 7, Interprofessional and Intraprofessional Collaboration in the Scholarly Project.

CURRENT TRENDS IN DOCTORAL EDUCATION

One of the concerns about beginning a practice doctorate for nursing was the ability of the profession to produce doctoral-level graduates. *The Future of Nursing* report (IOM, 2010) called for the doubling of doctorally prepared nurses by 2020. Rapid growth of DNP programs has occurred since

> IOM *Future of Nursing* report calls for a doubling of doctorally prepared nurses by 2020.

the AACN's work on defining and developing the practice doctorate *Essentials* in 2004. The number of DNP programs has increased from 20 in 2006 to 268 in 2015, with many more programs in development (AACN, 2015a). The concern that the practice doctorate would decrease the number of nurses pursuing a research doctorate in nursing appears to be unfounded. The AACN tracks the number of nursing education programs as well as graduates of those programs. The data show that since 2003, the number of PhD students enrolled in the United States has increased from 3,229 to 5,290 in 2014. During the same period, the enrollment in DNP programs increased dramatically, from 70 in 2003 to 18,352 in 2014 in 264 DNP programs across the country (AACN, 2015b). The number of PhD programs in nursing has also increased, from 106 in 2006 to 134 in 2014 (AACN, 2015a) (see **Figure 3-2**).

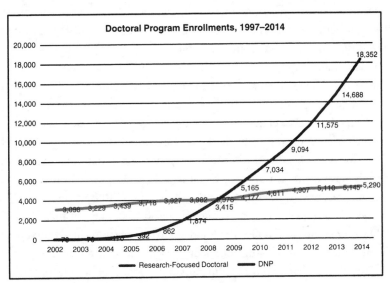

FIGURE 3-2 Doctoral program enrollments 1997–2014.

Reprinted with permission from American Association of Colleges of Nursing. (2015b). Custom report on doctoral Program Enrollments, 1997–2014. Washington, DC: AACN Research and Data Services.

REPORTS AFFECTING DNP EDUCATION

The Rand Corporation Report: The DNP by 2015: A Study of the Institutional, Political, and Professional Issues that Facilitate or Impede Establishing a Post-Baccalaureate Doctor of Nursing Practice Program.

In 2004, member schools of the American Association of Colleges of Nursing (AACN) voted to endorse the *Position Statement on the Practice Doctorate in Nursing*, which called for moving the level of preparation necessary for advanced nursing practice from the master's degree to the doctorate by the target year of 2015 (AACN, 2004). Over the past 10 years, colleges of nursing have made great strides in moving toward this target. Currently, the majority of schools with APRN programs, the largest subset of all advanced nursing practice programs, either offer or are planning to offer a DNP at the post-baccalaureate and/or post-master's level.

While the number of DNP programs for APRNs has grown significantly and steadily over this period, not all colleges of nursing have been able to fully transition their master's-level APRN programs to the practice doctorate by 2015 and many are electing to maintain both master's and DNP options to prepare APRNs. To better understand the issues facing colleges of nursing moving to the DNP, the AACN board of directors commissioned the RAND Corporation to conduct a national survey of nursing schools with APRN programs to identify the barriers and facilitators to offering a post-baccalaureate DNP (Auerbach et al., 2014). The report includes recommendations for next steps that AACN can take to help schools accelerate programmatic change and overcome challenges.

For the purposes of this study, the RAND Corporation was commissioned by AACN to focus on only the APRN master's degree program transition to the DNP. This study was undertaken between October 2013 and April 2014 to investigate schools' progress toward transitioning to the DNP for APRN programs as well as the barriers and/or facilitators to nursing schools' full adoption of the DNP. The RAND Corporation used a mixed-method approach, which included surveys and qualitative interviews to investigate schools' progress toward the adoption of the DNP. Data were analyzed from an online survey developed specifically for this project, as well as qualitative interviews with deans and directors of 29 nursing schools.

A summary of the report findings (Auerbach et al., 2014) showed:

- The number of schools with a DNP program has grown 10-fold in the past 7 years. Schools of nursing have made great progress in transitioning to the DNP by the target date of 2015. Currently, DNP programs, at either the post-baccalaureate (BSN-DNP) or post-master's (MSN-DNP) level, are offered at more than 250 schools nationwide.

- Approximately 30% of nursing schools with APRN programs now offer the BSN-DNP, and this proportion is anticipated to climb to greater than 50% in the foreseeable future.
- Schools in the West and Midwest and schools in states with a high density of existing nurse practitioners (NPs) were considerably more likely to offer BSN-to-DNP programs.
- Faculty enthusiasm and administrative support within the university are strong facilitators toward offering the BSN-to-DNP.
- The value of the added content of the DNP education is almost universally agreed on. Fully 93% of survey respondents offering or planning on offering the BSN-to-DNP cited the "value of the DNP education in preparing for future healthcare needs" as very important or critical to their decision.
- AACN endorsement and recommendation of the DNP also factored strongly in many schools' decisions to offer the BSN-to-DNP, as did a desire to expand into doctoral-level education.
- Schools continue to adopt the DNP, both as an option to be completed for practicing master's-level APRNs (the MSN-to-DNP) and as an entry-level APRN option for those with a bachelor of science in nursing (BSN) degree (the BSN-to-DNP).
- The schools interviewed perceived that employers are unclear about the differences between master's-prepared and DNP-prepared APRNs and could benefit from information on outcomes connected to DNP practice as well as exemplars from practice settings that capitalize on the capabilities of DNP-prepared nurses.
- Student demand for the DNP on the part of currently practicing APRNs appears robust, given the proliferation of MSN-to-DNP programs.
- Student demand for the BSN-to-DNP is growing.
- Schools cited faculty resources as constraints to the development of DNP programs.
- Costs and budgetary concerns are a key barrier to many schools, particularly those that are not freestanding or autonomous schools.
- Securing clinical sites and preceptors, similar to MSN APRN programs are cited as a restraining factor.
- Faculty resources for managing DNP projects were cited by schools as a potential barrier.
- Requirement of the DNP for certification and accreditation would accelerate the transition to BSN to DNP programs.

The Rand Corporation Report (Auerbach et al., 2014) recommended that the AACN should:

1. Conduct, and collaborate with others to conduct, outcome studies of DNP practice to better understand the impact of DNP graduates on patient care.
2. Provide outreach data to help employers and healthcare organizations understand the comprehensive competencies and capabilities of DNP-educated APRNs.
3. Focus on understanding and documenting successful strategies in overcoming barriers to offering BSN-to-DNP programs of departments or divisions within larger universities, since they may face greater hurdles to offering BSN-to-DNP programs.
4. Document and showcase examples of collaborative partnerships between schools and hospitals or other healthcare organizations for the purpose of providing clinical practice sites.
5. Provide greater clarity and guidance related to requirements for the DNP project.
6. Continue with ongoing efforts to assist schools in overcoming challenges to offering the BSN to DNP.

As a response to these recommendations, follow-up and active steps taken by AACN include the formation of two task forces to further improve DNP education: the Implementation of the DNP Task Force and the APRN Clinical Training Task Force. Each task force has produced white papers that address some of the barriers identified in the RAND Corporation study.

To find out more about these task forces and their charges, see www.aacn.nche.edu/about-aacn/committees-task-forces.

AACN Report on APRN Education: The APRN Clinical Training Task Force Report

Much attention has been paid to the Institute of Medicine's (IOM) 2010 *The Future of Nursing* report that APRNs be allowed to practice to "the full extent of their education and training" (p. 29). APRNs have a potential opportunity to contribute to the delivery of care to the additional 16.4 million *newly insured* patients due to healthcare reform (Office of the Assistant Secretary for Planning and Evaluation (ASPE), 2015). Nationwide, APRN education programs are experiencing increased demand for APRN enrollment and many programs report challenges in expanding enrollment to meet this demand. Colleges of nursing cite inadequate numbers and quality of clinical training sites and preceptors for APRN students.

In May 2013, AACN convened the APRN Clinical Training Task Force to develop a white paper that would re-envision clinical education and training for APRNs. Limited resources, including sufficient and diverse clinical sites, patients, and preceptors to prepare APRNs for contemporary practice is a frequently cited challenge. New regulatory requirements and changes in healthcare environments present increasing challenges for practitioners who serve as preceptors and for colleges of nursing preparing the next generation of providers.

Following nearly two years of consulting with experts within and outside the discipline of nursing, reviewing the literature, exploring new models of clinical education and competency development, reflection and discussion by the APRN Clinical Training Task Force, a report brief and a white paper were released in March, 2015 (AACN, 2015c).

The AACN Task Force (AACN, 2015c) concluded that the current methods of providing clinical education for APRNs needs to be re-envisioned in order to expand the pool of opportunities available to contemporary students and to reduce strictures in the pipeline to educating the APRN workforce in sufficient numbers to meet societal demand for these valuable services. Variability among APRN programs, particularly for Nurse Practitioners and Clinical Nurse Specialists, exists in the clinical competencies expected at various points throughout the curriculum and evaluation processes and tools. Increasingly, new models of care are emerging with a greater emphasis on interprofessional practice and education. Advances in technology both within healthcare delivery and education have created opportunities for APRNs to lead the effective integration of technologies into healthcare delivery. Academic practice partnerships are important to all APRN clinical education to ensure that students have access to patients, healthcare professional teams, and current data and experiences. Partnerships are increasingly important when considering interprofessional education, transition to practice for new graduates, implementation of new clinical education models, and the rapid changes that are occurring in healthcare systems. Across higher education, there is an increased interest and emphasis on examination and implementation of competency-based education and assessment models in a variety of disciplines and more specifically in the health professions (Carraccio et al., 2002; Carraccio & Englander, 2013).

The AACN Task Force made the following recommendations:

I. **Simulation should be used to enhance APRN clinical education, and the use of simulation to replace more traditional clinical experiences should be explored.**
   - Seek funding for five demonstration projects that are designed to study the impact of various methods along the continuum of simulation learning approaches as one component of APRN clinical education and assessment.
   - Funding and other resources should be provided at both the national and local levels for the development and use of simulation for learning and assessment, including funding for a national center of faculty innovation and faculty preparation and certification.
   - A national repository should be created and maintained for reliable/valid APRN simulation education materials.
   - Simulations should be developed and tested for assessment of the APRN common competencies.

II. **AACN-American Organization of Nurse Executives (AONE) principles for academic-practice partnerships should be adopted by all APRN programs.**
   - APRN programs, including face-to-face and distance education programs, should implement expectations described in Section II regarding the development and maintenance of APRN clinical experiences and student oversight.
   - Encourage and support the development of innovative partnerships for APRN clinical education as well as the use of a variety of incentives for practice sites and preceptors, e.g., adjunct faculty status, joint appointments, participation on curricular committees, research support, continuing education credits, and academic credit toward graduate degrees.
   - Support the development and testing of innovative APRN academic/practice regional consortia that reflect geographic and institutional diversity.
   - Develop and implement an accessible repository for APRN preceptor orientation materials.

III. **APRN clinical education and assessment should be competency based.**
   - Establish a common language or taxonomy by adopting definitions for competence, competencies, and competency framework that are recognized by APRN organizations and other health professions.

- Identify common, measurable APRN competencies that cross all four roles and build on or reaffirm the APRN core competencies (AACN, 2006).
- Progression of competence or milestones should be identified and defined across each of the common competencies.
- Develop a standardized assessment tool to be available to faculty and preceptors to use for formative and summative evaluation of the common APRN competencies.

IV. **Support the development of alternative or innovative APRN clinical education models**
- Encourage regulatory bodies to support or allow APRN education programs to develop and test innovative or less traditional clinical models.
- Encourage APRN programs to explore, implement, and test innovative or less traditional clinical models, including interprofessional learning experiences and use of technology.
- Seek funding to support the development and evaluation of alternative or innovative APRN clinical training models.

The Implementation of the DNP Task Force Report: Current Issues and Clarifying Recommendations

The *AACN Position Statement on the Practice Doctorate in Nursing* (AACN, 2004) changed the course of nursing education by recommending that advanced nursing practice education be transitioned to the doctoral level. A decade later, the Doctor of Nursing Practice (DNP) is widely accepted as the preferred pathway for those seeking preparation at the highest level of nursing practice. Considering the changing landscape in health care and higher education over the last ten years as well as the dramatic growth of DNP programs, the AACN Board of Directors convened the Implementation of the DNP Task Force to review the current state of DNP programs, and to provide recommendations to clarify curricular and practice expectations as outlined in the *Essentials of Doctoral Education for Advanced Nursing Practice [DNP Essentials],* AACN, 2006).

Growing evidence exists regarding variability among program requirements for the DNP final scholarly products including the scope of project, level of implementation, impact on system and practice outcomes, extent of collaborative efforts, dissemination of findings, and degree of faculty mentorship/oversight. Similar to other healthcare professions, nursing is faced with competition for practice sites and preceptors, complex affiliation agreements, and regulatory issues for distance learning modalities when obtaining practice experiences for DNP students. These issues were documented in the RAND report (Auerbach et al., 2014) and thoroughly explored by the task force. The white paper presents clarification as well as new and innovative ways to meet the DNP practice requirements.

The national dialogue reflects an ongoing need for clarification and restatement of the foundational concept of how *advanced nursing practice* is defined.

- *Advanced nursing practice* focuses on the provision of direct care to individual patients or populations, and the provision of indirect care such as nursing administration, executive leadership, health policy, informatics, and population health.
- The task force reaffirms that the discipline of education encompasses an entirely separate body of knowledge and competence (AACN, 2004, p. 13) and is not an area of advanced nursing practice.
- Also, it is important to remember that the DNP is an academic degree and not a role.

Implementation of the DNP Task Force Recommendations:

I. DNP Graduate Scholarship
- Graduates of both research- and practice-focused doctoral programs are prepared to generate new knowledge.
  - practice-focused graduates are prepared to generate new knowledge through
    1. innovation of practice change
    2. the translation of evidence
    3. implementation of quality improvement processes in specific practice settings, systems, or with specific populations to improve health or health outcomes.
- Organizational and systems leadership knowledge and skills are critical for DNP graduates to:
  - develop and evaluate new models of care delivery
  - create and sustain change at the organization and systems levels.
- The delineations in knowledge generation are not a hierarchical structure of importance; both are types of knowledge generating methods.
- DNP and PhD graduates have the opportunity to improve health outcomes.

II. **DNP Scholarly Project**
- The title of the final product to be "The DNP Project."
- DNP project elements include planning, implementation, and evaluation components.
- All DNP projects should:
    - focus on a change that impacts healthcare outcomes either through direct or indirect care
    - have a systems or population focus
    - demonstrate implementation in the appropriate area of practice
    - include a plan for sustainability
    - include an evaluation of processes and/or outcomes
    - provide a foundation for future practice scholarship.
- As mentioned, the discipline of education encompasses an entirely separate body of knowledge and competence; therefore, the focus of a DNP program, including practicum and DNP project, should not be on the educational process, the academic curriculum, or on educating nursing students.
- Integrative and systematic reviews alone are not considered a DNP project and do not provide opportunities for students to develop and integrate scholarship into their practice.
- A student's portfolio is not considered a DNP project but rather a tool to document learning.
- Group/team projects are acceptable when the project aims are consistent with the focus of the program.
    - Each member of the group must meet all expectations of planning, implementation, and evaluation of the project, and be evaluated accordingly.
    - Each student must have a leadership role in at least one component of the project and be held accountable for a deliverable.
- Dissemination of the DNP project should include a minimum of an executive summary or a written report that disseminates DNP project outcomes.
- Dissemination of the DNP project could take these forms:
    - publishing in a peer reviewed print or on-line
    - poster and podium presentations
    - presentation of a written or verbal executive summary to stakeholders and/or the practice site/organization leadership
    - development of a webinar presentation or video

- submission and publication to a non-refereed lay publication
- oral presentation to the public-at-large
- development and presentation of a digital poster, a grand rounds presentation, and/or a PowerPoint presentation.
- The DNP project team should consist of a student or a group of students with a minimum of a doctoral prepared faculty member and a practice mentor.
- The term "DNP Project Team" should be used to minimize confusion between the PhD dissertation committee and the faculty and mentors who oversee the DNP final project.
- Evaluation of the final DNP project is the responsibility of the faculty.
- A digital repository for the DNP final projects should be used to advance nursing practice by archiving and sharing outcomes.

III. **DNP programs:**
- Should provide evidence of meeting program outcomes delineated in the *DNP Essentials*.
- Should map student learning objectives to expected program outcomes and *DNP Essentials*.
- A post-baccalaureate full-time program of study should be 3 years including summers or four years on a traditional academic calendar.
- A post-master's program of study should be a minimum of 12 months full-time study to allow for acquisition of the doctoral-level outcomes and completion of the DNP project.
- Should be designed with attention to program efficiency.
- Consider new models and processes for implementing DNP project teams that provide efficient use of resources and support student learning.
- Adopt a process that allows for oversight and evaluation of DNP projects that ensures quality and equity of resources.
- Should provide faculty development to ensure quality student learning outcomes to include:
  - curricular design of DNP programs
  - development of new, innovative teaching strategies
  - development of innovative, new practice opportunities to support achievement of the DNP *Essentials* learning outcomes
  - strategies to support and evaluate the DNP project
  - implementation of quality improvement processes
  - interprofessional education and practice experiences.

- Preparation for the nurse educator role:
  - Requires additional coursework in pedagogies
  - Is not an area of advanced nursing practice.

IV. **DNP practice hours**

- Practice experiences should prepare the post-baccalaureate and post-master's DNP student with the outcomes delineated in all of the DNP *Essentials.*
- Opportunities to integrate all of the *Essentials* into one's practice are imperative for both post-baccalaureate and post-master's students.
- Faculty are responsible for assessing students' learning needs and designing practice experiences that allow students to attain and demonstrate the DNP *Essentials.*
- Programs are expected to demonstrate the synthesis and application of all DNP *Essentials.*
- All DNP students, including those in post-master's programs, are expected to complete a minimum of 1,000 post-baccalaureate practice hours.
- Practice immersion experiences afford the opportunity to apply, integrate and synthesize the DNP *Essentials* necessary to demonstrate achievement of desired outcomes in an area of advanced nursing practice.
- Practice experiences for the DNP student are not intended to be solely direct patient care focused but should include indirect care practices in healthcare related environments.
- Programs must demonstrate that graduates have attained all of the DNP *Essential* outcomes.
- Students who have completed more than 1,000 practice hours in their master's program will need to complete additional hours in the DNP program.
- Practice hours spent in master's nursing programs can be counted as post-baccalaureate practice hours, provided they can be verified.
- Practice experiences should have well defined learning objectives and provide experiences over and above the individual's job responsibilities or activities.
- Schools may credit practice hours to a post-master's DNP student who holds current national certification in an area of advanced nursing practice, as defined in the AACN 2006 *DNP Essentials*, and requires a minimum of a graduate degree.

- Post-master's students must have faculty supervised practice hours in the DNP program that provide the opportunity for the student to integrate all of the outcomes delineated in the DNP *Essentials*.
- DNP programs should not be preparing the nurse educator; therefore the focus of the practicum and DNP project should not be on the academic educational process, the academic curriculum, or on educating nursing students. Practice as a nurse educator should not be included in the DNP practice hours.

V. **Collaborative Partnerships**
- Programs should follow the Academic-Practice Partnership guiding principles developed by the AACN-AONE Task Force on Academic-Practice Partnerships (2012).
- Programs are encouraged to consider a broad range of academic-practice partnerships, e.g. with school systems, prison systems, public health departments, that afford students opportunities to engage in the full planning, implementation, and evaluation of a project that impacts healthcare outcomes.
- Academic and practice partners are encouraged to collect outcome data to demonstrate the added value of DNP graduates.

SUMMARY OF TRENDS

In summary, the trends identified confirm that DNP education is evolving, and change has occurred rapidly in recent years. The major trends relating to the practice doctorate identified are as follows:

- DNP programs are rapidly growing and changing. However, DNP student enrollments are not negatively affecting enrollment in research-focused PhD programs in nursing.
- There is a shift from programs offering only a post-master's level to DNP option to more programs adding the BSN to DNP option.
- The roles identified by DNP students are not only the traditional APRN clinical roles; students are also choosing a focus on nonclinical (indirect care) advanced nursing practice roles, such as nurse executive, health policy specialist, and informaticist.
- Most DNP programs are becoming accredited by organizations such as the CCNE, which ultimately should decrease variability in program standards.

- Academic rigor continues to be defined for the practice doctorate because the definition of rigor can be different from that applied to research-focused doctorates.

In response to the variability in DNP education, the AACN commissioned various task forces, including the Implementation of the DNP Task Force (2015d) to outline recommendations to define and clarify various aspects of DNP education.

SUMMARY

The demands of providing health care in our country to an increasingly complex population of patients require higher levels of nursing education and practice. The clinical doctorate in nursing, the DNP, has emerged to address the competencies that healthcare providers must have in order to apply evidence-based practice in the provision of high-quality patient-centered care in interdisciplinary teams, using such tools as information technology. There is an emerging model of generation of knowledge by both the research and practice nursing doctorates working in teams to develop clinical knowledge and translate that knowledge into practice in a timely fashion. Nonclinical roles (indirect care) for advanced nursing practice and the traditional roles of clinical advanced nursing practice benefit from the competencies attained through doctoral-level education.

With the rapid growth of DNP programs since 2004, standardization of DNP education is emerging along with an increased number of accredited programs. In response to variability in certain aspects of DNP programs, the AACN commissioned the Implementation of the DNP Task Force to clarify recommendations regarding the DNP project, DNP educational program characteristics, DNP practicum hour requirement and encouraging collaborative partnerships between academia and practice. Because the DNP project is the demonstration of attainment of the Essentials of Doctoral Education for Advanced Nursing Practice outcomes, these guidelines from the AACN are necessary to promote high-quality and rigorous standards. The challenges of dealing with complex disease states and the development of a subspecialty advanced practice role are illustrated in the following DNP project exemplar by Dr. Elizabeth Jensen. She describes how obtaining a DNP degree provided her with the knowledge and skill set to emerge as a provider, and nursing practice leader.

Improving the Care for Women with Vulvodynia
Elizabeth Jensen, CNM, APN, DNP Graduate
of the Frontier Nursing University

Vulvodynia is a serious women's health concern affecting millions of women in the United States. Many women are unable to find knowledgeable providers who treat vulvodynia, leaving women with vulvar pain disorders in the United States underserved. My DNP project was developed with the goal to improve the care for women with vulvodynia by increasing the numbers of APRNs who are comfortable and confident caring for women with vulvar pain disorders. A 19-item survey was deployed via SurveyMonkey to identify the educational needs of APRNs to care for women with vulvar disorders and determine the APRN's level of interest in addressing this important healthcare need. In total, 597 APRNs responded during the survey period. This national survey identified that APRNs are not comfortable diagnosing and treating vulvar disorders and need further education in vulvodynia, atypical vaginal infections, and vulvar skin disorders. More important, the majority of APRNs who responded expressed an interest in learning more about these topics.

The completion of this scholarly project fueled my interest to continue working in this subspecialty area as a practicing DNP with a goal to educate other APRNs. Shortly after graduation, I applied for a grant from the National Vulvodynia Association (NVA) to receive funds to open a dedicated vulvovaginal service. This grant was awarded to S.H.E. Medical Associates in Hartford, Connecticut, and I currently serve as the director of this service. In this role, I provide gynecological services to women who suffer with vulvar pain disorders, and our service is expanding rapidly. In addition, our service serves as a site for APRN providers and students who wish to expand their skills in this subspecialty. Obtaining a DNP degree provided me with the knowledge and skill set to emerge as a provider, and nursing practice leader in the subspecialty of vulvology.

Key Messages

- The DNP is a degree, not a role.
- Current educational preparation for the DNP is evolving but still reflects the *Essentials* of DNP education.
- The DNP is the practice-based doctorate.
- The PhD and DNS in nursing are the research-based doctorates
- The collaboration between the two doctoral levels of preparation will determine the future of nursing and its impact on health care.
- The definition of the DNP will continue to evolve, and the DNP graduate will be a part of the evolution.
- Nurses must have an understanding of the definition of the DNP and be able to clearly articulate it.
- The *Essentials* are intertwined within DNP education, and the DNP project is the culmination/demonstration of the DNP final product/skill set.

REFERENCES

American Association of Colleges of Nursing. (2004). *AACN position statement on the practice doctorate in nursing.* Washington, DC: Author.

American Association of Colleges of Nursing. (2006). *The essentials for doctoral education for advanced nursing practice.* Washington, DC: Author.

American Association of Colleges of Nursing. (2014). *Key differences between DNP and PhD/DNS programs.* Retrieved from: http://www.aacn.nche.edu/dnp/ContrastGrid.pdf

American Association of Colleges of Nursing. (2015a). DNP fact sheet. Retrieved from: http://www.aacn.nche.edu/media-relations/fact-sheets/dnp

American Association of Colleges of Nursing. (2015b). Custom report on doctoral Program Enrollments, 1997–2014. Washington, DC: AACN Research and Data Services.

American Association of Colleges of Nursing. (2015c). White paper: Current state of APRN clinical education. Retrieved from: http://www.aacn.nche.edu/APRN-White-Paper.pdf

American Association of Colleges of Nursing. (2015d). The doctor of nursing practice: Current issues and clarifying recommendations. Retrieved from: http://www.aacn.nche.edu/aacn-publications/white-papers/DNP-Implementation-TF-Report-8-15.pdf

American Association of Colleges of Nursing-American Organization of Nurse Executives (AACN-AONE) Task Force on Academic-Practice Partnerships. (2012). Guiding principles. Retrieved from https://www.aacn.nche.edu/leading-initiatives/academic-practice-partnerships/GuidingPrinciples.pdf

APRN Joint Dialogue Group. (2008). *Consensus model for APRN regulation: Licensure, accreditation, certification & education.* Retrieved from http://www.nonpf.org/associations/10789/files/APRNConsensusModelFinal09.pdf

Auerbach, D., Martsolf, G., Pearson, M., Taylor, E., Zaydman, M., Muchow, A., . . . Dower, C. (2014). The DNP by 2015: A study of the institutional, political, and professional issues that facilitate or impede establishing a post-baccalaureate doctor of nursing practice program. Retrieved from http://www.aacn.nche.edu/DNP/DNP-Study.pdf

Carraccio, C., & Englander, R. (2013). From Flexner to competencies: Reflections on a decade and the journey ahead. *Academic Medicine, 88*(8), 1067–1073.

Carraccio, C., Wolfsthal, S. D., Englander, R., Ferentz, K., & Martin, C. (2002). Shifting paradigms: From Flexner to competencies. *Academic Medicine, 77,* 361–367.

Chism, L. A. (2016). *The doctor of nursing practice: A guidebook for role development and professional issues.* Sudbury, MA: Jones and Bartlett.

Institute of Medicine. (2001). *Crossing the quality chasm: A new health system for the 21st century.* Retrieved from http://www.iom.edu/~/media/Files/Report%20Files/2001/Crossing-the-Quality-Chasm/Quality%20Chasm%202001%20%20report%20brief.pdf

Institute of Medicine. (2003). *Health professions education: A bridge to quality.* Retrieved from http://www.nap.edu/openbook.php?record_id=10681&page=45

Institute of Medicine. (2010). *The future of nursing: Leading change, advancing health.* Washington, DC: National Academies Press.

Lamb, G. (2012, January). *Interprofessional initiatives in doctoral nursing education: The ASU experience.* Presented at the AACN Doctoral Conference, San Diego, CA.

Office for the Assistant Secretary for Planning and Evaluation (ASPE). (2015). *Health insurance coverage and the affordable care act, September 2015.* Retrieved from https://aspe.hhs.gov/pdf-report/health-insurance-coverage-and-affordable-care-act-september-2015

CHAPTER 4

Scholarship in Practice

Rosanne Burson

CHAPTER OVERVIEW

To appreciate the scholarly project, there must be an understanding of both practice and scholarship. This chapter reveals the history of scholarship as it supports the developing nature of the practice doctorate and knowledge generation. The purpose of the doctor of nursing practice (DNP) project is defined, and the current view of potential projects is presented. Several exemplars highlight the process of developing the DNP project and the impact of the process on the DNP student. Finally, recommended action steps are offered in considering project topics.

CHAPTER OBJECTIVES

After completing the chapter, the learner will be able to:
1. Have an understanding of scholarship as it relates to the practice doctorate
2. Explore the historical underpinnings that have evolved nursing's view of knowledge generation
3. Understand the critical nature of the DNP project to have an impact on the evolution of the DNP and practice outcomes
4. Review the current state of DNP projects
5. Conceptualize the types of projects that can and are being considered
6. Begin to examine potential topics of interest in relation to the appropriate level of scholarship

WHAT IS SCHOLARSHIP?

An investigation of scholarship as it relates to history, and specifically to nursing practice, contributes to the understanding of the scholarly project. "Scholarship" is defined in *Merriam-Webster's Learner's Dictionary* as "serious formal study or research of a subject" ("Scholarship," 2015, para. 2). The nursing literature confirms that scholarship is a critical feature of our continuing survival and implies a unique knowledge base (Bunkers, 2000; Fawcett, 1999). Magnan (2016) identified "three recurring themes in the literature regarding nursing scholarship as (a) breadth and depth of knowledge within a defined area, (b) innovation and creativity, and (c) exposure of the scholarly project to public scrutiny and peer review" (p. 125). As the DNP student considers topics for scholarly work, an assessment of the topic in relation to these themes will assist in ensuring a project that meets the expectations of scholarly work.

> Scholarship is the mechanism that provides knowledge development within a discipline.

Scholarship is the mechanism that provides knowledge development within a discipline. The understanding and acceptance of where knowledge development comes from are evolving. It is increasingly understood that knowledge production is measured according to its contribution to improved outcomes rather than its contribution to generalizable knowledge (Rolfe & Davies, 2009). What this means for the DNP student is that the work that is done in relation to improving outcomes for patients and healthcare systems is increasingly viewed as important knowledge that will be accrued and shared to produce further improvements. This is a big change in what historically has been accepted as knowledge generation.

Ferguson-Pare predicted in 2005 that future nurses would be scholar-practitioners driven by emerging trends of patient-centered care. She stated, "This is the time for nursing to embrace scholarly activities and to engage in continuous teaching-learning, research, and scholarly inquiry in our practice. The emergence of scholar-practitioners in nursing will assure a future for the profession" (p. 120). That future is here, driven by forces internal and external to nursing that are demanding nursing's full contribution to improving health. It is a time of opportunity and potential.

Important external forces have contributed to the movement of incorporating practice more deeply in scholarship. As has been discussed in earlier chapters, the Institute of Medicine (IOM) has been a key driver to instrumental change in health care. The IOM reports have identified the lack of quality and safety within our health systems and a need for fundamental change that supports a redesigned system focused on quality outcomes that use evidence, information technology, organizational support, and the alignment of payment policy (IOM, 1999, 2001). In 2010, the IOM produced the report *The Future of Nursing*, which stated that nurses should practice to the full extent of their training and be full partners in redesigning health care. Evidence-based care, high-quality outcomes, and cost containment are required components of healthcare reform.

Nursing's expertise and input are critical at this time but must be provided at an appropriate level of scholarship to be an optimal and valued contribution. It is time to expand the nursing repertoire to incorporate a broader base of knowledge that includes, but reaches beyond, the clinical focus. In 2006, Kitson reflected on her 1999 article regarding scholarship in practice in

> It is time to expand the nursing repertoire to incorporate a broader base of knowledge that includes, but reaches beyond, the clinical focus.

the *Journal of Advanced Nursing*: "But what we need now is the political and business acumen to improve and integrate our academic and practice infrastructures to enable nursing scholarship and nursing innovation to flourish" (p. 545). The *Essentials* of DNP education serve to further drive the nature of the practice doctorate to lead healthcare systems. Each of the DNP *Essentials* contributes by strengthening the student's core knowledge skill set. The ability to develop innovations specific to health incorporates all the components of DNP practice, including collaboration, informatics, and business and political aspects. As the DNP student develops a scholarly project, identifying the specific *Essentials* that will be demonstrated in the project can confirm evidence of doctoral-level work.

> The ability to develop innovations specific to health incorporates all the components of DNP practice, including collaboration, informatics, and business and political aspects.

The demonstration of doctoral work is important to the validation of the educational degree and the potential for leadership and effective knowledge development that affects healthcare outcomes.

HISTORY OF SCHOLARSHIP AND NURSING PRACTICE

Nursing has explored and struggled with critical aspects of practice as they relate to scholarship over many years. The doctor of nursing science (DNSc) was presented in 1970 with an emphasis on advanced clinical practice and was an early effort to give nursing parity with other disciplines. The DNSc required both clinical competence *and* demonstrated ability to perform scholarly research. In 1979, the doctor of nursing (ND) degree emerged. Again, parity with other health professional doctoral programs, such as medicine, dentistry, optometry, and others, was sought. However, the ND focused exclusively on the advanced clinical aspects rather than research (AACN, 2004). The doctorate of nursing practice (DrNP) evolved to also focus on advanced clinical expertise and was geared toward preparing nurse practitioners for independent primary care roles. Today, the DNP concentrates on evidence-based practice (EBP) for improved delivery of care, patient outcomes, and clinical systems management (AACN, 2004). The DNP is considered a practice doctorate and is inclusive of all advanced nursing practice roles: nurse practitioner, nurse-midwife, nurse anesthetist, and clinical nurse specialist, as well as nurse administrator, nurse informaticist, and nurse policy expert.

Over the years, there have been many barriers to full implementation of the practice doctorate. One barrier was the lack of a broader view of scholarship beyond generalizable knowledge. Previously, it had been assumed that knowledge generation could only be elicited from a quantitative research process. However, today, societal needs are driving scholarship to develop knowledge that affects outcomes. Although challenges to the acceptance of the DNP continue, the current healthcare environment is in need of leaders to pave the way, and the DNP prepared nurse is equipped with the skill set to take on this challenge. The need for leadership and transition to a patient-centered, cost-effective system provides a mechanism for acceptance. The DNP-prepared nurse is required to rapidly demonstrate ability and effectiveness to impact health care. This demonstration begins with the DNP-prepared nurse project and will expand as the DNP-prepared nurse continues to impact practice.

> Societal needs are driving scholarship to develop knowledge that affects outcomes.

SCHOLARSHIP EVOLUTION

It is important for the DNP prepared nurse to have an understanding of the evolution of scholarship. Many brilliant minds have paved the way for this progression. The significance of this evolution has been critical to the current state of the practice doctorate in nursing and the ability to have an impact on population outcomes.

During the early to middle part of the 20th century, empirical science was viewed as the only way to generate knowledge. Quantitative research was regaled as the highest level of truth. This had been demonstrated in the hierarchy of types of research and in the predominance of quantitative research. However, the scientific/laboratory view of controlling for variables has been difficult to transition to practice. This separation of research and practice has limited our ability to integrate new knowledge into practice and for practice to have an important influence on research. Increasingly, it is understood that the complexities of health care cannot always be explained via a single model of research. Nursing's holistic history implores a view of knowledge through multiple lenses.

A broadening of the view of scholarship has occurred over the last quarter century. For example, qualitative research added to the understanding of many phenomena and became more relevant and accepted as a format to generate new knowledge. One of the most significant contributions to the broadening of scholarship was developed by Ernest Boyer. In his classic book, *Scholarship Reconsidered: Priorities of the Professoriate* (1990), Boyer established an inclusive view of scholarship consisting of discovery, teaching, practice, and integration. He asked, "How can the role of the scholar be defined in ways that not only affirm the past but also reflect the present and adequately anticipate the future?" (p. 75). This reflective quote should guide scholars in respecting knowledge generation of the past.

> "How can the role of scholar be defined in ways that not only affirm the past but also reflect the present and adequately anticipate the future?" (Boyer, 1990, p. 75).

At the same time, the scholar should be encouraged to develop and accept new methods to meet the needs of new knowledge generation. Boyer suggested moving beyond the usual way of looking at scholarship in a narrow view of original research and to consider *how useful the work is for society*. It is no longer enough to develop knowledge for knowledge sake; now the requirement is to investigate how the scholarship relates to the world.

Although Boyer was considering the view of scholarship within academia, traditional thinking about knowledge generation began to be questioned in all areas of scholarship. Dirks (1998) discussed the new scholarship that must incorporate both the conceptual and analytical with the concrete and practice components that also include reflection. This view recognizes that different types of scholarship work together to drive fully formed knowledge generation that has an impact, from the conceptual thought through to practice and back to the conceptual process. New ideas are evolving about this relationship between theory and practice that defines truth for a discipline (Reed & Shearer, 2011). The outcome of scholarship and knowledge generation should be a positive result

> Scholars with a variety of strengths and perspectives will be required to participate in these more complex approaches, using each other's strengths as in a network.

for society. Scholars with a variety of strengths and perspectives will be required to participate in these more complex approaches, using each other's strengths as in a network.

In 1999, the AACN published the position paper *Defining Scholarship for the Discipline of Nursing.* The paper confirms a view of the evolution of scholarship to include discovery, teaching, application in clinical practice, and integration of ideas. The report identified that the four areas of scholarship developed by Boyer were important to the values of the profession of nursing. These values include a commitment to scientific advancement and recognition of its significance for society. This argument is very applicable in nursing because of the demands of practice and the commitment to the public to incorporate the latest research in the delivery of care. In addition, these values highlight the integrated relationship between theory, research, and practice. All areas of knowledge generation need to support each other in order to have an impact on science advancement and society. Reed and Shearer (2011) discussed the relationship between theory and practice, stating that "theory will not so much be applied or disseminated from research to practice as it will emerge from scholarly thinking in practice, and then continue to be transformed as practice contexts change" (p. 30). **Figure 4-1** visually captures the integration of knowledge generation through research, practice, and theory. Note that all aspects affect the others and are affected by each other. This depiction suggests that various types of scholars need to interact at their highest level of skill to allow the network to function at its highest capacity and have the greatest societal impact.

Within this model, the role of the practitioner-scholar (DNP) is problem solving and producing positive outcomes in a local context. In contrast, the role of the scientist-scholar (PhD) is to develop theories about large areas of reality. Both

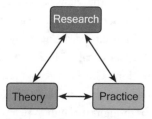

FIGURE 4-1 The relationship between theory, research, and practice.

Modified from McEwen, M., & Wills, E. M. (2014). *Theoretical basis for nursing.* Philadelphia, PA: Wolters Kluwer Health/Lippincott Williams & Wilkins.

types of scholars contribute to knowledge generation and are interdependent to fully impact health.

TYPES OF SCHOLARSHIP

Boyer defined the scholarship of *discovery* as original research. Discovery scholarship typically reflects the historical view of knowledge generation of research and theory development, which has been the work of the PhD research nurse. Four phases of knowledge development have been described by Velasquez, McArthur, and Johnson (2011) in an effort to qualify all aspects of scholarly activity within the doctoral work of both PhD and DNP. The first two phases tease out different aspects of discovery. The *exploration phase* incorporates knowledge discovery in both quantitative and qualitative avenues. This terminology aligns with AACN's (1999) applied definition of discovery scholarship to include empirical and historical research, theory development, methodological studies, and philosophical inquiry and analysis. The term *explication* is described as theory evaluation, also identified by AACN within the discovery component of scholarship. The first two phases of knowledge development fit well with the definition of discovery scholarship and suggest an overlap between practice and research nursing doctorates.

The scholarship of *integration* (Boyer, 1990) is "serious, disciplined work that seeks to interpret, draw together, and bring new insight to bear on original research" (p. 19). Within nursing, the scholarship of integration includes interfaces between nursing and other disciplines. Some products of this level of scholarship include integrative reviews of the literature, analysis of health policy, development of interdisciplinary educational programs and service projects, studies of systems in health care, original interdisciplinary research, and integrative models or paradigms across disciplines (AACN, 1999). Nursing's history as a collaborator and team player makes scholarship of integration a natural fit. Nursing's understanding of theory based in multiple disciplines also contributes to this fit.

> Nursing's history as a collaborator and team player makes scholarship of integration a natural fit. Nursing will need to continue to step up to the table, using higher levels of analysis to be considered a *team leader*.

However, nursing will need to continue to step up to the table, using higher levels of analysis to be considered a *team leader* who can fully develop as the IOM has envisioned.

The scholarship of integration refers to writings and other products that use concepts and original works from nursing and other disciplines in creating new patterns. Integration places knowledge in a larger context and illuminates data in a more meaningful way. The scholarship of integration emphasizes the interconnection of ideas and brings new insight to bear on original concepts and research (Boyer, 1990). Original work in the scholarship of integration takes place between two or more disciplines. Integration combines knowledge in new creative applications that change paradigms and offer keen insights to solve problems. The scholarship of integration has great potential to be a key aspect of practice scholarship because of its collaborative nature and outcome focus.

The scholarship of *application* focuses on these questions: "How can knowledge be applied to consequential problems? How can it be helpful to individuals as well as institutions? Can social problems themselves define an agenda for scholarly investigation?" (Boyer, 1990, p. 22). Thoun (2009) encouraged a look beyond Boyer's work in defining practice scholarship and suggested, "This pattern of scholarship involves systematic inquiry of professional practice that is imaginative, artistic, and resourceful" (p. 555).

Application scholarship is related to practice issues. Some of the works included in application scholarship are analysis of patient or health services outcomes, reports of clinical demonstration projects, and policy papers related to practice. Other examples include the measurement of quality-of-life indicators, the development and refinement of practice protocols and strategies, the evaluation of systems of care, and the analysis of innovative healthcare delivery models (AACN, 1999).

> Within the conceptual model of knowledge generation, there is an understanding that overlap and mutual support will exist within doctoral scholarship.

Velasquez et al. (2011) further described levels of knowledge development that can be identified with integration and application. The terms used to describe aspects of knowledge development related to integration and application are *engagement* and *optimization*. Engagement incorporates implementation, evaluation, and dissemination of knowledge. Types of work within engagement include program evaluation and quality improvement. Optimization is described as a revising and refinement of interventions. Within the conceptual model of knowledge generation, there is an understanding that overlap and mutual support will exist within doctoral scholarship. Knowledge generation is not hierarchal but is shared with contributions from practice and research.

> Knowledge generation is not hierarchal but is shared with contributions from practice and research.

Scholarship activities will continue to develop within integration and application and will begin to converge because both aspects are needed in a scholarly practice environment. The complex nature

Scholarship activities will continue to develop within integration and application and will begin to converge because both aspects are needed in a scholarly practice environment.

of health systems as they affect patient outcomes will require an integrated, interdisciplinary approach within the application of practice. The DNP prepared nurse, focused in these areas of scholarship, is expected to participate within this environment.

As the research scholar (PhD) defines and tests new theories that are generalizable to populations, the practice scholar (DNP) will apply them within a local context and measure their applicability within settings (translation and implementation science). The PhD-prepared nurse generates external evidence through rigorous research to extend science and theory and guide practice. The DNP-prepared nurse generates internal evidence through outcomes management, quality improvement and EBP projects that translate external evidence into practice and policy to improve care and outcomes (Melnyk, 2013).

PRACTICE SCHOLARSHIP AND NURSING THEORY

Practice scholarship has been infused in nursing throughout nursing history. Early nursing scholars include Florence Nightingale, who used data in her clinical explanations to improve patient care. "Nurses such as Virginia Henderson brought nursing education and practice closer by concentrating on the relationship between nurses and patients rather than on the intricacies of procedures and manual skills" (Fairman, 2008, p. 4). Scholarship has been intricately woven with societal needs as well. Nursing knowledge continued to be framed by clinical experience. Patients who would not have survived previously began to suffer from chronic diseases. "Much of the practice scholarship that emerged in the 1950s through the 1970s was . . . a response to nurses' demands for knowledge to safely care for patients, experientially based to organize the complexity of clinical situations" (Fairman, p. 4).

In the past few years, clinical inquiry has become a first step in development toward EBP. Clinical inquiry identifies knowledge gaps. Expert nurses ask questions that relate to patient outcomes. This process involves questioning and evaluating. "In the EBP paradigm, clinical expertise is combined with best scientific evidence, patient values and preferences and the clinical circumstance" (Salmond, 2007, p. 114).

It is clear that links between practice, nursing theory, and research need to be further developed and that practice is a key source of knowledge application and knowledge development. If credence is given to practice knowledge generation, there will be new descriptions of what occurs within situation-specific theory to affect outcomes for patients.

> If credence is given to practice knowledge generation, there will be new descriptions of what occurs within situation-specific theory to affect outcomes for patients.

Reed and Shearer (2011) explained new strategies for theorizing that include concepts such as guerilla theorizing, *bricoleur*, and improvisation. *Guerilla theorizing* is making something that is innovative, flexible, and impermanent, derived from the practitioner's inspiration and knowledge, ethical concern, and interaction with the immediate world. The practitioner-scholar knows that understanding the context of the care delivery directly affects the impact on outcome. Consideration of each unique situation creates a specific plan of action that is inclusive. *Bricoleur* is creating a new coherent structure from what is at hand. Drawing on knowledge and experiences, the practitioner-scholar considers multiple sources to create an innovation that improves care delivery. *Improvisation* is creation out of existing elements in the moment. Just as the jazz musician improvises in the moment to create a beautiful sound, the practitioner-scholar creates a strategy from known elements to effect success within a local context. These strategies are rooted in the scholarship of integration and application and are examples of knowledge generation within practice. Nursing practice has often used strategies to affect outcomes. However, there is newfound power in the description of the processes that occur in practice-based knowledge generation. The scholarly nature of this application also demands dissemination of the local knowledge. Dissemination will be further discussed in Chapter 15, Disseminating the Results.

Table 4-1 shows combined similar descriptions of types of scholarship and knowledge generation in an effort to assist the DNP student in considering types of scholarship for the DNP project and differentiating PhD scholarship.

To demonstrate the ability of the DNP student in using clinical expertise, EBP, and the *Essentials* of DNP education to create an innovation, the following project is described.

Two DNP students proposed an innovation of care within the primary care arena for patients with diabetes. This short story illustrates how the students progressed in the development of the scholarly project. Their extensive clinical background as advanced practice nurses, diabetes program managers, and

Table 4-1 Types of Scholarship and Knowledge Generation

Types of Scholarship/ Knowledge Generation	Definition	Examples
Discovery	Original research	Empirical and historical research
Exploration	Quantitative/qualitative	Theory development and testing
Explication	Theory testing	Methodological studies Philosophical inquiry and analysis
Integration	New insight on original research Interfaces between nursing and a variety of disciplines Creating new patterns, placing knowledge in a larger context, or illuminating the data in a more meaningful way	Integrative reviews of the literature Analysis of health policy Development of interdisciplinary educational programs and service projects Studies of systems in health care
Bricoleur	Creating knowledge or combining knowledge in applications that offer new paradigms and insights	Original interdisciplinary research Integrative models or paradigms across disciplines
Application	Related to practice issues and outcomes Knowledge applied to problems	Analysis of patient or health services Outcomes reports of clinical demonstration projects
Engagement	Implementation/evaluation dissemination of knowledge	Policy papers related to practice Assessment and validation of patient care outcomes
Optimization	Revising and refinement of interventions	Measurement of quality-of-life indicators
Guerilla theorizing	Local interaction to make something innovative and flexible	Development and refinement of practice protocols/strategies Evaluation of systems of care
Improvisation	Creating something new in the moment out of preexisting elements	Analysis of innovative healthcare delivery models Program evaluation Quality improvement Clinical inquiry Translation of EBP

(Continued)

Table 4-1 Types of Scholarship and Knowledge Generation (*Continued*)

Types of Scholarship/ Knowledge Generation	Definition	Examples
Teaching	Centers on student learning/ entices future scholars	Research related to teaching methodology or learning outcomes
	Dissemination of existing knowledge	Learning theory development
	Creation of new knowledge through interaction	Development or testing of educational models or theories
		Successful applications of technology to teaching and learning
		Design of outcome studies or evaluation/assessment

Data from concepts in AACN, 1999; Boyer, 1990; Melnyk, 2013; Reed & Shearer, 2011; Velasquez, McArthur, & Johnson, 2011.

certified diabetes educators (CDEs) had given them a deep understanding of diabetes care, education, and management. The skill set at their disposal included knowledge of the scope and standards of care of diabetes education and care, proven competencies as diabetes educators, years of team interdisciplinary collaborations, experiences in the field around the country observing the primary care environment, and finance and management skills from experience in industry, entrepreneurial efforts, and management. Personal experiences with diabetes and family members also added to the conglomeration of strengths.

As the two students progressed through doctoral education, they continued to build on their original strengths and developed new skills, particularly in the areas of data mining, implementation science, outcome management, and policy. They continued to examine their phenomena of interest through multiple, varied lenses, and they explored their topic of interest within the literature. The students began to integrate (connect the dots) all of what they knew and were continuing to learn. Gaps and needs were identified that could support a primary care innovation that had the potential for clinical and cost-effectiveness. All the pieces of the intervention were built from known parts but redesigned in a new way.

The DNP project was titled *Exploring the Cost and Clinical Outcomes of Integrating the Registered Nurse, Certified Diabetes Educator in the Patient-Centered Medical Home* (Moran, Burson, Critchett, & Olla, 2011).

The type of scholarship described is one of integration and application. It was interdisciplinary and focused on practice outcomes that included financial and clinical viability. The project interfaced nursing with multiple disciplines and exemplified teamwork and collaboration. Multiple theories were used to build the framework of the innovation. These included chaos theory, caring science, and Donabedian's quality improvement model. The project was specific to practice issues and outcomes reporting on a multiplicity of clinical and psychological measures, as well as cost features. The term *bricoleur* accurately explains this process of combining knowledge applications to offer new paradigms and insights. The success of this project moved the scholarship team into an entrepreneurial business venture to further expand and develop the innovation.

It is important to understand that this process occurred over 2 years of study. The DNP student will bring personal strengths and experiences to the table and will expand the possibilities through new knowledge, skill sets, and views.

> The DNP student will bring personal strengths and experiences to the table and will expand the possibilities through new knowledge, skill sets, and views.

The process takes time, and ideas will change and develop as the scholarly project takes shape. Patience and perseverance are important characteristics of the DNP student as doctoral education is experienced and transforms the student.

The previous exemplar can be reviewed in the context of the Actualized DNP Model (see **Figure 4-2**). The Actualized DNP Model explores how the unique skillset of the nurse prepared with a practice doctorate is able to apply advanced practice knowledge in existing and new nursing roles that lead to achievement of healthcare outcomes (Burson, Moran, & Conrad, 2016).

Advanced nursing knowledge refers to achievement of the DNP *Essentials* that prepares experts in advanced nursing practice, implementation science, and leaders in applying research in order to improve practice (AACN, 2006; Burson et al., 2016; Cary & George, 2011; Levin & Slyder, 2012). Clinical knowledge includes leadership abilities, a focus on nursing theory, clinical management, coordination of care, information technology utilization, interprofessional collaboration, and business and policy acumen (Burson et al., 2016; Draye, Acker, & Zimmer, 2006; Swanson & Stanton, 2013).

In enacting advanced nursing roles incorporating this unique skillset, the practice doctorate uses an EBP application component that generates new knowledge in practice (practice-based evidence) (Burson et al., 2016). Implementation science is used to promote the integration of research science and evidence into healthcare policy and practice (National Institutes of Health, 2015).

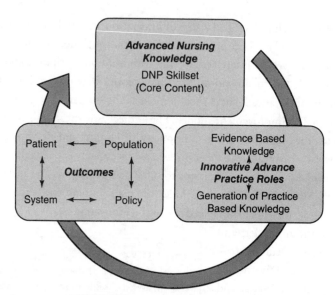

FIGURE 4-2 Actualized DNP model

Reproduced from Burson, R., Moran, K. J., & Conrad, D. (2016). Why Hire a DNP Prepared Nurse? The Value Added Impact of the Practice Doctorate. *Journal of Doctoral Nursing Practice, 9*(1).

As the DNP-prepared nurse functions within organizations using a unique skill set and advanced knowledge bases, data are used to drive innovation and measure outcomes, not only for individuals and populations but also systems and policy outcomes. This demonstrates practice scholarship achieving healthcare reform goals to improve healthcare quality while decreasing costs (Burson et al., 2016).

This figure depicts the DNP project; demonstrating many of the *Essentials* in the development, implementation, and evaluation of the project. Note that each sphere identifies the collaborative work that was required for this project and its connection to the appropriate *Essential*.

WHAT IS THE PURPOSE OF THE DNP PROJECT?

In 2006, the AACN defined the purpose of the DNP project as a deliverable of accumulation of knowledge and summative evaluation of DNP education process. The scholarly project also adds to nursing knowledge and has value that goes beyond the program deliverable. The DNP curriculum contributes to each of the competencies that are then demonstrated in the DNP project. Within the process of education and knowledge synthesis, the *Essentials* are integrated and demonstrated (AACN, 2006). The *Essentials* exemplify a thoughtful contribution and roadmap of the competencies the nursing scholar must exemplify to have an

> The DNP *Essentials* exemplify a thoughtful contribution and roadmap of the competencies the nursing scholar must exemplify to have an impact on health care from a nursing perspective.

impact on health care from a nursing perspective. The DNP *Essentials* are presented and described in Chapter 3, Defining the Doctor of Nursing Practice: Current Trends, and are listed in **Table 4-2**. Doctoral coursework supports the DNP *Essentials* and the development of the new knowledge and skill set for the DNP student. The coursework also offers the student an opportunity to explore his or her topic of interest within each *Essential*.

Taking the preceding example, the patient-centered diabetes project, to the next step demonstrates the connection to the DNP *Essentials*. See **Figure 4-3**, which depicts the DNP project plan and the facilitation of multiple team collaborations. In the center is the patient, depicting patient-centered chronic disease management related to DNP Essential I: Scientific Underpinnings for Practice. This *Essential* drove the development of the intervention based on empirical knowledge of disease process, educational principles, and caring science.

Table 4-2 Doctor of Nursing Practice *Essentials*

I	Scientific Underpinnings for Practice
II	Organizational and Systems Leadership for Quality Improvement and Systems Thinking
III	Clinical Scholarship and Analytical Methods for Evidence-Based Practice
IV	Information Systems/Technology and Patient Care Technology for the Improvement and Transformation of Health Care
V	Health Care Policy for Advocacy in Health Care
VI	Interprofessional Collaboration for Improving Patient and Population Health Outcomes
VII	Clinical Prevention and Population Health for Improving the Nation's Health
VIII	Advanced Nursing Practice

Data from American Association of Colleges of Nursing. (2006). The essentials for doctoral education for advanced nursing practice. Washington, DC: Author.

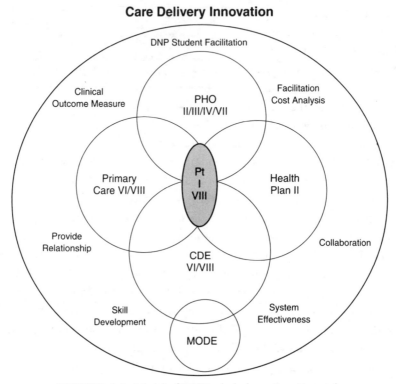

FIGURE 4-3 Model of DNP scholarly project *Essentials*.

This core also incorporates DNP Essential VIII: Advanced Nursing Practice. The DNP connects the dots between practice, organizational, population, fiscal, and policy issues to develop the intervention.

The top icon, Physician Health Organization (PHO), illustrates multiple *Essentials*. Within this collaboration, the DNP demonstrates organizational and systems leadership in order to develop the innovation (Essential II: Organizational and Systems Leadership for Quality Improvement and Systems Thinking). It was also at this level that Essential IV: Information Systems/Technology was used to assess data before and after intervention, as well as population health data that were used specific to each practice (Essential VII: Clinical Prevention and Population Health for Improving the Nation's Health).

Moving clockwise, health plan collaboration occurred to evaluate the current reimbursement and revenue-generating contributions that could assist in making the project viable in the long term (Essential II). Collaboration also occurred with CDEs, primary care providers, and staff within the primary care setting using Essential VI: Interprofessional Collaboration for Improving Patient and Population Health Outcomes. The Michigan Organization of Diabetes Educators (MODE) was a part of the networking that occurred tᴏ identify interest in and the knowledge base of CDEs in the patient-centered medical home (PCMH) strategies.

Of course, the process of developing the proposal, achieving institutional review board (IRB) status, and analyzing the data is evidence of Essential III: Clinical Scholarship and Analytical Methods for Evidence-Based Practice. Advanced nursing practice (Essential VIII) was demonstrated in mentoring registered nurses and the office staff, as well as the providers, in transforming care within the practice.

Seven of the eight *Essentials* were identified in this project plan. The completion of the project and the knowledge derived could then be used to promote Essential V: Health Care Policy. Although not every project will exemplify all the *Essentials,* the student should consider the elements that will be used in order to effectively develop and implement the scholarly project. It is the systems approach—focused on data, outcomes, finance, and clinical measures—that will promote both the skills of the DNP-prepared nurse and attainment of healthcare transformation.

The scholarly project incorporates practice and scholarship. There is an emerging realization that scholarship requires the integration of practice in a practice discipline. The defining feature of practice is that it incorporates an intervention that influences an outcome. The expansive view of the AACN definition of nursing practice allows for the full impact of contributions from all avenues of advanced practice in order to positively influence the nation's health system. The AACN definition of *advanced nursing practice* is "any form of nursing intervention that influences health outcomes for individuals or populations, including the provision of direct care or management of care for individual patients or management of care populations, and the provision of indirect care such as nursing administration, executive leadership, health policy, informatics and population health" (AACN, 2015a). Advanced nursing practice includes nurse practitioners, clinical nurse specialists, nurse anesthetists, nurse-midwives, nurse administrators, policy specialists, and informaticists.

Earlier discussion in this chapter focused on the critical nature of scholarliness in contributing to the knowledge base of nursing from a practice perspective. It becomes clear that the DNP project is much more than a mere demonstration of what the student has learned; it is a demonstration of how practicing scholarly nurses

> The DNP project is a demonstration of how practicing scholarly nurses can build new knowledge.

can build new knowledge. The DNP project is an effort to build the bridge between research and practice and narrow the gap that has existed there. This gap has prevented nursing from contributing fully to the body of knowledge that is desperately needed to achieve the clinical effectiveness and fiscal benefits so sorely needed in our healthcare system. The DNP project is a demonstration of how practicing scholarly nurses can build new knowledge.

The DNP project contributes to the DNP's understanding of practice knowledge generation by the lived experience. The experience of the scholarly project fulfills the transformation of the student to adopting a scholarly way of thinking. The transformed student approaches issues with a new and developed view that incorporates a broad skill set.

This new approach to knowledge generation is a critical feature of how the DNP will move forward. It is practice scholarship that is embraced in the DNP project. "The practice doctorate in nursing has helped stimulate movement away from strict adherence to traditional methods of research with new models of clinical knowledge generation and practice being envisioned" (Reed & Shearer, 2011, p. 40). Practice scholarship demonstrates that new knowledge is built on both sides of the bridge. While PhD researchers generate external evidence, such as extending science and theory to guide practice, the DNP expert clinician generates internal evidence via outcomes management, quality improvement, EBP projects and translational evidence to improve health care, patient outcomes, and organizational or health policies (Melnyk, 2013). Implementation science is highlighted in the scholarship of the DNP-prepared nurse. DNP scholarship generates new knowledge through practice change innovation, translation of evidence, and quality improvement processes that may be transferable to other contexts but not generalizable. PhD scholarship generated new knowledge through research and statistical methodologies that may be broadly applicable (AACN, 2015a).

WHAT IS THE POTENTIAL IMPACT OF THE DNP PROJECT?

If the DNP project is to have an impact on our healthcare system and the quality of care, it must be done within the context of outcomes. In considering projects worthy of such study, several questions can be asked: Is there a contribution to comprehensive quality health care? Are there specific benefits for a group, population, community, or policy? Does the project advance nursing practice at the local, state, and national levels?

Reed and Shearer (2011) stated that "quality improvement initiatives spearheaded by DNP graduates exemplify building knowledge about local care and methods for improving practice to increase quality and safety within their health care systems" (p. 39). Practice scholarship encompasses all aspects of the delivery of nursing interventions to have a direct impact on outcomes. "Practice scholarship in nursing is identified as when patient health care problems are solved or community health problems are identified" (Smith & Liehr, 2005, p. 272). See Chapter 16, The Rest of the Story—Evaluating the Doctor of Nursing Practice, for a framework for evaluation of the DNP degree and outcomes.

WHAT QUALIFIES AS A DNP PROJECT?

The DNP project should encompass multiple aspects of the DNP *Essentials*. The project should be broadly practice based (refer back to the AACN definition of "practice"). A few topic examples include a project based on a population, health system, or policy issue. Some formats for the DNP project include quality improvement, demonstration projects, clinical inquiry, or translation of EBP and program evaluation. The DNP student should reflect on life experiences both professionally and personally to understand the strengths and the passions that are already owned and can be used in building a strong scholarly project. Developing an understanding of the needs of the stakeholders within the context of an organization must also be considered (see information on conducting an assessment in Chapter 6, Developing the Scholarly Project).

The DNP project has been reviewed in the literature and within various venues. The variability of projects has been noted, with the developing understanding that DNP projects must incorporate evidence synthesis, leadership, and measurement of outcomes (Brown & Crabtree, 2013; Grey, 2013; Kirkpatrick & Weaver, 2013).

There has been further inquiry by the AACN in the development of appropriate criteria for DNP scholarship that will include particular aspects of practice knowledge generation and DNP accountability. In response to the variability in DNP education, the AACN commissioned the Implementation of the DNP Task Force (2015c) to outline recommendations for the DNP project (see Chapter 3, Defining the Doctor of Nursing Practice: Current Trends).

CURRENT VIEWS OF THE DNP PROJECT

Rigor of the DNP Project

The DNP project elements include planning, implementation, and evaluation components. Projects should focus on changes that impact healthcare outcomes either through direct/indirect care with a system or population focus.

Implementation should be demonstrated in an appropriate area of practice and include an evaluation of processes and/or outcomes and a plan for sustainability (AACN, 2015a). As the student considers development of the DNP project, it is helpful to have consistent criteria applied. Waldrop, Caruso, Fuchs, and Hypes (2014) suggest an acronym of "EC as PIE" as criteria that include Enhancing outcomes (health/practice/policy), Culmination of practice inquiry, Partnership engagement, Implementing evidence, and Evaluation of outcome. The results of the work from the AACN task force on the DNP project has given new direction to the criteria of the project, which serves to clarify consistency and rigor without strangling creativity. Elements of the project should include planning, implementation, and evaluation components (AACN, 2015a).

In addition, there is new clarity with what the project is called. Previously, it was recognized that programs called the DNP scholarly project a variety of names that exemplified variability in focus (Moran et al., 2014). Nineteen project titles were identified (N=39). The AACN has recommended that the title of the DNP scholarly project be "DNP Project." Each of these steps forward serves to bring us toward consensus and continued evolution.

It is clear that DNP knowledge generation and scholarship are in the early stages of development and will continue to evolve in response to society's needs. As students contemplate the significance of the project for themselves, they should also consider the work that has been done to get nursing to this important crossroad. The DNP project not only will contribute to the student's successful transition but also will add to the knowledge base of nursing and impact nursing's work as we move to the future.

SCHOLARSHIP BEYOND THE DNP PROJECT

DNP student enrollment and graduation rates continue to increase (AACN, 2015b). With the increase in DNP graduate numbers, we are now at a point in the DNP degree trajectory where society is beginning to see the impact of practice scholarship and the associated benefit of the practice doctorate. Therefore, defining the practice scholarship of the DNP is critical to ensure the impact of the work in clinical, political, administrative, and academic venues.

The DNP project is the beginning of the work that will be continued by the DNP graduate. Because the DNP-prepared nurse is becoming part of the fabric of

> The DNP-prepared nurse is becoming part of the fabric of systems within organizations, universities, and entrepreneurial efforts.

systems within organizations, universities, and entrepreneurial efforts, practice scholarship will need to be further developed in the multiple arenas where the DNP interfaces.

The DNP-prepared nurse within organizations is beginning to drive scholarship to implement institutional policy change, funnel EBP to the bedside, and direct practice-based evidence to research. This DNP graduate works in teams and employs high-level interdisciplinary competencies to improve health systems and populations. Roles will continue to evolve to incorporate the knowledge and skill set that the DNP prepared nurse brings to quality efforts within organizations. It is crucial that the DNP prepared nurse demonstrate the ability to successfully impact outcomes related to leading system change, implementing policy change, and management of persons with multiple chronic conditions across sites and that the impact is evaluated (Brown & Crabtree, 2013, Redman, Pressler, Furspan, & Potempa, 2015). The DNP prepared nurse within academia is beginning to incorporate a practice model that influences tenure track (see Chapter 16, The Rest of the Story–Evaluating the Doctor of Nursing Practice). The scholarship of integration and application is becoming a part of this model. As more and more of these DNP-prepared faculty members encounter organizational appointments and are asked to provide consultation services, there will be a need to balance competing priorities. This is where the value of the scholarship team is recognized. PhD/DNP collaborative teams will continue to evolve to further all of nursing's work.

Finally, the DNP prepared nurse within health policy scholarship is beginning to enhance the vision of emerging healthcare systems. The rigor of practice scholarship gives credibility to the DNP prepared nurse and influences policy.

RECOMMENDATIONS

It is critical that the outcome-focused nature of practice scholarship be recognized as an effective means of knowledge development that contributes to the changes needed in our healthcare system. To reach these goals, utilization of all skill sets of DNP prepared nurses is needed to effect change in populations, healthcare organizations, and policy. A word of caution is exercised in focusing too heavily on one advanced practice role or another. The strengths of nurse practitioners, nurse midwives, clinical nurse specialists, nurse anesthetists, nurse administrators, informaticists, and policy experts will be required to meet the challenges that are before us.

There will be ongoing challenges to continue scholarship after attainment of the DNP degree to continue to impact health care. The DNP-prepared nurse will need to more clearly define practice scholarship for organizations and academia to carve out time for scholarship in their clinical role—which ultimately is the purpose of the DNP prepared nurse.

There is a need to develop ways to categorize our knowledge development to further disseminate and build on practice-based knowledge. This work is already under way and is further discussed in Chapter 16, The Rest of the Story—Evaluating the Doctor of Nursing Practice.

There is great value in the work of teams. Interdisciplinary and intradisciplinary relationships will be required to impact complex issues. Development of scholarship teams will increase creativity, impact, and production. There is movement to accept group/team DNP projects. Each member of the group must meet all expectations of planning, implementation, and evaluation of the project and have a leadership role in at least one component of the project and accountability for a deliverable (AACN, 2015a). Working closely with PhD colleagues to further the work of scientific inquiry will build a nursing repository of knowledge that can be used to solve issues and is further discussed in Chapter 7, Interprofessional and Intraprofessional Collaboration in the Scholarly Project.

The DNP nurse is prepared to answer the charge from the IOM for nurses to take their place at the decision-making table and to collaborate with other healthcare professionals to improve the health and health care of our nation. Scholarship is the driving force that will disseminate practice-based evidence and support the developing success of the practice doctorate to close the gap between research and practice, thereby meeting societal needs of improved health for our populations. Dissemination of outcomes related to DNP prepared nurses' work will propel the influence and the impact forward. This dissemination is an obligation of the DNP prepared nurse to society and will result in a positive effect on health care.

The following excerpt by Dr. Angela McConachie describes the impact that the process of completing the scholarly project has had on her perspective and her practice.

Completing the Scholarly Project: Impact on Perspective and Practice
Angela McConachie, DNP, NP

DNP education is a journey, learning many different aspects along the way, culminating with the scholarly project. The voyage through doctoral classes provided me the opportunity to grow as much as the final project itself. Each class taught me something new and pushed me to get involved and meet professionals within a variety of areas.

My scholarly project had a major impact, not only on my outlook on nursing but also on my entire professional career path.

When I first started my studies, I was a nurse practitioner in an acute care medicine division in a major medical/academic setting, and I enjoyed my position. During this time, there was a push to bring EBP to the bedside nurse, and the hospital already had an educational program in place. My scholarly project focused on the facilitators and barriers the bedside RN faced related to the use of EBP on a daily basis, after completing the established educational program.

During the data collection and analysis of my project, I started to recognize differences between EBP education and the expectations of EBP use on the nursing division. Glancing back on my scholarly assignments and personal experience with new nursing graduates, I was astonished at the gap between nursing education and the RN, as well as how EBP is used in the educational setting. This sparked an entirely new direction for my professional career as I went back and spoke with the deans of several local colleges and universities to get their opinions on the topic. The passion displayed for change in the nursing education setting was contagious. Change was discussed related to classroom, lecture, books, simulation, and clinical experiences. What is the best way to do things? What does the evidence show? How can we bring EBP to the nurses as soon as possible? How can we incorporate EBP into not only the nursing curriculum of a program but also the classroom, simulation, and clinical setting? How can we lead by example as nursing professionals and stress the critical component of EBP? I wanted to know these answers!

I completed my capstone project as planned, but a flame ignited within me in regard to nursing education. Therefore, before I graduated with my DNP, I took a leap of faith, entered the field of nursing education, and became full-time, scholarship-track faculty. It has been a few years since the transition, and I teach in a very interactive style. I (plus the students) bring in recent articles related to disease processes, and we discuss how things change on a daily basis, all while integrating nursing interventions and patient safety. My class evaluations are excellent, and the students embrace the learning environment I have created. I hope the ideas I have planted in them will continue to grow as they seek initial employment and throughout their careers.

Key Messages

- Scholarship is the mechanism that provides knowledge development within a discipline.
- A broadening of the view of scholarship includes integration and application.
- Practice scholarship embodies all aspects of nursing interventions that affect outcomes in individuals, populations, systems, and policy.
- The DNP project integrates and demonstrates the *Essentials* of DNP education.
- DNP project elements include planning, implementation, and evaluation components.
- The DNP project is also a demonstration of the effectiveness of the DNP prepared nurse.

Action Plan—Next Steps

Use the topic assessment format that follows to consider your ideas for a DNP project:

Topic Assessment	Your Topic Interest
1. DNP *Essentials* covered (I–VIII)	
2. Breadth and depth of knowledge	
3. Innovation and creativity	
4. Potential for peer review	
5. Type of scholarship	
6. Aspect of practice	
7. Potential contribution	

1. Which DNP *Essentials* could be demonstrated in your idea for a scholarly project?
2. Does your project idea consist of breadth and depth of knowledge within a defined area?
3. Is there the potential for innovation and creativity to affect an outcome?
4. Will you be able to expose the DNP project to public scrutiny and peer review?

5. What type of scholarship is evidenced within your project idea—discovery/integration/application?
6. What aspects of practice are you focused on—individual, population, system, policy?
7. Is there a contribution to comprehensive quality health care? Are there specific benefits for a group, population, community, or policy? Does the project advance nursing practice at the local, state, and national levels?
8. Is this topic of interest a need at the organizational level?
9. Is there a planning, implementation, and evaluation component?
10. What areas of expertise and passion do you bring that you can build on?
11. What skill sets do you need to develop in order to successfully implement your DNP project?

REFERENCES

American Association of Colleges of Nursing. (1999). *American Association of Colleges of Nursing position statement: Defining scholarship for the discipline of nursing.* Retrieved from http://www.aacn.nche.edu/publications/position/defining-scholarship

American Association of Colleges of Nursing. (2004). *Position statement on the practice doctorate in nursing.* Retrieved from: http://www.aacn.nche.edu/publications/position/DNPpositionstatement.pdf

American Association of Colleges of Nursing. (2006). *The essentials of doctoral education for advanced nursing practice.* Retrieved from: http://www.aacn.nche.edu/DNP/pdf/Essentials.pdf

American Association of Colleges of Nursing. (2012). *2012 Data on doctoral programs.* Retrieved from: http://www.aacn.nche.edu/membership/members-only/presentations/2012/12doctoral/Potempa-Doc-Programs.pdf

American Association of Colleges of Nursing. (2015a). The doctor of nursing practice: Current issues and clarifying recommendations. Retrieved from http://www.aacn.nche.edu/aacn-publications/white-papers/DNP-Implementation-TF-Report-8-15.pdf

American Association of Colleges of Nursing. (2015b). DNP fact sheet. Retrieved from: http://www.aacn.nche.edu/media-relations/fact-sheets/dnp

American Association of Colleges of Nursing. (2015c). *Implementation of the DNP task force.* Retrieved from http://www.aacn.nche.edu/news/articles/2015/dnp-white-paper

Boyer, E. (1990). *Scholarship reconsidered: Priorities of the professoriate.* The Carnegie Foundation for the Advancement of Teaching. New York, NY: Wiley.

Brown, M. A., & Crabtree, K. (2013). The development of practice scholarship in DNP programs: A paradigm shift. *Journal of Professional Nursing, 29*(6), 330–337. doi:10.1016/j.profnurs.2013.08.003

Bunkers, S. S. (2000). The nurse scholar of the 21st century. *Nursing Science Quarterly, 13*(2), 116–123.

Burson, R., Moran, K., & Conrad, D. (2016). Why hire a DNP? The value added impact of the practice doctorate. *Journal of Doctoral Nursing Practice, 9*(1).

Cary, A. H., & George, G. (2011). The Doctor of Nursing Practice (DNP). *Oregon State Board of Nursing Sentinel, 30*(1), 10–11.

Dirks, A. L. (1998). *The new definition of scholarship: How will it change the professoriate?* Retrieved from: http://webhost.bridgew.edu/adirks/ald/papers/skolar.htm

Draye, M., Acker, M., & Zimmer, P. (2006). The practice doctorate in nursing: Approaches to transform nurse practitioner education and practice. *Nursing Outlook, 54*, 123–129. doi:10.1016/j.outlook.2006.01.001

Fairman, J. (2008). Context and contingency in the history of post World War II nursing scholarship in the United States. *Journal of Nursing Scholarship, 40*(1), 4–11.

Fawcett, J. (1999). The state of nursing science: Hallmarks of the 20th and 21st centuries. *Nursing Science Quarterly, 12*(4), 311–315.

Ferguson-Pare, M. (2005). What is a community of scholars in the practice environment? *Nursing Science Quarterly, 18*(2), 120. doi:10.117/0894318405275863

Grey, M. (2013). The doctor of nursing practice: Defining the next steps. *Journal of Nursing Education, 52*(8), 462–465. doi:10.3928/01484834-20130719-02

Institute of Medicine. (1999). *To err is human: Building a safer health system.* Washington, DC: National Academies Press.

Institute of Medicine. (2001). *Crossing the quality chasm.* Washington, DC: National Academies Press.

Institute of Medicine. (2010). *The future of nursing: Leading change, advancing health.* Washington, DC: National Academies Press.

Kirkpatrick, J. M., & Weaver, T. (2013). The doctor of nursing practice capstone project: Consensus or confusion? *Journal of Nursing Education, 52*(8), 435–441. doi:10.3928/01484834-20130722-01

Kitson, A. (1999). The relevance of scholarship for nursing research and practice. *Journal of Advanced Nursing, 29*(4), 773–775.

Kitson, A. (2006). From scholarship to action and innovation. *Journal of Advanced Nursing, 56*(5), 435–572.

Levin, R. F., & Slyder, J. (2012). Evidence-based practice on the DNP. *Research and Theory for Nursing Practice: An International Journal, 26*(1), 6–9.

Magnan, M. A. (2016). The DNP: Expectations for theory, research and scholarship. In L. Chism (Ed.), *The doctor of nursing practice: A guidebook for role development and professional issues* (3rd ed., pp. 117–148). Burlington, MA: Jones & Bartlett Learning.

McEwen, M., & Wills, E. M. (2014). *Theoretical basis for nursing.* Philadelphia, PA: Wolters Kluwer Health/Lippincott Williams & Wilkins.

Melnyk, B. M. (2013). Distinguishing the preparation and roles of doctor of philosophy and doctor of nursing practice graduates: National implications for academic curricula and health care systems. *Journal of Nursing Education, 52*(8), 442–443.

Moran, K., Burson, R., Critchett, J., & Olla, P. (2011). Exploring the cost and clinical outcomes of integrating the registered nurse-certified diabetes educator in the patient-centered medical home. *The Diabetes Educator, 37*(6), 780–793.

National Institutes of Health. (2015). Fogarty International Center: Advancing Science for Global Health. Retrieved from: http://www.fic.nih.gov/researchtopics/pages/implementationscience.aspx

Redman, R. W., Pressler, S. J., Furspan, P., & Potempa, K. (2015). Nurses in the United States with a practice doctorate: Implications for leading in the current context of health care. *Nursing Outlook, 63*, 124–129.

Reed, P. G., & Shearer, N. B. C. (2011). *Nursing knowledge and theory innovation: Advancing the science of practice.* New York, NY: Springer.

Rolfe, G., & Davies, R. (2009). Second generation professional doctorates in nursing. *International Journal of Nursing Studies, 46,* 1265–1273.

Salmond, S. W. (2007). Advancing evidence based practice: A primer. *Orthopaedic Nursing, 26*(2), 114–123.

Scholarship. (2015). *Merriam-Webster's Learner's Dictionary.* Retrieved from: http://www.learnersdictionary.com/search/scholarship

Smith, M. J., & Liehr, P. (2005). Story theory: Advancing nursing practice scholarship. *Holistic Nursing Practice, 19*(6), 272–276.

Swanson, M., & Stanton, M. (2013). Chief nursing officers' perceptions of the doctorate of nursing practice degree. *Nursing Forum, 48*(1), 35–44. doi: 10.1111/nuf.12003

Thoun, D. S. (2009). Toward an appreciation of nursing scholarship: Recognizing our traditions, contributions, and presence. *Journal of Nursing Education, 48*(10), 552–556.

Velasquez, D. M., McArthur, D. B., & Johnson, C. (2011). Doctoral nursing roles in knowledge generation. In P. G. Reed & N. B. C. Shearer (Eds.), *Nursing knowledge and theory innovation: Advancing the science of practice* (pp. 37–50). New York, NY: Springer.

Waldrop, J., Caruso, D., Fuchs, M. A., & Hypes, K. (2014). EC as PIE: Five criteria for executing a successful DNP final project. *Journal of Professional Nursing, 30*(4), 300–306.

The Scholarly Project

CHAPTER 5

The Phenomenon of Interest

Katherine Moran and Rosanne Burson

CHAPTER OVERVIEW

Nursing practice is guided by science and theory. Nursing, as a profession, historically has been considered a practice discipline that is complex, varied, and underdetermined. There is an inherent societal obligation for the nurse to use good clinical judgment based on evidence-based practice that is informed by research. The nurse must "attend to changing relevance as well as changes in the patient's responses and nature of his clinical condition over time" (Benner, Tanner, & Chesla, 2009, p. xiv). However, because practice in the individual case is open to variations that are not necessarily accounted for by science (underdetermined), the nurse must use clinical reasoning to select and use relevant science (Benner et al., 2009). This means that the nurse must be able to recognize important changes and/or trends in the patient's condition and use good clinical judgment when providing nursing care.

> The nurse must be able to recognize important changes and/or trends in the patient's condition and use good clinical judgment when providing nursing care.

CHAPTER OBJECTIVES

After completing the chapter, the learner will be able to:

1. Understand the meaning of nursing phenomena in relation to the identification of issues that are in need of change
2. Consider personal practice interests and expertise in contemplating phenomena
3. Scan the literature for potential areas of interest
4. Evaluate potential nursing theories as a framework for the nursing phenomenon
5. Explore the phenomenon through patterns of knowing
6. Apply the process of concept analysis to the phenomenon or a characteristic of the phenomenon

This complex nature of nursing practice provides many opportunities to explore nursing phenomena. The focus of this chapter is to explore phenomena of interest for the doctor of nursing practice (DNP) project. Nursing theory and nursing knowledge are briefly explored to help the DNP student understand the significance of nursing phenomena. Along with the guidance received from his or her advisor a variety of strategies are introduced to help the DNP student select a phenomenon of interest for the DNP project.

> In this day of attention to patient-centered care and outcomes, the aspects of care delivery that nurses provide by their inherent understanding of phenomena require further examination, demonstration, and dissemination.

THE EXPERTISE OF NURSING PRACTICE

In 2011, the Institute of Medicine and the Robert Wood Johnson Foundation put forth a report that highlights the value of nursing and outlines the central role that nurses will play in the future health of our nation. In this report, *The Future of Nursing: Leading Change, Advancing Health,* nurses are called to lead and manage collaborative efforts with other healthcare practitioners to improve health care. Understanding the unique attributes of the expert nurse and expert nursing practice will help the nursing profession meet the challenges set forth by the Institute of Medicine (2011).

According to Morrison and Symes (2011), expert nursing practice includes a degree of involvement and engagement with patients that demonstrates intuitive knowledge and skilled know-how through knowing the patient, reflective practice, and risk taking. According to Benner et al. (2009),

> "Expert nursing practice occurs when the nurse is able to see the situation in alternative ways, either through introspection or by consulting others; allowing the nurse to realize the true meaning of the present and past events. The nurse reflects on the goal or perspective that seems evident to them and on the action that seems appropriate to achieving their goal; referred to as deliberative rationality" (p. 16).

This unique skill set places the practicing scholar in the best position to identify those areas of clinical concern that require further research/improvement and to help ensure that the healthcare needs of patients within the community, organization, or healthcare unit are being addressed.

The ability of the nurse to be tuned in to the meaning of the event *to the patient* and to choose individualized interventions that are unique for this patient at this time are the ultimate contributions that he or she offers. This *hidden work* is what influences the patient's experience of the relationship and often affects clinical outcomes. The profession has not articulated well the skill set nurses bring to the table that enhances the work that is done. This is partly because the relationship and caring aspect of nursing has been seen as the *soft side* of nursing and historically is not valued as much as the science-based technical aspects. For example, within the advanced practice role, the perceived value from organizations and other practitioners has been the utilization of the medical model in providing care. Nursing care is not measured, although in fact that may be the very thing that assists patients in meeting outcomes. In this day of attention to patient-centered care and outcomes, the aspects of care delivery that nurses provide by their inherent understanding of phenomena require further examination, demonstration, and dissemination. These processes will serve to highlight the hidden work of nursing and to validate its importance to the patient's healthcare experience and outcome.

> The hidden work of the nurse is what influences the patient's experience and often positively affects clinical outcomes.

IDENTIFYING THE PHENOMENON OF INTEREST

What are the phenomena that are of interest to the DNP student? When asked this question individually, DNP students may have difficulty adequately articulating the details of their interest. Perhaps it is because they have not been able to get their arms around a specific area of focus, or maybe their interests are too broad and not sufficiently narrowed to begin to articulate intent. Although the student's advisor provides direction and support as the student considers a variety of phenomena, it is a question that each student must answer individually. The scholarly project phenomenon of interest must center on a topic that is meaningful to the practice doctorate student and is *valued* by the practice setting. Further, as mentioned, practicing scholars are in the best position to identify those areas of clinical concern that require further research and/or improvement. Identifying the phenomenon of interest is the first step in developing the DNP project.

What Is a Phenomenon?

While some students may start the DNP program with a good understanding of the phenomenon they want to explore, as mentioned, others may not yet have a phenomenon in mind or they may not have a full understanding of what is meant by the term *nursing phenomenon*. To better understand what constitutes a phenomenon, it is important to understand the meaning of the word. According to Merriam-Webster, *phenomenon* is defined as "a fact or event of scientific interest susceptible to scientific description and explanation; an exceptional, unusual, or abnormal person, thing, or occurrence" ("Phenomenon," 2015, para. 1). *Nursing phenomenon*, on the other hand, is described as "a type of factor influencing health status with the specific characteristics: Aspect of health of relevance to nursing practice" (International Classification for Nursing Practice [ICNP], n.d., para. 1). Hence, the phenomena within the realm of nursing are complex in nature. These phenomena incorporate humans and their environment and relate to all aspects of human function as an individual, family member, or member of community—within the context of the physical or biological environment and human-made environments of norms, attitudes, and policy (ICNP, n.d.). Consequently, it is not surprising that many DNP projects deal with complex health-related issues (Christenbery, 2011).

One way to approach identifying the phenomenon of interest is to consider the areas of the DNP student's clinical expertise. Phenomenon identification derives from a practice situation that resonates. Practice experience occurs between the nurse and the patient. Further, reflecting on aspects that the student has observed within a particular patient population may give some direction. The expert nurse draws on this understanding and has developed specific interventions that align with the known phenomenon. For example, in working with patients with diabetes who are in need of insulin initiation, the nurse notes that there are often multiple barriers. Patients may experience fear of insulin related to injections or hypoglycemia. The patient may have insidious thoughts related to feelings of failure and guilt for having not been *perfect* in his or her approach to lifestyle behavior change and other recommendations from the healthcare provider. Patients may have decreased self-efficacy or empowerment issues that limit their ability to self-manage and maintain motivation. There may be family history whereby a family member started insulin, and this appeared to contribute to his or her demise. Misunderstanding the other factors related to the family member's experience can exacerbate the difficulty the patient experiences as he or she tries to overcome this new hurdle. The expert nurse has the skill set to help the patient explore the specific barriers that are contributing to his or her inability to move forward, toward better glucose control and improved health. The identified phenomenon of barriers to insulin initiation may be the beginning of an intense exploration of the topic, resulting in an intervention that improves outcomes for patients.

When considering potential topics or phenomena of interest for the DNP project, it may be helpful to begin by casting a wide net and to think about areas of interest from a broad, general perspective. Multiple methods can be used to help the student identify a pertinent topic. For example, it may be helpful to review research reports found in the Cumulative Index to Nursing and Allied Health Literature (CINAHL) database. Reviewing published reports could help the DNP student identify topics that need further exploration or studies that could be replicated on a smaller scale (to validate findings or increase generalizability). Scanning the table of contents of professional journals or even a professional organization's website may help the student identify topics of concern relevant to nursing. By way of example, a website to peruse regarding pertinent topics is the Doctors of Nursing Practice (http://doctorsofnursingpractice.ning .com/), an online community of DNP graduates and DNP students that highlights practice innovation and professional growth.

However, remember that the goal is to identify an area of interest specifically for the DNP project; therefore, the project should include subject matter in which the student has some expertise, such as his or her area of practice or specialty. The student should ask himself or herself if *there is something about this practice setting that needs further inquiry.* Perhaps a population of patients is not reaching their healthcare goals because of some common barrier, or maybe a current healthcare policy (organizational or legislative) is interfering with optimal patient care. In both of these examples, a clinical problem results in a trigger that leads to identifying a phenomenon worth exploring. This is what is meant by identifying a clinical problem in the *context of the needs of the organization or population*. To better understand how to determine the needs of an organization or population see Chapter 6 for more information on conducting an assessment.

At this beginning stage of discernment, a question the student should ask is, *What is interesting to me?* Consider not just areas of interest but areas of passion that will take the student through the journey and energize him or her to complete the process. Another important understanding for the student is that doctoral study is transforming and takes time. The initial topics of interest will most likely *morph* as the student is exposed to new concepts in his or her educational program. The student will view the phenomenon through many new lenses, which will change the appearance of the original idea. This is a normal part of the process. The student will reflect continuously on the phenomenon, and it will gradually evolve into the scholarly project.

Examples of DNP phenomena of interest are provided in **Table 5-1**.

Once a broad category or area of interest is identified, the next step is to drill down to a more specific focus. This is crucial. *Areas of interest* that are too broad or vague may become unmanageable, causing frustration and wasted time. Narrowing the focus gives the student the opportunity to demonstrate a comprehensive

> *Areas of interest* that are too broad or vague may become unmanageable, causing frustration and wasted time.

Table 5-1 DNP Phenomenon Topics

Examples of DNP phenomena of interest

- Endoscopic performance for colorectal cancer prevention
- Influenza vaccination rates in children
- Vessel health and preservation
- Enhancing patient satisfaction using a Web-based patient-provider messaging system
- Evidence-based depression care for homeless women
- Acute care nurse practitioner cost effectiveness and patient outcomes in rapid response teams
- Hypothermia in neurocritical care
- Diagnosis and treatment of mild traumatic brain injury
- Palliative care/end-of-life education program

Data from Vanderbilt University School of Nursing. (2014). 2014 Doctor of Nursing Practice Scholarly Projects. Retrieved from http://www.nursing.vanderbilt.edu/dnp/pdf/dnp_scholarlprojects_2014.pdf

understanding of the topic. Remember, the DNP student must be able to successfully complete the project; an incomplete project does not inform nursing practice, and it does not equate to a valid program deliverable, which is required for graduation!

To effectively narrow the focus, it is helpful to start by reviewing what is already known about the topic and, conversely, what is not known about the topic. For example, perhaps the DNP student has a good understanding of the healthcare needs of the immigrant population, but now the student wants to focus on health promotion activities used by recent immigrants. This topic could be further narrowed to *health promotion strategies used by Latino women who emigrated to the United States from Latin America*. One method used to narrow a topic is to ask the following questions: Who, what, where, and when? *Who* is the population of interest? *What* is it about this population that is interesting? *Where* is the population found? *When* did the observation occur? Is it a current or historical observation or related to a specific period of life?

As the subject matter moves from a broad category to a more focused topic, multiple potential elements of interest will begin to emerge. One word of caution is needed regarding narrowing the project focus: care should be taken to prevent the focus of the project from being narrowed too much. If the topic is narrowed to very specific criteria, there is a very real risk that there will be no (or very little) information available in the literature to inform the project.

IDENTIFICATION OF A PROBLEM/CONCERN

Now that a topic has been identified, it is time to think about *why* this topic is important or what is it about this topic that is a concern. Is there a need to change nursing practice to improve patient outcomes in an organization or for a specific population? Is there an unmet societal need? Does this concern occur frequently enough to warrant further exploration? What does the literature reveal about this topic?

When reviewing the literature at this point in the project development process, the goal is really only to *browse* the literature in order to gain a general understanding of the topic, determine how much work has been done, and determine if this is indeed something worth exploring further. If very little information is available in the literature to support the need for investigation, an exploratory study may be needed to determine the incidence/prevalence of the phenomenon, to ascertain who is affected by the phenomenon, and to determine how this population has been affected (Siedlecki, 2008). The information gleaned from an exploratory study could provide the foundation for future postdoctoral scholarly work for the DNP scholar, making this an appealing project worth embarking on as a DNP student.

If one determines that the topic is interesting, it is time to take it one step further—to begin to think about *how* to address this or *if* anything can be done about it. Finally, remember to consider the resources that will be needed to investigate this phenomenon.

Reviewing the idea with an advisor will help the student identify potential barriers and help him or her determine the feasibility of implementing the project. Remember, if the student is able to clearly articulate the value of the topic, implementing the project is feasible, and there are nursing strategies that could be explored to address the concern, the topic is worth further investigation (see **Figure 5-1**).

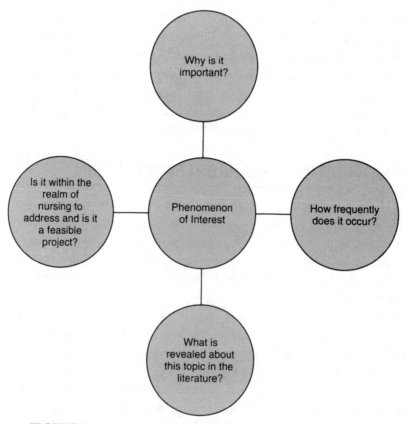

FIGURE 5-1 Process used to identify the phenomenon of interest.

USING NURSING THEORY TO EXPLORE A PHENOMENON

Theory provides an orderly way to view phenomena. Nursing theory was initially developed to guide practice through the clarification of the nursing domain. Theory

> *Theory* is used to guide nursing practice, and it provides an orderly way to view phenomena.

provided a way for nurses to convey professional convictions and gave nurses a means of systematic thinking about nursing practice (McEwen & Wills, 2014).

Nursing theory is made up of concepts (words or phrases used to describe the concept) and propositions (statements that describe the relationship among the concepts) that help to explain a phenomenon of interest (Jensen, 2015). Sometimes the term *construct* is also included in the description of a theory. A construct is used to describe something that is not directly or indirectly observed, such as social support (Schmidt & Brown, 2015). Theory can be classified based on scope/level of abstractness or type/purpose, as depicted in **Figure 5-2**.

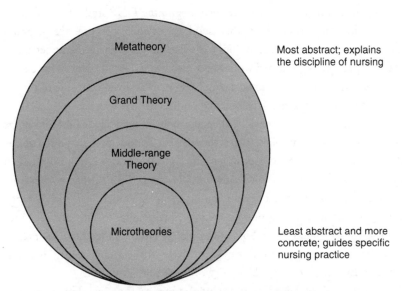

FIGURE 5-2 Levels of abstraction in nursing theory.

Modified from McEwen, M., & Wills, E. M. (2014). *Theoretical basis for nursing.* Philadelphia, PA: Wolters Kluwer Health.

Level of abstractness refers to the complexity of the theory and the specificity or concreteness of the concepts and proposition (McEwen & Wills, 2014). For example, grand theories are most abstract because they are used to explain the discipline of nursing and include very broadly defined concepts. The concept of *health*, for example, is broad, with potentially broad interpretation. Nursing recognizes that the concept of health encompasses more than simply the absence of disease. Health is a dynamic process that changes over time and can vary based on the individual's circumstances, experiences, and exposures to internal and external environments.

Because this concept is complex and broad in scope, it is not easily tested. A few examples of grand theories include Dorothea Orem's self-care deficit theory, Rosemarie Parse's theory of human becoming, and Imogene King's open system theory. These theories provide a philosophical umbrella under which nursing practice functions. Many of these theories were developed in the last century and serve to create paradigms that support nursing practice.

Grand theories are often the theories learned at the bachelor's level of nursing. Unfortunately, the abstractness of the grand theory is often difficult for the novice nurse to integrate intentionally within his or her practice. For some nurses, the disconnect between theory and practice may start here and continue even as nurses advance in their clinical experience. Beginning DNP students often comment that they are unsure about the usefulness of theory to practice. If grand theories were presented as philosophies to novice nurses, perhaps the understanding of how practice is grounded would become clearer. Grand theories have been very important to nursing's knowledge development and will continue to form a base on which theories specific to practice can build.

The next level of abstraction in theory classification includes middle-range theories. As the name implies, these theories are found in the middle of the ladder of abstraction (between abstract and concrete) and are more limited in scope than grand theories. As a result, middle-range theories tend to be more generalizable to nursing practice and can be tested. The focus for middle range theories is on understanding nursing-related phenomena, so they are very useful for the scholar-practitioner. Some examples of middle-range theories include Nola J. Pender's health promotion model, Merle Mishel's uncertainty in illness theory, and E. Lenz and L. Pugh's theory of unpleasant symptoms.

The final level of abstraction includes practice theories. These theories are used to guide specific areas of practice; therefore, they are very concrete and narrow in scope, and they include concepts that are measurable and easily tested (McEwen & Wills, 2014). "Situation-specific theory" is another term that

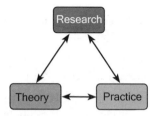

FIGURE 5-3 This figure depicts the reciprocal relationship between theory, research, and practice.

Modified from McEwen, M., & Wills, E. M. (2014). *Theoretical basis for nursing.* Philadelphia, PA: Wolters Kluwer Health.

highlights practice theory, which focuses on the context in which the theory is being used. This type of theory, as the name implies, is specific to the situation and encompasses the particular needs of a unique group of patients. An example of a situation-specific theory is Ramona Mercer's conceptualization of maternal role attainment/becoming a mother. Because situation-specific theory is within a local context and supports the use of evidence-based research that is appropriate to the situation at hand, DNP students find this appealing in practice.

There is a fluid relationship between theory, research, and practice that is important to understand. Each informs and impacts the other (see **Figure 5-3**). Theory is validated through research, which can lead to further theory development.

Both theory and research are used to inform practice. Similarly, information gleaned through theory application in practice can inform theory development and/ or continued research. The symbiotic relationship between theory, research, and practice is important to recognize because of the potential opportunities for further study that can emerge when using theory to explore a phenomenon. This type of exploration is valuable to nursing because of the potential to add to nursing knowledge.

For example, complex patient care and social issues can be identified and subsequently addressed through the use of theory. From the perspective of a scholarly project, the DNP student can use theory to recognize the antecedents to health-related events that negatively impact a population (e.g., those events that lead to colon cancer in women or to prostate cancer in men). Theory can help the DNP student recognize health and illness patterns within a population and the subsequent implications (Christenbery, 2011).

In addition to helping the DNP student recognize health patterns, theory also helps the student develop patient-centered nursing interventions to promote health and wellness and a framework to evaluate the effectiveness of these interventions (Christenbery, 2011).

For many DNP students, there are "a-ha!" moments related to the realization that nursing theory has been there all along in their practice. Nursing theories have continued to evolve, and the exploration of theories that are relevant to each student's practice is an important aspect of the process of doctoral education. Connecting appropriate theory to the DNP project will offer a supporting framework and will deepen the understanding of the chosen phenomenon.

LOOKING AT A PHENOMENON THROUGH A DIFFERENT LENS

Theoretical Framework

Clearly, theories can and should be used to study a phenomenon of interest. As mentioned previously, using one or even several theories to view a phenomenon is a valuable exercise because it helps the DNP student better describe or explain the phenomenon. However, sometimes just the process of identifying a theory to help inform the project can be a daunting task.

Several strategies can be used to make this process more manageable. First, it is helpful to begin by identifying the concepts (and relationships among the concepts) that describe the phenomenon of interest under consideration. This can be accomplished by reviewing the literature. Look for published articles that include the phenomenon of interest and then identify the concepts used to describe the phenomenon, as well as the theory or theories chosen to inform the work. The DNP student can then select a theory to use as a framework that best represents the concepts that describe his or her phenomenon of interest. A concept analysis can also begin to further inform the understanding of the phenomenon and will be discussed later in the chapter. In addition to reviewing the literature, there are multiple resources, both electronic and in print, that can provide the DNP student with an overview of the numerous theories available for use (see Helpful Resources). Finally, technology will be an asset as the student considers reviewing the huge amount of data involved in the exploration of various theories. A great start is the use of websites to begin looking at all the nursing theories available.

As the DNP student considers various theories for use, keep in mind a series of questions to evaluate each theory. These questions should reflect the student's perception of practice and include:

1. Does this theory reflect the student's personal nursing practice?
2. Does this theory help to describe, explain, and predict the phenomenon that the student is interested in?

3. Can this theory be used as a guide in the framework of the scholarly project?
4. Does the theory offer a way to develop, assess, implement, and evaluate innovations that the project explores?
5. Will the use of this theory help to support excellent nursing practice?

For example, the student who is looking at phenomena focused on interpersonal relationships may consider nursing theories that give a framework to the relationship that develops between nurse and patient. The student may consider Hildegard Peplau's theory of interpersonal relations in nursing, Jean Watson's caring science, or Rosemarie Parse's human becoming theory, in which there are interpersonal effects on both the nurse and patient.

Theories outside of nursing are also worthy of consideration as the phenomenon is evaluated. Interdisciplinary aspects of DNP work encourage the review of theories specific to the phenomenon. For example, if the phenomenon is related to health behavior, an exploration of the various theories within this framework is recommended. Examples of health behavior theories from other disciplines include the health belief model, the theory of planned behavior, and the social cognitive theory. Another example is a phenomenon related to societal aspects where there may be congruence with complexity science, critical, feminist, or environmental theory. During this period of immersion, it is important for the student to develop a broad understanding of the available theories to identify links to the phenomenon of interest. A thorough and updated text will give the DNP student a starting place for this review and professional development (see Helpful Resources). Examination of the phenomenon within a specific theoretical framework will clarify aspects of the phenomenon and give direction to the DNP project. This process takes time and is often incorporated in theory coursework, which supports DNP Essential I: Scientific Underpinnings for Practice and DNP Essential III: Clinical Scholarship and Analytic Methods for Evidence-Based Practice.

Ways of Knowing

Another way to explore and understand the phenomenon of interest is to view it through the multiple lenses of the *patterns of knowing*. The fundamental patterns of knowing in nursing were initially identified by Carper in 1978 as part of her doctoral work. The patterns of knowing were developed in an attempt to help nursing as a profession better understand the characteristic ways that nurses think about phenomena that are a concern of nursing. This was done not to extend the range of knowledge but rather to understand what it means to *know* and what types of knowledge are important to nursing (Carper, 1978).

The ways of knowing are important concepts in the development and application of nursing theory. They also provide a holistic framework designed to direct practice, education, and research. The DNP student can further explore a specific phenomenon of interest by viewing it through the lens of one or several patterns of knowing. Again, this process will give the student insight, aids in informing the project, and helps the student better describe or explain the phenomenon of interest.

Carper's original four fundamental patterns of knowing are *empirical knowing*, referred to as the science of nursing; *esthetics*, referred to as the art of nursing; *personal knowledge*, allowing for a therapeutic use of self; and *ethical knowledge*, or the moral knowledge in nursing (see **Figure 5-4**). These patterns are separate but interdependent and interrelated; they are not mutually exclusive.

> *Empirical knowledge* is systematically organized into general laws and theories for the purpose of describing, explaining, and predicting phenomena of concern to nursing.

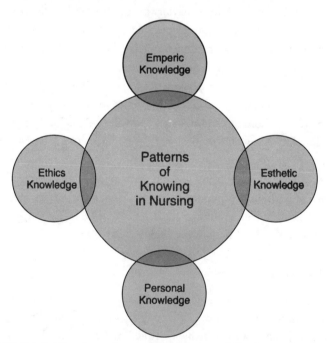

FIGURE 5-4 This figure depicts the four original fundamental patterns of knowing by Barbara A. Carper.

Data from Chinn, L. P., & Kramer, M. K. (2015). *Integrating theory and knowledge development in nursing.* St. Louis, MO: Mosby Inc. an affiliate of Elsevier, Inc.

Empirical knowledge includes knowledge that is objective and quantifiable. It is tested, replicated, and proved through scientific methods.

Empirical knowledge is systematically organized into general laws and theories for the purpose of describing, explaining, and predicting phenomena of concern to nursing (Cody, 2013). Evidence-based practice is just one example of empirical knowledge that informs nursing practice. The nurse using evidence to inform practice develops a skill set and knowledge base from well-documented scientific knowledge that has been rigorously tested. Chinn and Kramer (2011) clarified the conceptualization of this pattern by asking the critical question, "What is this, how does it work?" (p. 14). The DNP student can apply this questioning process to determine aspects of the pattern of knowing for the phenomenon of interest. Critical questions defined by Chinn and Kramer (2011) will be asked in each subsequent pattern of knowing to substantiate the pattern in relation to the phenomenon.

> *Esthetic knowledge* implores the nurse to use skills of empathy, caring, and engagement to care for individual patients.

Esthetic knowledge is used by nurses to better understand each patient's unique health experience; the nurse is able to sense the meaning in the moment and tailor the patient's nursing care without conscious deliberation. Esthetic knowledge encompasses the lived experience and is expressive in nature. The nurse is able to assist the patient in coping with the experience through perceived insight that is gleaned from *being in the moment* with the patient.

It is important to note that the *perception* referred to in esthetic knowledge is more than simple recognition; it is the gathering of important details and nuances that together create the experience as a whole (Carper, 1978). It gives meaning to variables that cannot be quantitatively formulated (McEwen & Wills, 2014). The nurse understands what is *significant in the patient's experience* and, as a result of this perception, is able to determine what is needed to help the patient move forward. By using esthetic knowledge, the nurse is able to see the holistic needs of the patient and act appropriately. Activities that have been considered as simple or basic nursing care can have a profound effect on patient outcomes. Unfortunately, the true value of these acts is often overlooked. Esthetic critical questions include, "What does this mean, how is this significant?" (Chinn & Kramer, 2011, p. 14).

Personal knowledge encompasses the way nurses view themselves and the patient (McEwen & Wills, 2014). Personal knowledge is largely expressed in

> Using *personal knowledge*, the nurse is able to view the patient from a holistic perspective rather than from a strictly biological or medical perspective, promoting wholeness and integrity.

personality; it is subjective and incorporates experience and reflection. Using personal knowledge, the nurse is able to view the patient from a holistic perspective rather than from a strictly biological or medical perspective, promoting wholeness and integrity. These interpersonal contacts and relationships with patients are examples of what is meant by *therapeutic use of self.* Through personal knowledge, the nurse may come to understand that there is something sacred in the relationship between the patient and the nurse, that what nurses do involves more than providing protection, promotion, and optimization of health and abilities; nurses facilitate healing and wellness through that human connection. Critical questions related to the personal lens include, "Do I know what I do, do I do what I know?" (Chinn & Kramer, 2011, p. 14).

Ethical knowledge is based on obligation to service and respect for human life. Nurses draw on ethical knowledge when moral dilemmas arise to address conflicting norms

> *Ethical knowledge* is based on obligation to service and respect for human life.

and interests and to provide insight into areas that cannot be tested (McEwen & Wills, 2014). Ethical knowledge requires rational examination and evaluation of what is good, valuable, and desirable as it relates to the maintenance or restoration of health. Ethical issues could arise from situations involving consent, distributive justice, or personal integrity, to name a few. In these cases, the nurse may be challenged to overcome fear because of uncertainty of outcomes or have conflicting feelings resulting from personal core values or beliefs. The nurse must act with *moral courage* and address the situation with conviction and confidence, doing what is right for the patient. Ethical critical questions include, "Is this right, is this responsible?" (Chinn & Kramer, 2011, p. 14).

Now, consider a phenomenon of interest viewed through the lens of the ways of knowing: caring for the adult patient with chronic obstructive pulmonary disease (COPD) who continues to smoke cigarettes. When viewing this phenomenon using empirical knowledge, the data are clear: smoking cigarettes is detrimental to one's health. It damages lung tissue and is certainly a concern for the patient with COPD.

Using esthetic knowledge, however, the nurse is able to recognize the forces driving a patient's decision to smoke. Perhaps through structured interviews or focus groups with patients with COPD, the nurse is able to use skills of empathy, caring, and engagement to better understand the needs of the patient with COPD who smokes. Perhaps the nurse identifies the long smoking history, extraordinary family or work stressors, and the desire to quit, but the lack of perceived coping strategies available to use to be successful in this endeavor.

The nurse reflects on what is learned and incorporates information from previous experiences or similar situations. This personal knowledge helps inform the nurse. The nurse should recognize personal biases and how personal values and beliefs can either help the patient move forward or serve as a roadblock that sabotages all efforts. In the latter case, the DNP student should carefully consider whether this is a phenomenon that he or she is comfortable pursuing. Remember, the key in all patient–nurse relationships is a *therapeutic* use of self.

Finally, using ethical knowledge, the nurse examines the situation and evaluates what is good, valuable, and desirable as it relates to the maintenance or restoration of health from the *patient's perspective*. The nurse has a moral obligation to inform the patient of the risks of smoking but also to consider quality of life and what is required to maintain or improve that quality.

It is imperative to look at your phenomena through each lens. The student may have a bias toward one lens or another. In the preceding example, a nurse who looks only through the empiric lens will not be able to incorporate the patient perspective from the esthetic and ethical lens or the impact of the nurse's personal knowing on the situation. This is known as "patterns gone wild," and the impact is a stunted view of the phenomena that does not allow the full view and experience of the phenomena (Chinn & Kramer, 2011). Patterns gone wild predictably limits the ability of the nurse to understand each unique human interaction within all patterns and may prevent the development of specific patient-centered interventions and positive outcomes that would have been attained.

In 2008, Chinn and Kramer added a final pattern of knowing termed *emancipatory knowing* (see **Figure 5-5**). This pattern incorporates equity, justice, and transformation and questions what is, while wondering what could be. "The dimensions of emancipatory knowing surround and connect with the four fundamental patterns of knowing" (Chinn & Kramer, 2011, p. 64). Critical questions include: What are the barriers to freedom? What is hidden? What is invisible? Who is not heard? Who benefits? What is wrong with this picture? Emancipatory knowing examines the "social, cultural, and political status quo" and vision changes that need to occur (Chinn & Kramer, 2011, p. 12). Having the ability to look at the power structures in place that contribute to social problems and being able to consider other options are at the root of this pattern—to create a new lens to view the world.

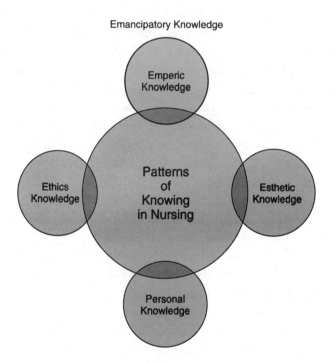

FIGURE 5-5 This figure depicts the revised fundamental patterns of knowing by Barbara A. Carper that includes Chinn and Kramer's addition of emancipatory knowing.

Data from Chinn, L. P., & Kramer, M. K. (2015). *Integrating theory and knowledge development in nursing*. St. Louis, MO: Mosby Inc. an affiliate of Elsevier, Inc.

> *Emancipatory knowing* is expressed in praxis, whereby the nurse reflects on issues that are not fair and initiates changes to eliminate the injustices.

Emancipatory knowing is *expressed* in praxis, whereby the nurse reflects on issues that are not fair and initiates changes to eliminate the injustices. This is also termed *reflection in action* (Chinn & Kramer, 2011). The phenomenon of interest may be framed by emancipatory knowing, while the scholarly project is also a demonstration of praxis.

Concept Analysis

Another lens to examine the phenomenon of interest through is a concept analysis. The purpose of a concept analysis is to allow the student to match the phenomenon with concepts. A concept categorizes information and contains defining characteristics called attributes. In performing a concept analysis, the scholar may distinguish between similar concepts, explain a term, or refine ambiguous concepts. An example will be discussed related to a published analysis of the concept of "overcoming" (Brush, Kirk, Gultekin, & Baiardi, 2011). The aim of the analysis was to "develop an operational definition of overcoming and explicate its meaning, attributes, and characteristics as it relates to homeless families" (Brush et al., 2011, p. 160). As described in the article, the process used is based on Walker and Avant's (2011) concept analysis method, which is an excellent resource to review prior to initiating a concept analysis.

The result of the concept analysis will provide a precise operational definition or help to more clearly define the problem. Concept analysis also helps to define standardized nursing language and to develop new tools. The concept analysis is a formal exercise to determine the defining attributes of the phenomenon. Although the analysis is precise, the end product is variable. Precision occurs because of the specific process that is used to analyze the concept. Variability occurs because people see things differently, knowledge changes over time, and the understanding of the concept may change.

The first step is identifying a critical concept within the phenomenon. This step will keep the analysis manageable and will be helpful in the overall understanding of the phenomenon, which will benefit the eventual project. Frame the concept of interest within an introduction that describes the concept of interest and provides definition. Avoid umbrella terms; the more specific the definition of your concept, the more manageable it becomes. For example, in the article reviewed, the authors noted that in a previous qualitative study of homeless mothers, *overcoming* their situation was frequently mentioned as a desired outcome. Through concept analysis, the authors were able to explore definitions of overcoming in dictionaries and the literature. Using all sources of definition, from dictionaries and colleagues to ordinary and scientific sources, gives a broad view of the concept. This process is important because identifying the uses of the concept from practice and literature further defines the concept.

Defining attributes of the concept is the primary work of concept analysis. The student should look at characteristics that appear consistently. In the previous example, three key attributes were identified from the literature that allowed for the development of a clear definition. "Overcoming is thus defined as a deliberate and thoughtful process of changing or conquering a self-perceived problematic circumstance, challenge or adversity in order to live a healthier and happier future existence" (Brush et al., 2011, p. 162).

The authors then identified antecedents to and consequences of the concept overcoming. Antecedents are events that must occur prior to the concept, whereas consequences are outcomes of the concept. This process allows for a deeper and more specific understanding of the concept. Antecedents in the example of overcoming include recognition of the need to change, demonstrated readiness to change, and determination to change. Possible consequences of overcoming include a return to a more stable, better quality of life (Brush et al., 2011).

Once the antecedents and consequences are recognized, the empirical referents are identified that allow for measurement of the concept and demonstrate that it has occurred. The authors in this example mentioned that there are no direct measurements but suggested using measures of related constructs such as resilience, hope, optimism, self-efficacy, and perceived support (Brush et al., 2011).

Finally, a model, a borderline, and a contrary case are discussed. This allows one to clearly define what the concept *is* (model), to recognize a case that has *some* of the characteristics of the concept (borderline), and to clearly recognize what the concept *is not* (contrary). Each type of case study serves to highlight and clarify characteristics. In the continuing example of overcoming, each case compared the characteristics of the person with the previously discussed antecedents and the resultant consequences.

A concept analysis of a phenomenon or a characteristic of a phenomenon can assist the scholar in defining a problem or distinguishing between similar concepts. This is a creative process. Having just considered the process of concept analysis, what concepts of interest come to mind in relation to practice and phenomena of interest?

Foundational Tenets of Nursing Knowledge

One part of the scholarly process involves considering personal and professional philosophies that are a framework for one's practice. The scholar will likely identify a framework that has been in place in the background, but perhaps not with full awareness. Bunkers (2000) described 16 foundational tenets that are grounded in nursing theory and conceptual frameworks. As the following tenets are reviewed, reflect on frameworks that have had the most meaning for one's practice.

1. Honoring human freedom and choice
2. Cultivating an attitude of openness to uncertainty and difference
3. Appreciating the meaning of lived experiences of health
4. Understanding the nature of suffering
5. Committing to social justice
6. Believing in the imagination as a source of knowledge
7. Recognizing the significance of language in structuring meaning and reality
8. Understanding health as a process
9. Understanding community as a process
10. Believing in the power of personal presence

11. Participating in scientific inquiry
12. Asserting the ethics of individual and communal responsibility
13. Emphasizing living in the present moment
14. Respecting life and nature
15. Acknowledging mystery
16. Focusing on quality of life (Bunkers, 2000, p. 123. Reprinted by permission of SAGE Publications, Inc.)

As one ponders phenomena of interest, consider the aspects of practice that impact both the nurse and the patient in the delivery of care. **Table 5-2** is a worksheet for the student to use when contemplating a phenomenon of interest.

Table 5-2 Phenomenon Assessment Worksheet

Aspects of the Phenomenon	Phenomenon of Interest What is my phenomenon of interest?
Personal:	
Interest	What is my interest level in relation to this phenomenon?
Expertise	What is my level of expertise in relation to this topic?
Literature	What does the literature document regarding this phenomenon? Are there gaps in the literature related to this topic?
Patterns of Knowing	What knowledge do I have of the phenomenon looking through each pattern?
Empirical Esthetic Personal Ethical Emancipatory	
Applicable Theories	What theories may support the structure of a project utilizing this phenomenon?
Nursing Theories Nonnursing Theories	
Related Concepts/ Concept Analysis	What concepts are part of the phenomenon that need further definition?
Foundational Tenets	Which of the foundational tenets are important aspects of this phenomenon? How important are the identified tenets to my professional practice?
Peer Contributions	What do my peers think about my thoughts about this phenomenon?
Faculty Consultation	What input has faculty provided regarding the phenomenon?

KEEPING YOUR OPTIONS OPEN

> *Selecting a phenomenon of interest* is a fluid process, informed by the literature and flexible to change.

Selecting a phenomenon of interest for the DNP project is a fluid process, informed by the literature and flexible to change. The scholar will spend considerable time mulling over the potential ideas. Conversations with fellow students and faculty will also add to the richness of the experience. Having said that, certainly time constraints will play an important part in the decision-making process, such as the timeline to graduation! Therefore, it is important to carefully consider the options and discuss them with an advisor. However, remember that the ultimate decision should be made by the DNP student. When the student is passionate about the topic, and the topic is personally meaningful, the time and work involved in completing the project successfully become a labor of love.

Once the DNP student has considered the phenomenon of interest, ideas will evolve and may develop into potential scholarly projects. Review Chapter 4, Scholarship in Practice, to consider types of scholarship that can develop the project. To illustrate an in-depth exploration of a phenomenon of interest, the following excerpt is presented by Dr. Katherine A. Marshall.

Identifying the Project Topic
Katherine A. Marshall, DNP, RN, PMHCNS-BC

My clinical practice involves the assessment, treatment, and planning of care for community-bound psychiatric and dementia patients for a Metro-Detroit home healthcare agency. This terminal and vulnerable population has challenged the healthcare system with unique needs and rapidly growing costs for care. Hospitalizations are frequent, futile, and often conclude with decreased functional ability and poor quality of life. My expertise in this arena fueled my passion to address the need for clinical staff to identify impending dehydration and malnutrition and impact futile hospital admissions. The agency, like many other healthcare facilities, has felt the impact of the growing dementia population and identified an interest in making changes related to the care of this population. A match between my interests and that of the organization became evident.

A review of the agency's hospital admission records for dementia patients revealed that these patients had higher rates of admission for dehydration and malnutrition than other admission diagnosis. Overall agency admission rates for these diagnoses were 21% compared to the national average of 16% (Centers for Medicare and Medicaid, 2014). State of Michigan records indicated that the percentage of dementia patients admitted for dehydration and malnutrition in the counties served by the agency had consistently increased over the last several quarters (MPRO, 2014). The data were alarming and, trending toward increased hospital admissions, increased costs and undesirable outcomes for dementia patients. In addition, patients and families were impacted negatively with each and subsequent admissions. Upon hospital discharge, patients were physically weaker from being bed-bound and presented with greater confusion; all of this ultimately decreasing the patient's quality of life.

Identifying clinical phenomena and characteristics that place this population at risk for hospitalization would provide possible opportunities to decrease hospitalization rates and improve quality of life by developing best practice guidelines and system improvements related to preventive interventions, care, and treatment of the dementia patient in home health care. A literature review identified a gap in standards of care related to this population. After realizing this gap, the first step was to explore and describe retrospectively the incidence and correlations of variables or factors that predict or precede dehydration and malnutrition in the home care agency's dementia patients hospitalized for dehydration and malnutrition—in order to give attention to opportunities for improvement related to the care of this population.

The Outcome and Assessment Information Set (OASIS) Start of Care document, a comprehensive assessment tool completed at the start of care, provided the data on the identified variables. Through the literature review, variables were identified that have a potential influence on the condition of dehydration and malnutrition. Potential variables of influence that were identified and extracted from the OASIS were primary residence and degree of support, co-morbidities, basal metabolic rate, incidence of urinary tract infections (UTIs), and nutrition score. Demographic data included gender, ethnicity, and age. Forty-four subjects with dementia had been admitted to the hospital with an admission diagnosis of dehydration and malnutrition over a 2-year period. While a single variable or collection of variables were not identified that would predict risk for hospitalization for dehydration and malnutrition, there were areas identified that would benefit from increased clinical attention and process improvement.

This first step prompted an early intervention by a multidisciplinary team within the agency to assess and educate the patient and family on dementia progression including the signs and symptoms of dehydration and malnutrition. Further, clinicians now have an increased awareness that dehydration and malnutrition are likely and common events in the dementia patient. A high priority is placed on education, prevention, and early intervention to avoid the unnecessary and taxing hospitalization of the dementia patient. Patients and families are introduced to and provided palliative care and hospice resources earlier in their home care experience, thus avoiding unnecessary hospitalizations and invasive futile treatments.

It is critical to identify a phenomenon of interest where the student has expertise and knowledge and then to match this to an organization's need to move the topic from an area of interest to an identified area of improvement. Using the literature helped me develop an understanding of the current state of the art, while the data from my organization framed the topic within the local context. These first steps set the stage for a project that is both evidence-based and effective within the specific organization.

Key Messages

- Nursing practice is guided by science and theory, and conversely practice ultimately informs science and theory.
- The complex nature of nursing practice provides many opportunities to explore nursing phenomena.
- The *hidden work* of the nurse is what influences the patient's experience and often positively affects clinical outcomes.
- The DNP project phenomenon of interest must center on a topic that is meaningful to the practice doctorate student and is *valued* by the practice setting.

- A *nursing phenomenon* is "a type of factor influencing health status with the specific characteristics: Aspect of health of relevance to nursing practice" (ICNP, n.d., para. 1).
- As the scholar ponders phenomena of interest, he or she should consider the aspects of practice that impact both the nurse and the patient in the delivery of care.
- When the value of the phenomenon of interest can be clearly articulated, there is an identifiable need within society, implementing the project is feasible, and nursing strategies could be explored to address the concern, the topic is worth further investigation.
- Examining a phenomenon within a specific theoretical framework will clarify aspects of the phenomenon and give direction to the DNP project.
- The DNP student can examine a phenomenon of interest by viewing it through the lens of one or several patterns of knowing, which will help the student describe or explain the phenomenon of interest and give the student deeper insight.
- Conducting a concept analysis may help the DNP student to match the phenomenon with concepts, distinguish between similar concepts, explain a term, or refine ambiguous concepts.
- After the DNP student thoughtfully reflects on the phenomenon of interest, the phenomenon will gradually evolve into the DNP project.

Action Plan—Next Steps

1. Identify your areas of clinical expertise, patient populations, and interests.
2. Consider phenomena that you have noted in patient experiences.
3. Become immersed in the literature related to the phenomenon.
4. Observe the phenomenon through multiple lenses, such as the patterns of knowing.
5. Contemplate your nursing framework as evidenced by the foundational tenets.
6. Review potential applicable theories within and outside nursing.
7. Discuss your ideas with your advisor, faculty, peers, and colleagues.
8. Allow your ideas to develop and gel.
9. Identify potential organizations/arenas that could support your area of interest.
10. Enjoy the creativity and the potential of the DNP project.
11. Begin to think about a plan for the project in relation to the phenomenon.
12. Begin to consider the resources you will need to develop your project.

REFERENCES

Benner, P., Tanner, C. A., & Chesla, C. A. (2009). *Expertise in nursing practice: Caring, clinical judgment and ethics.* New York, NY: Springer.

Brush, B., Kirk, K., Gultekin, L., & Baiardi, J. (2011). Overcoming: A concept analysis. *Nursing Forum, 46,* 160–168.

Bunkers, S. S. (2000). The nurse scholar of the 21st century. *Nursing Science Quarterly, 13*(2), 116–123.

Carper, B. A. (1978). Fundamental patterns of knowing in nursing. *Advances in Nursing Science, 1*(1), 13–24.

Chinn, L. P., & Kramer, M. K. (2011). *Integrating theory and knowledge development in nursing.* St. Louis, MO: Mosby-Elsevier.

Christenbery, T. L. (2011). Building a schematic model: A blueprint for DNP students. *Nurse Educator, 36*(6), 250–255.

Cody, W. K. (Ed.). (2013). *Philosophical and theoretical perspectives for advanced nursing practice* (5th ed.). Burlington, MA: Jones & Bartlett Learning.

Institute of Medicine. (2011). *The future of nursing: Leading change, advancing health.* Washington, DC: National Academies Press. Retrieved from: http://www.nap.edu/catalog/12956.html

International Classification for Nursing Practice. (n.d.). *Nursing phenomena classification.* Retrieved from: http://www.omv.lu.se/icnpbeta/dbrun/hierarchies/1A_Nursing_Phenomena.htm

Jensen, E. (2015). Linking theory, research, and practice. In N. A. Schmidt & J. M. Brown (Eds.), *Evidence-based practice for nurses: Appraisal and application of research* (pp. 133–149). Burlington, MA: Jones & Bartlett Learning.

McEwen, M., & Wills, E. M. (2014). *Theoretical basis for nursing.* Philadelphia, PA: Wolters Kluwer Health/Lippincott Williams & Wilkins.

Morrison, S. M., & Symes, L. (2011). An integrative review of expert nursing practice. *Journal of Nursing Scholarship, 43*(2), 163–170.

Phenomenon. (2015). *Merriam-Webster.* Retrieved from: http://www.merriam-webster.com/dictionary/phenomenon

Schmidt, N. A., & Brown, J. M. (2015). *Evidence-based practice for nurses: Appraisal and application of research.* Burlington, MA: Jones & Bartlett Learning.

Siedlecki, S. (2008). Making a difference through research. *Association of PeriOperative Registered Nurses Journal, 88*(5), 716–729.

Walker, K. C., & Avant, L. O. (2011). *Strategies for theory construction in nursing* (5th ed.). Upper Saddle River, NJ: Prentice Hall.

Helpful Resources

Butts, J. B., & Rich, K. L. (2013). *Philosophies and theories for advanced nursing practice.* Sudbury, MA: Jones & Bartlett Learning.

Meleis, A. I. (2010). *Transitions theory: Middle range and situation specific theories in nursing research and practice.* New York, NY: Springer.

nurses.info. (2010). *Theories*. Retrieved from: http://www.nurses.info/nursing_theory_ midrange_theories.htm

Nursing theories: A companion to nursing theories and models. (2012). Retrieved from: http://currentnursing.com/nursing_theory/introduction.html

Parker, M. E., & Smith, M. C. (2010). *Nursing theory and nursing practice*. Philadelphia, PA: F.A. Davis.

Peterson, S. J., & Bredow, T. S. (2012). *Middle range theories: Application to nursing research*. Philadelphia, PA: Wolters Kluwer Health/Lippincott Williams & Wilkins.

Developing the Scholarly Project

Katherine Moran

CHAPTER OVERVIEW

The DNP project involves rigorous scholarly inquiry with a focus on advancing nursing knowledge by identifying issues related to clinical practice, helping influence change that will lead to an improvement in clinical practice, and/or contributing to solutions. As one can imagine, developing the DNP project requires considerable thought and planning. The experience can easily become overwhelming without some direction to guide the DNP student who is beginning the process. The goal of this chapter is to introduce the DNP student to elements of a scholarly project that need to be considered early in the development phase.

CHAPTER OBJECTIVES

After completing the chapter, the learner will be able to:

1. Conduct a literature search
2. Write a literature review
3. Conduct an assessment
4. Formulate a problem statement

5. Identify key stakeholders
6. Define the project goal
7. Outline the project scope
8. Develop a project framework
9. Describe the project type

DEVELOPING THE DNP PROJECT

In preparation for the development of the DNP project, the student should spend time exploring phenomena that he or she finds interesting. In Chapter 5, The Phenomenon of Interest, the doctor of nursing practice (DNP) student learned the definition of *nursing phenomenon*, explored a variety of strategies to use to identify a phenomenon of interest for the DNP project, and undoubtedly recognized the value of utilizing multiple methods to explore the phenomenon comprehensively. It is important that the DNP student allow enough time to go through this process because it helps him or her gain deeper insight into the phenomenon of interest and identify a direction for the DNP project.

Once the student identifies a phenomenon of interest for the DNP project, he or she is ready to begin the scholarly project development process.

Conducting a Literature Search and Writing the Literature Review

As mentioned in Chapter 5, a literature review is conducted to sum up what is known and what is not known about the topic of interest, but it can also help refine clinical questions, illuminate the value of the phenomenon of interest, or identify the appropriate methods to use to examine the phenomenon (Polit & Beck, 2014). However, at this point in the process, instead of browsing the literature to better understand or describe a phenomenon, it is time to carefully review the literature to support the value and/or the need to study the phenomenon of interest. For example, the literature review can help identify a void in knowledge

> The literature review is a method used to support the value and/or the need to study the phenomenon of interest.

or a gap between the current state of the phenomenon of interest and the desired state.

The ability to perform a comprehensive literature review and articulate the findings effectively is essential. Today, technology has made it possible to access information quickly and efficiently using a computer and the Internet. However, there is more to a literature review than the process involved in performing a search. Therefore, it is beneficial to learn key strategies for conducting a literature review as well as interpreting the results.

According to Timmins and McCabe (2005), an effective literature search is a "crucial stage in the process of writing a literature review, the significance of which is often overlooked" (p. 41). Certainly, the process can be very labor intensive, especially if time has not been taken to develop an organized search strategy. To ensure a successful outcome, a literature search should be based on a systematic, thorough, and rigorous approach that is unbiased, up-to-date (within the last 5 years is ideal), and reproducible (Polit & Beck, 2014; Timmins & McCabe, 2005). There are several effective approaches to reviewing the literature. One method includes looking through databases, journals, and books to develop a list of relevant material. Another useful method involves identifying a relevant article and using the reference list to identify other potentially useful articles, books, or other sources of pertinent data (Timmins & McCabe, 2005). Both methods provide a means to begin gathering relevant information and set the parameters for the search.

When using a database to begin a search, it is important to identify a database that contains information relevant to the phenomenon of interest. A database is a large collection of information organized to allow users rapid search and retrieval ("Database," 2015). The information contained in a database or repository is stored in a form that is quickly searchable and readily retrievable, based on the words used in the query. A variety of databases exist; some require a subscription to access, and some are freely available to all. Databases may contain general information, cross-disciplinary topics, or subject-specific citations. Even databases that contain the same subjects may be different from one another. For example, PubMed is a comprehensive resource for biomedical literature, and the Cumulative Index to Nursing and Allied Health Literature (CINAHL) is a comprehensive resource for nursing and allied health literature. See **Figure 6-1** for a list of common databases.

It is important to develop a thorough yet logical search strategy. Taking time to choose appropriate search terms, whether keywords or subject headings, will help to organize the inquiry and defend the interpretation of the results once

- *CINAHL®*, the Cumulative Index to Nursing and Allied Health Literature, is a comprehensive resource for nursing and allied health literature. *CINAHL* has expanded to offer four databases, including two full-text versions. The *CINAHL* databases are available on EBSCO*host* (EBSCO, 2011, para 1).

- *PubMed/MEDLINE,* established by the National Library of Medicine, indexes biomedical literature to help provide health professionals access to information necessary for research, health care, and education. PubMed comprises more than 21 million citations for biomedical literature from MEDLINE, life science journals, and online books. Citations may include links to full-text content from PubMed Central and publisher websites (PubMed, n.d., para 1).

- *Business Source Premier* is a business research database. This is the industry's most popular business research database and features the full text for more than 2,100 journals. Full text is provided back to 1965, and searchable cited references back to 1998 (Business Source Premier, 2012, para. 1).

- *Emerald Fulltext* is a collection of management and information science journals. The database covers all major management disciplines.

- *Cochrane Collaboration/Cochrane Nursing Care Network* develops and distributes systematic reviews of interventions for many healthcare professionals.

FIGURE 6-1 Examples of databases used when conducting a literature search.

the review is complete. It is helpful to consult a librarian at this stage in the process. Librarians can help identify the appropriate keywords, subject headings, and limits for the search so that the information received is not overwhelming and is relevant to the topic.

Consider, for example, the following keywords: *asthma* and *children*. A search of the CINAHL database (2010 to present) identified 1,395 references. It is clear that the keywords are too broad to identify any specific, relevant information regarding this population. In this case, the librarian can help identify a more appropriate search strategy to use, along with the proper Boolean (or logical) operators and limits to further narrow the search.

The method used to organize the literature should be logical to the user and allow for easy retrieval. A variety of methods can be used to achieve the same outcome. Some individuals find it helpful to use index cards to capture pertinent information about an article, and others rely on electronic reference or citation management software to record and organize references, such as EndNote, ProCite, or RefWorks; one of these products may be available for use through the university at no cost to the student (see Helpful Resources). Because many people have a personal computer today, more and more people are managing the data electronically in files created on the computer. The information can be categorized under major headings and then further categorized in subfolders within the major headings. Consider, for example, a diabetes management case scenario. A major heading for a literature review category could be *diabetes management*, and within that folder could be subfolders for *fasting blood glucose* or *cholesterol*. To further organize the information captured in the electronic folders, some individuals develop a literature summary table. A summary table is used to organize the literature based on information that is important to the user, that is, the year of publication, author, name and type of the work, sample size, methods, and results (if the work is research). See **Table 6-1** for an example of a literature summary table.

Irrespective of the method used, the value here is to capture the reference information, the key ideas, and/or a brief summary of the literary work to refer to when writing the literature review.

When conducting the literature search, it is important to keep in mind the need to attain primary source material whenever possible. Primary sources are original materials that have not been filtered through interpretation or evaluation from another author (secondary source). Primary sources present "original thinking, report a discovery, or share new information" (University of Maryland Library, 2014, para. 1). The problem associated with secondary sources relates to the interpretation of the intent of the original author. Therefore, when information is found through a secondary source, it is important to take the time to search for the primary work. Generally, reference information regarding the primary source can easily be obtained from the secondary source reference list.

Once the literature is compiled, the information gathered must be interpreted. This is a very important step in the process. It involves selecting information that is most applicable to the phenomenon of interest and then interpreting and synthesizing the information. Unfortunately, sometimes knowledge about a subject may be incomplete, or there may even be opposing views expressed in the literature. Therefore, interpreting and synthesizing the literature can be a difficult process. The reality is, there may not be one single truth about a phenomenon because a multitude of individuals are contributing to the knowledge base. Further, each contributor has a specific purpose in mind for that contribution, which adds in some way to the value of the overall knowledge base. The task at hand, then, is to articulate where the literature is congruent, where and how it differs, and the overall message based on the review. The review should offer a summary of knowledge currently available. Price (2009) stated, "Even where more is

Table 6-1 Example of a Literature Summary Table

Year	Author, Title, Journal	Purpose	Design (descriptive, systematic review, observational etc.)	Sample	Result
2008	Kelleher and Andrews. An observational study on the open-system endotracheal suctioning practices of critical care nurses. *Journal of Clinical Nursing*	Compare endotracheal suction (ETS) practices of critical care nurses with recent research recommendations	Nonparticipant structured observational design	45	Participants varied in their ETS practices. They did not follow best practice recommendations, resulting in lower quality ETS treatment.
2008	Evangelista, Moser, Westlake, Pike, Ter-Galstanyan, and Dracup. Correlates of fatigue in patients with heart failure. *Progress in Cardiovascular Nursing*	1) To determine how prevalent fatigue is in patients with systolic heart failure (HF). 2) To identify clinical and psychological states associated with HF.	A cross-sectional, correlational design	150	Fatigue levels were moderately intense and highly prevalent in the sample population. Fatigue had predictable clinical dimensions and psychosocial correlates. Fatigue may influence patients' adherence to their medical regimen, social relationships, and quality of life.
2008	Jacobson, Myerscough, DeLambo, Fleming, Huddleston, Bright, and Varley. Patients' perspectives on total knee replacement. *American Journal of Nursing*	To describe patients' pre- and postoperative experiences with total knee replacement (TKR).	Qualitative descriptive design	27	Four overarching themes: 1) Many patients delayed having surgery for months to years, even though they had pain. 2) Once they decided to have surgery, they spent time waiting and worrying about the outcome. 3) Patients struggled with the need for independence and to accept the new knee. 4) Postoperatively, patients experienced pain after surgery and with rehabilitation but were hopeful they would regain function.

Reproduced from Brown, S. J. (2014). *Evidence-based nursing: The research-practice connection* (3rd ed.). Burlington, MA: Jones & Bartlett Learning.

debated than agreed it is possible to point to the richness and the complexity of the literature available" (p. 49).

Remember, from the perspective of the phenomenon of interest, the interpretation and summary of the literature review offers an opportunity to substantiate the need for the original inquiry by identifying the void in knowledge or a gap between the current state of the phenomenon of interest and the desired state. Further, it offers a lead-in to why the phenomenon is important, or it describes the benefits of investigating the phenomenon.

Therefore, it is essential that the concluding points of the review refer back to the purpose and focus of the literature review (Price, 2009).

Organizational Assessment

As mentioned in Chapter 5, practicing scholars are in the best position to identify those areas of clinical concern that require further research and/or improvement, which allows them to develop the clinical question in the context of the needs of an organization or population. When the DNP student is considering a quality improvement project, this is of critical importance to the success of the project because the project must be *valued* by the practice setting. In other words, the student should avoid identifying a project then looking for an organization to welcome a change initiative. The DNP student should first take the time to complete an assessment at the organization of interest to enhance project implementation, organizational change and determine the potential for sustainability.

To *assess* involves estimating or determining the importance, value, or significance of the object of interest. In this context, performing an assessment in relation to a phenomenon of interest involves a comprehensive analysis that could be used to highlight the variance from what is found in the *current state of being* to what could be found in a *future or desired state of being*. In some situations an organization may have a desired state in mind and may enlist the DNP student to help the organization achieve the desired state. Even in this scenario, it is important to begin with an assessment to confirm the organization's prediction. Once the assessment is complete, the difference between the current and desired state is then *measured* to determine if there is an actual need. In other words, an *assessment* of the organization, department, or unit of practice conducted by the DNP student will help (1) identify the gap between the current and desired state of being but also will (2) provide data that supports the need for change. Using data to drive change is essential in the healthcare arena today. This process can also help to secure project funding; because financial resources are often limited, projects are often prioritized within the system and implemented only when there is compelling evidence that supports the need for change. The assessment can also help identify what resources are currently being used and what resources exist to address the current needs. Simply stated, a comprehensive assessment provides a means to easily identify where opportunities exists. This process serves a significant purpose when conducting a scholarly project.

SWOT Analysis

An assessment can be used to evaluate the strengths and weaknesses of a variety of phenomena, such as the strengths and weaknesses of a community, organization, program, project, or even a process. One tool used to perform an assessment is called a strengths, weaknesses, opportunities, and threats (SWOT) analysis. The SWOT analysis looks at both internal and external attributes and threats to the phenomenon of interest. For example, perhaps the focus of the assessment is on evaluating a diabetes education program. The *internal* attributes of the program are those traits that are helpful to the program. They may include efficient processes, experienced staff, or an aesthetically appealing environment. These intrinsic factors have a positive influence on the program outcome. On the other hand, weaknesses of the program include any *internal* traits that could be harmful to the program. Perhaps there is underlying tension between key stakeholders (registered nurses, dietitians, social workers, psychologist, exercise physiologist, etc.), ineffective communication, or gaps in critical knowledge. These intrinsic factors can disrupt the program and potentially interfere with the ability of the program to meet its objectives. Together, these two evaluations provide a general perspective of the current situation.

The external factors are then examined to identify any potential *external* opportunities that could help the program. Perhaps there are opportunities to collaborate with other community members, or maybe key stakeholders are willing to provide additional support in an area identified as a program weakness. Finally, those external factors that may threaten or potentially harm the program or interfere with the program's ability to achieve objectives are also examined. External threats may include significant external competition (that is changing the marketplace), or perhaps there is a very real threat that the primary program funding source will be withdrawn. Either of these external factors or others like these could have a catastrophic effect on program outcomes if left unaddressed.

Once this process is complete, a determination can be made regarding how to proceed. This could include using the identified strengths to take advantage of the identified opportunities, or, in contrast, it may include using the identified strengths to minimize internal weaknesses or even overcome identified external threats.

The evaluation of the internal strengths and weaknesses, in conjunction with the evaluation of the external opportunities and threats, provides a broad view of the current situation. However, remember that the SWOT analysis is just one of many assessment tools that can be used to assess the phenomenon of interest. Chapter 12, The Scholarly Project Toolbox, includes examples of additional assessment tools the student may find helpful. See **Figure 6-2** for an illustration of the SWOT analysis model.

Conducting a Needs Assessment

Once the broad-view or "macro-level" assessment is complete, the DNP student can drill down to the "micro level" to determine the most important or immediate needs of the organization. Conducting a *needs assessment* is fairly straightforward. First, determine what it is that you want to know (which may have been identified through the SWOT analysis), who

> The assessment . . . can lead to the identification of a gap in the current state of a phenomenon or help validate current perceptions.

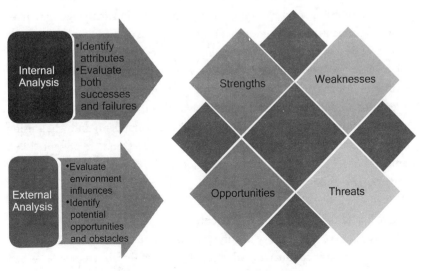

FIGURE 6-2 An example of a SWOT analysis chart.

the best person(s) is to answer the question(s), and how the data will be gathered; then, outline the data analysis plan and determine how you will share the findings with the organization.

One very important first step in performing a needs assessment is to create an assessment plan. To begin the process, have a clear objective in mind. As mentioned, think about what needs to be determined. The answer to this question establishes the direction the assessment will take and the questions that need to be asked to obtain the pertinent information. Finally, it also helps narrow the target audience. The next step involves identifying who would be best prepared to answer the assessment questions. Is it an individual or a group of individuals? If several individuals need to provide input, how will those individuals be chosen? Choosing the appropriate individuals is important because a representative sample of the population is necessary to ensure that the data captured are valid. A more detailed discussion related to identifying key stakeholders follows this section.

Finally, once the DNP student identifies who is best equipped to answer the assessment questions, a decision will need to be made regarding how the data will be collected, such as via interviews, focus groups or surveys; and how the results will be evaluated.

Interviews can be conducted in person, over the telephone, or through an Internet resource, such as Skype. The advantages of interviews are that (1) the response rates tend to be higher compared to surveys, (2) respondents have an opportunity to ask questions to gain clarity on a question that they may have otherwise left blank, and (3) additional information is gained by observing the respondent, which can help in interpreting responses (Polit & Beck, 2014). Regardless of the technique used, the student will want to have a structured set of questions prepared that may include both closed-and/or open-ended questions. The key is to carefully construct the questions so that they are clear to the respondent, are sensitive to the psychological state of the respondent, and when using questionnaires or surveys, are the appropriate grade level, and are presented in a meaningful order that encourages cooperation (Polit & Beck, 2014). Developing appropriate questions can be a labor-intensive process. Therefore, the DNP student should allow time in the project schedule for survey development and testing to assure the best outcomes are achieved.

A focus group or community forum serves the same purpose as an individual interview, except it is conducted with a small group of five to ten people. When selecting individuals to participate in the focus group, care should be taken to attract a diverse population with a broad view of the phenomenon of interest.

The DNP student can choose to send an invitation to potential participants or may choose to invite participants in person; however, he or she should also send a reminder prior to the event with the date, time, and location identified. During the focus group the DNP student should guide or facilitate the discussion using the structured questions. It may be helpful to solicit additional help to conduct the focus group in order to capture the responses from the participants and/or help facilitate the discussion.

Surveys are used to gain quantitative data that are primarily closed-ended, such as yes-or-no answers, but may include a few open-ended questions to add clarity. As mentioned, the DNP student should allocate sufficient time for survey development and testing in the project plan. The advantages of using a survey format are that it provides anonymity for the respondent and can easily be dispersed via the postal service or electronically via email. Another advantage is that respondents can then answer the survey at their convenience; but the downside is the response rates tend to be low.

Once the information is obtained, the data are analyzed. The data analysis method used will be dependent on the types of questions that are asked, such as quantitative (closed-ended) or qualitative (open-ended) questions. The DNP student will want to consult with his or her advisor to determine the best method to use for data analysis. See Chapter 14 for more detailed information on this topic. Once complete, the results of the analysis should be shared with the organization. Communicating the assessment results can be accomplished using a formal (presentation or white paper) or informal process (verbal communication) depending on the student's relationship with the organization and the preference of the organization's key stakeholders (see Chapter 15, Disseminating the Results).

> The process of conducting a needs assessment is fairly straightforward. First, determine what it is that you want to know, who the best person(s) is to answer the question(s), how the data will be gathered, then outline the data analysis plan and determine how you will share the findings with the organization.

Keep in mind that when the purpose of the assessment is simply to verify that the phenomenon of interest is worth exploring or to identify the perceived state of the phenomenon, a DNP scholar–created questionnaire will suffice. As mentioned, this type of assessment could be accomplished fairly quickly by conducting a small focus group or community forum or by surveying a convenience sample of the target population. When the results of the assessment are the central purpose for the project, measures need to be taken to ensure that a valid and reliable tool is used to conduct the assessment and that appropriate statistical methods are used to analyze the data. This type of assessment takes a considerable amount of time and resources to complete and may require institutional review board (IRB) approval (discussed later in this chapter). However, a comprehensive assessment, such as a community or organizational *needs assessment*, provides valuable data that describe the current state of the phenomenon of interest, how the proposed project could address the findings, as well as the potential project impact ("Methods for Conducting," 2008).

Developing the Problem Statement

The definition of a *problem*, according to Merriam-Webster, is "a question raised for inquiry, consideration or solution . . . [or] an intricate unsettled question" ("Problem," 2015, para. 1). Both definitions are fairly straightforward; they indicate that a question is involved. However, defining a *problem statement* has not been quite as forthcoming. In fact, it has not been consistently described in the literature. Some consider the purpose of the project and problem statement as one in the same, whereas others lump together the objective, hypothesis, or summary of the content as the problem statement (Hemon & Schwartz, 2007). In an attempt to bridge this gap, for the purposes of this discussion and in the context of the DNP project, a problem statement will encompass a *phenomenon in need of inquiry that is examined in order to develop a potential solution.*

> The problem statement encompasses a phenomenon in need of inquiry that is examined in order to develop a potential solution.

The problem statement is an introduction to the intent of the project. It should include enough information for the reader to gain an understanding of the issues surrounding the phenomenon of interest and the reason the project was selected as an area of focus. The problem statement provides the background to the problem and justification for investigating the phenomenon of interest, as demonstrated through the literature review.

Hemon and Schwartz (2007, p. 308) indicated that a problem statement should include four components:

1. Lead-in
2. Declaration of originality
3. Explanation
4. Indication of the central focus

Using this definition as a guide to formulate a problem statement, the *lead-in* should include information that helps to set the stage; it is the first introduction to the problem. To illustrate this concept, consider the following lead-in:

> Articulating the problem statement . . .
> The goal is to identify an issue, describe it clearly but succinctly, and adequately articulate why it is important that the problem be addressed.

Successful diabetes management in the primary care setting is a difficult, costly, and labor-intensive process that requires proven skills in lifestyle counseling (Moran, Burson, Critchett, & Olla, 2011). The information provided in this lead-in introduces the audience to the phenomenon of interest: diabetes management in primary care. It also highlights the area of concern: multiple factors that make it difficult to provide successful diabetes management in this care setting.

The lead-in statement is then followed by the *declaration of originality*, supported by information from the literature review. The intent here is to substantiate the need for the inquiry by identifying the void in knowledge or the gap between the current state of the phenomenon and the desired state. Continuing with the previous case example, consider the following: *Although many studies have proved the value of addressing the needs of the diabetes population in this care setting, there is a paucity of studies that look at clinically effective interventions or strategies in relation to cost* (Moran et al., 2011). In this case, the need for the investigation or declaration of originality is substantiated by the paucity of studies available that look at interventions or strategies in relation to cost in this care setting.

Next, the *explanation* of the phenomenon should highlight the value of the project and/or the benefits of investigating the phenomenon. The explanation of the purpose in the example centered on the need to improve diabetes clinical and cost outcomes in the primary care setting. Finally, the *indication of central focus* should tie all the previously mentioned components together to form a complete package, which is accomplished by articulating and/or defining what the project will accomplish. To clearly communicate the central focus, consider beginning this concluding statement by simply proclaiming the purpose of the project or study: "The purpose of this study was to implement and evaluate a care delivery model integrating the Registered Nurse-Certified Diabetes Educator in the Patient Centered Medical Home to assist in achieving positive clinical and cost outcomes in diabetes care" (Moran et al., 2011, p. 783).

Another approach that may be used to facilitate writing the problem statement is to begin by defining *who, what, where, when,* and *why*. In other words, *who* the problem involves, *what* the issue is, *when* and *where* the problem is oc-curring, and *why* it is important to investigate.

It is important to clearly define *who* is affected by the problem; this informa-tion will be included in the lead-in. Using the previous example, the specific group identified in the problem statement is primary care providers and their patients. The *what* and the *where* in this statement involve providing successful diabetes management for patients with diabetes within the primary care setting. This defines the boundaries of the problem. One can conclude that providing diabetes management for patients with diabetes in this specific care setting is dif-ficult and possibly not effective. Discussing the impact of the issue or why this problem is important would also be appropriate here. For example, one could link the phenomenon of interest with patient outcomes. In this case, including information in the literature regarding less than optimal overall glucose control in this care setting could be considered. This introduces the reader to the po-tential negative impact on the stakeholders, that is, patients with diabetes and their healthcare providers. One could even link the less than optimal clinical outcomes in this setting to the current cost of care of patients with diabetes. Regardless of the approach used, the goal is to identify an issue, describe it clearly but succinctly, and adequately articulate why it is important that the problem be addressed. Remember, a well-written problem statement will engage the audience and leave them with a desire to read more.

Identifying Key Stakeholders

Once the problem statement for the potential project is developed, it is critical to identify and reach out to the key stakeholders. Stakeholders are those individuals or groups who touch the project in some way or have an interest in the project outcome. These individuals can affect or could be affected by the outcome of the project. The student should consider those individuals or groups who are invested from the micro and macro level because they can provide in-formed and unique perspectives on issues that may have otherwise been overlooked.

> Key stakeholders . . . are those in-dividuals or groups who touch the project in some way or have an in-terest in the project outcome.

To begin, list all the individuals or groups who may be interested in the proj-ect. Who the potential stakeholders are depends on the project, of course, but a few examples may include service users, mentors, colleagues, organizational leaders, and community organizations. In the diabetes management example, the key stakeholders could include patients, families, healthcare providers, healthcare staff, healthcare institutions, payers, and even the community. Think about stakeholders who could benefit from the project, those who may have to make changes to current processes as a result of the project, and those who have something to lose. Determining the type of influence a stakeholder may have on the project's success is critical. Positive influence stakeholders may be willing to champion the project or support the project in some way, whereas negative influence stakeholders may be a restraining force.

Once all stakeholders are identified, consider which stakeholders are vital to the success of the project. These are the key stakeholders. The task at hand now is to determine what can be done to get stakeholder support or to reduce stakeholder resistance. This may include identifying the potential benefits of the project for certain stakeholders, such as outlining the project costs and benefits and developing strategies to minimize any perceived negative impact by other stakeholders.

This process may seem cumbersome and time consuming, but it is a valuable use of time because it helps to garner support for the project and minimize potential roadblocks. Remember Pareto's principle, or the 80–20 rule? It is very applicable to planning the DNP project: 20% of the work consumes 80% of the needed time. Furthermore, identifying and engaging key stakeholders is a good use of time because stakeholders can provide objective guidance on project implementation, identify options and/or solutions to address identified issues, provide input in areas in which there is an information gap, or help identify specific resources that are available to support the project.

Determining Project Goals

A goal is the end toward which effort is directed ("Goal," 2015, para. 1). In the case of the DNP project, it is what the student strives to achieve. Project goals describe what the student intends on delivering within the context of the project. Generally, a project's overall goal is relatively high level, though it should provide enough information to define when the project is complete. The project goal is the underpinning for decision making.

> Project goals describe what the student intends on delivering within the context of the project.

When considering potential project goals, think visionary! Perhaps the goal is to achieve a specific milestone, to test a hypothesis, to share insights or discoveries learned through the process, or to improve a process or outcome within an organization. For example, perhaps after conducting an organizational needs assessment the student identifies that there has been a steady increase in the number of medication administration errors occurring in the medical intensive care unit (MICU) over the past 9 months. After sharing this information with the organization, a decision is made to investigate the cause, determine the best course of action, and finally implement a quality improvement project with the aim of reducing the medication error rate in the MICU. The possibilities are limited only by imagination and available resources, including time. To this last point, it is crucial that the chosen project goal be achievable within the prescribed DNP program time frame; otherwise, there is a very real risk of not meeting program deadlines, which could result in failure to progress.

Once the goal has been identified, the next step is to define it. When articulating the goal of the project, clarity is the key. It is vital that the goal be clearly identified to ensure that everyone knows what event will mark the completion of the project. From here, the student can work backward to identify the interim goals (or objectives) that must be met in order to achieve the final desired outcome.

Defining the Project Scope

The project scope includes all the work that needs to be accomplished in order to fulfill the project goals. It helps to define when the project begins and when the project ends. To define the project scope, the student will need to consider the boundaries of the project. This includes identifying what will and will not be included (features and functions), along with identi-

> The project scope includes all the work that needs to be accomplished in order to fulfill the project goals.

fying the deliverables. Defining the project scope early on in the process helps the student during the implementation process. It is much easier to determine what is relevant to the project and what is not when clear boundaries have been identified up front. In the medication administration error scenario, the scope is defined by unit (MICU) and only includes medication errors. In this case, the scope may also include all three shifts, and it may include parenteral and oral medications, etc. To this last point, it may be easier for the student to understand all the dimensions of the project if the various components are diagrammed or graphed; this gives a visual representation of the project scope.

When defining the project scope, consider the following: What will make this project personally meaningful? Certainly the ultimate goal of the DNP project is to provide a medium for the student to demonstrate achievement of the DNP *Essentials,* which translates to an outcome that directly or indirectly benefits society. This is of great significance, and as such, what is and is not included in the project should be determined by the student after assessing what he or she believes is of most value. This process fosters personal investment in the outcome and makes the entire project more meaningful to the student. After all is said and done, the student owns the project and is responsible for achieving the deliverables.

Once the scope of the project is clear, the objectives of the project should be defined. This will help keep the project on track, clarify any assumptions, and avoid any unintended surprises. Objectives should describe what will be done (a measurable component) and when it will be completed. There may be a wide variety of types of objectives, depending on the type of DNP project. For example, in the medication administration error scenario the DNP student conducts a root cause analysis and determines that there is a system issue that is contributing to the increase in medication administration errors in the MICU. As a result of these findings a plan is developed, based on best practice, to address the problem. An example objective for this quality improvement project could be: *Amend the current medication administration policy and procedure to include safety checks and medication administration safe zones to decrease medication administration errors within 3 months after the new policy has been implemented.* An objective could include cost metrics, technical processes, or other measurable success criteria as indicated by the project. The key is to be as specific as possible. The student must accurately capture the conditions that are necessary to achieve the project's overall goal. One final point, the student will want to carefully consider the DNP program deliverables in the project goals and objectives. See Chapter 15, Disseminating the Results, for more information on program deliverables.

Determining the Theory and Framework

The next step in the process is to articulate the necessary features or functions that are required to meet the objectives. To begin, the student will need to outline the implementation process. Using a conceptual framework may be helpful in this phase of project development because it assists in identifying and categorizing the various components of the project. A conceptual framework is a "group of concepts that are broadly defined and systematically organized to provide a focus, a rationale, and a tool for the integration and interpretation of information" ("Conceptual Framework," 2015, para. 1). The Donabedian model is an example of a conceptual framework that focuses on three main categories: structure, process, and outcome (Donabedian, 1988). Using this framework, the student is able to identify all the concepts that affect the project structure (the setting in which the project will be implemented and who will be involved in the project), the process (what will be done and how it will be delivered), and, finally, the outcome (what will be measured, reviewed, or assessed). In Chapter 16, The Rest of the Story—Evaluating the Doctor of Nursing Practice, the Donabedian model is used as a framework to evaluate the practice doctorate.

The Donabedian model is just one example of a conceptual framework; there are many to choose from. In addition to a conceptual framework, the student will also need to consider a theoretical framework to help inform and/or guide the project. As indicated in Chapter 5, a theoretical framework is used to guide the student's perspective by further defining the project variables, identifying the known relationships among variables, and providing a framework for examining outcomes. Theory helps to explain or predict the relationships around the phenomenon of interest. If this is the case, the student and the student advisor need to determine the framework(s) that best captures the components of the student's scholarly project. More detailed information regarding the implementation process is covered in Chapter 13, Project Implementation.

Quality Improvement

Since many DNP projects are focused on improving processes and outcomes in practice it is important to understand what is meant by quality improvement and how implementation science may be used to impact these outcomes. The Health Resources and Services Administration (HRSA) (2011) defines quality improvement as a systematic and continuous process that leads to measurable improvement in healthcare services and the health status of targeted groups. Further, because a health organization's quality is linked to the organization's service delivery approach or underlying systems of care, the principles of quality improvement should focus on the systems/processes of care, the patients, the care team, and the use of data to drive change (p. 1).

Using the prior discussion of Donabedian's (1988) framework to address the medication errors in the MICU, the key components of the organization's systems, processes, and outcomes of care can be depicted. For example, the organization's *system or structure* would include resources (infrastructure, people, materials, technology), the *process* would include what is done and how it is done, and the *outcome* would include the results of the care provided (patient satisfaction, change in health behavior and health status). The organization's resources and processes need to be evaluated together in order to improve the end result.

While the structure and resources for an organization are generally easy to recognize, it may be difficult for some organizations to identify their processes because of the complex nature of health care. To better understand the processes used within an organization and the subsequent impact on outcomes, a process map can be used to diagram the events that lead to an outcome. A process map typically includes identifying and mapping the sequence of activities involved in a particular outcome; which includes identifying what is performed, who performs it, when it is performed, etc.). Following this process allows one to visualize opportunities for improvement (see Chapter 12 for an example of a process map).

When evaluating outcomes, one measure of quality that is of particular importance in health care is the degree of which the patient's needs are met; such as, access to care, culturally sensitive care, and patient safety. It should be no surprise that in order to meet the patient's needs effectively and to continue to improve quality it takes an inter-professional team. According to HRSA (2011) the healthcare team has the knowledge, skills and experience to make needed and long-lasting improvements. It is because of the unique perspectives from each team member that creativity and innovation evolve. The DNP student engaged in this process will have an opportunity to demonstrate his or her leadership competencies in facilitating the work of the inter-professional team. The importance of this role cannot be understated, because behind every effective team is an equally effective leader who is able to organize and facilitate the work of the team.

Finally, the team will need to use data to drive the change. This will include quantitative data (frequencies) for measurement of change but also qualitative data to provide context for the needed improvements (HRSA, 2011). Determining what is most important to measure can be difficult. For this reason HRSA (2011) recommends beginning with standardized performance measures, which are derived from practice guidelines that are designed to measure systems of care (see AHRQ Clinical Guidelines and Recommendations, http://www.ahrq.gov/ professionals/clinicians-providers/guidelines-recommendations/). Good performance measures should be relevant, measureable, accurate, and feasible. The data should be collected at established intervals and then analyzed to determine opportunities for change.

Implementation Science

A new and developing interprofessional research field in healthcare is *implementation science research*, also known as dissemination science or health services research. The focus of implementation science research is identifying and implementing best-practice approaches to health care in a variety of healthcare settings with an ultimate goal of improving outcomes. According to the Fogarty International Center (2013) implementation science is:

> the study of methods to promote the integration of research findings and evidence into healthcare policy and practice. It seeks to understand the behavior of healthcare professionals and other stakeholders as a key variable in the sustainable uptake, adoption, and implementation of evidence-based interventions . . . the intent of implementation science and related research is to investigate and address major bottlenecks (e.g. social, behavioral, economic, management) that impede effective implementation, test new approaches to improve health programming, as well as determine a causal relationship between the intervention and its impact (para. 3).

There is an increasing need for this type of research in health care to improve outcomes. It is well known that there is a gap that exists between research and practice; which has resulted in a delay in adopting evidence-based approaches that have been proved to positively impact healthcare outcomes. Implementation science research holds promise for bridging this gap. This can be accomplished in a variety of ways, such as by using scientific methods to compare evidence-based interventions, identify strategies that promote the integration of evidence into practice, develop new approaches to improve healthcare delivery, evaluate a population based intervention, or improve program quality and performance, to list a few.

However, because this field is still in its infancy, there is a need to recognize how implementation science research differs from other forms of research. Scientific rigor must be balanced with the need to conduct research in real world settings. Therefore, it is important to keep in mind that implementation science research may not produce results with the same precision as other forms of research; however, that does not mean that implementation science research is not of high quality. Implementation science researchers will need to use both quantitative and qualitative methods with some modification to include approaches used in economics and business fields to evaluate health interventions (Fogarty International Center, 2013). Further, quality improvement methods, such as rapid cycle improvement techniques, should also be considered when implementing effective innovations. Undoubtedly, DNP prepared nurses as well as DNP students will be included as part of implementation science research teams in the near future; as the DNP competencies (which are rooted in quality improvement) are in perfect alignment with the requirements for implementation science research.

DEFINING THE PROJECT TYPE

The DNP project can take many forms (see **Figure 6-3**). The boundaries for the project are determined by the DNP program requirements. While all projects will exemplify some of the DNP *Essentials,* such as interprofessional collaboration or use of data and informatics, they may not exemplify all of the *Essentials.*

Quality Improvement

The definition of *quality* as it relates to health care is subjective; it differs based on who is defining it. For the patient, quality may include accurate, skillful, and compassionate care. Healthcare providers, on the other hand, may define quality as achievement of the desired health outcome, whereas healthcare payers (health insurance companies) are likely to include some aspect of cost-effectiveness. Quality improvement projects in health care encompass those efforts that seek to improve services for the future. According to the Institute of Medicine (IOM), *healthcare quality* is defined as "The extent to which health services provided to individuals and patient populations improve desired health outcomes. The care should be based on the strongest clinical evidence and provided in a technically and culturally competent manner with good communication and shared decision making" (Peerpoint, 2012, para. 1).

The IOM (2001) summary report *Crossing the Quality Chasm* outlines six aims for improvement that are built on the need for health care to be:

1. *Safe:* avoiding injuries to patients from the care that is intended to help them.
2. *Effective:* providing services based on scientific knowledge to all who could benefit, and refraining from providing services to those not likely to benefit.

- Quality improvement
- Translating evidence into practice
- Clinical or practice-based inquiry
- Healthcare delivery innovation
- Program development and evaluation
- Demonstration project
- Healthcare policy
- Generating new evidence or knowledge

FIGURE 6-3 Examples of DNP projects.

3. *Patient-centered:* providing care that is respectful of and responsive to individual patient preferences, needs, and values, and ensuring that patient values guide all clinical decisions.

4. *Timely:* reducing waits and sometimes harmful delays for both those who receive and those who give care.

5. *Efficient:* avoiding waste, including waste of equipment, supplies, ideas, and energy.

6. *Equitable:* providing care that does not vary in quality because of personal characteristics such as gender, ethnicity, geographic location, and socioeconomic status (p. 3).

Quality Improvement Focus

As mentioned, healthcare quality improvement projects generally focus on analyzing elements of specific areas of performance in order to gain some measure of improvement. Given the current focus on healthcare quality by the IOM, the DNP scholar is well positioned to influence healthcare quality at the micro level (reducing medical errors on a specific care delivery unit) and/or macro level (leading efforts to reduce infant morbidity and mortality at the state level).

Quality Improvement Methods

Several different quality improvement methods have been used effectively in the healthcare arena. A few of the most common tools used in quality improvement projects are presented in Chapter 12. The following are a few examples of the quality improvement methods used by DNP scholars:

- FADE model—*Focus* (define the process that needs improvement), *Analyze* (collect the data and analyze), *Develop* (determine the plan of action), Execute (implement the plan), and *Evaluate* (measure the change and continue to monitor).

- Model for Improvement—a framework developed by Associates in Process Improvement (Langley et al., 2009) that is used by the Institute for Healthcare Improvement (IHI) to guide improvement work. The model includes three focus questions:
  1. What are we trying to accomplish?
  2. How will we know that a change is an improvement?
  3. What changes can we make that will result in improvement?
  By asking these questions, the organization is actually setting aims, establishing measures, and selecting changes. The changes are then tested using

several PDSA cycles (see later). After refining the change using the PDSA cycle, the change is then implemented on a broader scale and is eventually spread through other parts of the organization.

- Shewhart Cycle—uses rapid cycles of improvement until an optimal process is reached. This model uses the PDSA cycle to test change—*Plan* (plan a change), *Do* (implement the plan), *Study* (analyze the results), and *Act* (take action based on the results).
- Six Sigma—focuses on identifying and eliminating defects in a process in order to reduce variability and improve outcomes. This model uses the DMAIC strategy—*Define* (define the opportunity for improvement, the project goals, and the key stakeholders), *Measure* (determine what to measure and collect the data), *Analyze* (analyze the data to determine the root cause), *Improve* (implement a solution and continue to collect data to evaluate the outcome), and *Control* (develop and initiate a monitoring plan).

Other Quality Improvement Considerations

The goal of this chapter is to provide a broad overview of the types of DNP projects currently being developed, not to provide specific instruction on how to conduct these types of projects. Students who choose to complete a quality improvement project as evidence of their scholarly work need to be aware of quality improvement requirements. Selecting a mentor with expertise in quality improvement is desirable.

Nursing Research

While it is recognized that DNP students will primarily be focused on projects that improve practice and will therefore be using quality improvement frameworks, there is also a recognition that some students will choose to engage in *implementation science research* or other forms of research to improve practice. For this reason, information that is important for the DNP student to consider related to research is included. *Research*, in general, is defined as an "investigation or experimentation aimed at the discovery and interpretation of facts, revision of accepted theories or laws in the light of new facts, or practical application of such new or revised theories or laws" ("Research," 2015, para. 1). When considering the more specific nature of *nursing research*, Houser (2015) defined it as a "systematic process of inquiry that uses rigorous guidelines to produce unbiased, trustworthy answers to questions about nursing practice" (p. 5).

Research Focus

The National Institute of Nursing Research (NINR), an organization dedicated to improving the health and health care of Americans through funding of nursing research, is focusing on research that "promotes and improves the health of individuals, families, and communities across the lifespan, in a variety of clinical settings and within diverse populations" (NINR, 2011, p. 5). This could be accomplished through clinical problem analysis, knowledge generation (especially when collaborating with PhD colleagues), or translating evidence into practice.

Research Question

A method often used to develop a good research question is the PICO approach, which stands for *Population* (describes the patient population, i.e., age, gender, etc.), *Intervention, influence or exposure* (names the clinical intervention or therapies of interest; or identifies the potentially harmful influences or exposures of concern), *Comparison* (identifies a comparison intervention or the intervention is compared with usual care), and *Outcomes* (describes the outcome or consequences). With some clinical questions it may also be helpful to use a PICOT question, which includes the *Timeframe* (describes the timing in relation to the intervention and/or duration for data collection). For example, a clinical question using the PICOT format could be: Do patients with type 2 diabetes who attend a 6-week diabetes management program experience lower HbA_{1c} results than those patients who do not attend the program? In this case, the P indicates patients with type 2 diabetes, the I is a diabetes management program, the C represents patients who do not attend the program, the O is the HbA_{1c} results, and the T is 6 weeks. This format helps the scholar focus on elements of the question that are of interest (Brown, 2014; Polit & Beck, 2014).

Research Method

The research methods may be qualitative (when the goal is to understand the lived experience around the phenomenon of interest), quantitative (when the goal is to test a hypothesis, measure a phenomenon, or examine how the phenomenon of interest works), or a mixed method (both quantitative and qualitative).

Research Design

The research design may be nonexperimental (descriptive, correlational, predictive, or quasi-experimental design) or experimental (used to test cause and effect) in nature. The design is determined based on the research question or purpose, the availability of subjects and time frame, the skills of the researcher, ethical factors, amount of control required, the resources available to conduct the study, and expectations of the audience for research (Houser, 2015). The overall study plan, the details of how the study will be conducted, will be determined by the research design.

Other Research Considerations

The institutional review board. Before beginning a research project, approval is required from the university's IRB and/or from the review board where the study is conducted. The IRB, an independent ethics committee, comprises a group of individuals who "oversee all research involving human subjects and ensures studies meet all federal regulation criteria, including ethical standards" (Houser, 2015, p. 61). Applying for and receiving IRB approval can be a labor-intensive and time-consuming process. Once the application for IRB approval is submitted, it can take any-

> The institutional review board . . . oversees all research involving human subjects and ensures that studies meet all federal regulation criteria and ethical standards.

where from several weeks to several months to receive approval, depending on the type of review (expedited or full review). See Chapter 9, Creating and Developing the Project Plan, for more information regarding submitting for IRB approval.

Time and resources. Because of the short time frame associated with the typical DNP program, the student will need to choose a project with a fairly well-defined scope to complete the DNP program requirements on time. Not only does the actual study need to be completed on time, but the analysis and interpretation of the results need to be conducted and the final documentation (i.e., a research report) produced. In cases in which the project is large or complex, some DNP programs have allowed DNP students to complete the project together, with each student being responsible for specific elements of the project.

Expertise. If research is the focus of the DNP scholarly work, the student should work with a study team and/or individual researcher with expertise in conducting research. See Chapter 14, Aligning Design, Method, and Evaluation with the Clinical Question, for information on collecting and mining the data.

Pilot Study

A pilot study, also known as a feasibility study, is a smaller study that is done to determine if a larger study is practical and/or achievable. A pilot study could be done to ensure validity and reliability of instruments and to assess costs, efficiency, and/or accuracy (Houser, 2015). A pilot study conducted to determine feasibility should replicate the larger study as close as possible (i.e., setting, intervention, data collection, and analysis).

Pilot Study Focus

A pilot study is useful because it can identify areas of concern around a study design that can then be fixed before implementing the study on a larger scale. For instance, there may be issues with the randomization process of participants or with the data collection procedure. A pilot study can also be used to determine if the level of intervention is appropriate (for example, length of the intervention) or to see if the intervention causes adverse effects. Using the case example presented earlier, a pilot study was used to determine if providing diabetes education, management, and support using a registered nurse–certified diabetes educator would be cost-effective and improve clinical outcomes.

Pilot Study Methods and Design

The methods and design used in a pilot study are analogous with those of a larger research study.

Other Pilot Study Considerations

A pilot study can be especially helpful for a student because it gives him or her some experience. It also allows for preliminary testing of a hypothesis, and, as mentioned previously, it can help reduce unanticipated problems in the main study; this may save time and/or money if procedural issues inherent in the study design are discovered before it is implemented on a larger scale.

The institutional review board. If the pilot study involves human subjects, approval from the university and study setting IRB may be required. Remember that it may take anywhere from several weeks to several months to receive IRB approval (depending on the type of review), so careful planning is essential.

Time and resources. Although a pilot study can be completed in significantly less time than a large study, a fair amount of time is still required to complete the study in its entirety, including the analysis and interpretation of the results and final documentation. Again, careful planning is essential.

Expertise. As mentioned, if research is the focus of the DNP scholarly work, the student should work with a study team and/or individual researcher with expertise in conducting research.

Healthcare Delivery Innovation

The current U.S. healthcare system is at a crossroads. New methods for care delivery and approaches to disease management are being evaluated to determine if there is a more cost-effective means to meet the healthcare needs of the population. The focus is beginning to shift from acute, episodic care to prevention. Clinical teams are exploring the benefits of redefining care around medical conditions. For these and other reasons, DNP healthcare delivery projects are also popular choices for scholarly work. These projects often include an intervention or innovative approach to healthcare delivery that has an ultimate goal of positively affecting outcomes.

Healthcare Delivery Innovation Focus

The focus may include designing and evaluating new models of care, implementing and evaluating evidence-based practice guidelines, integrating telehealth into chronic disease management, or even redesigning care delivery systems in resource-poor settings. The potential projects in this category are extensive. The DNP student may consider using an implementation science or quality improvement approach when addressing these types of practice projects.

Healthcare Delivery Innovation Methods

The method used to deliver the project is dependent on the focus. For example, a DNP student embarking on a quality improvement project may use quantitative methods to answer the clinical question but may also want to consider qualitative methods to provide additional clarity. Projects that organize care using a team approach are gaining momentum because payers are looking for ways to improve clinical outcomes and efficiency. For example, the DNP student could choose to partner with a hospital- or community-based organization to coordinate delivery of care. Certainly, collaborating with other healthcare providers in the area or even health payers can be an effective approach when implementing a scholarly project.

Other Healthcare Delivery Innovation Considerations

When considering implementation of a healthcare delivery innovation, regardless of the specific type of project or methods used to implement the project, there should be a focus on the cost-effectiveness of the innovation as well as the clinical effectiveness. For instance, in the case study that was used to illustrate how to write a problem statement, the focus of the study was on implementing clinically effective interventions or strategies in the primary care setting to address the needs of a diabetes population. However, the authors chose to also include the cost associated with implementing this type of intervention. The results were that the model was both clinically and cost-effective in the population studied (Moran et al., 2011). In the end, the authors were able to make a business case for implementing the registered nurse–certified diabetes educator in the patient-centered medical home.

Healthcare Policy Analysis

Healthcare policies must be evaluated frequently to ensure that they are still relevant to society, that is, they continue to meet societal needs. Policy analysis helps with this process. The DNP student who engages in healthcare policy analysis within a scholarly project works to evaluate the historical evolution of the policy and determines if there is still congruence within the current social context. If there is incongruence, the results of the analysis may be used for policy modification recommendations (Porsche, 2012). The policy analysis may be the first step in formulating a project plan to address the healthcare needs identified. The DNP project should include planning, implementation, and evaluation components to address policy needs identified in the analysis to impact healthcare outcomes (AACN, 2015).

Healthcare Policy Analysis Focus

The intent of the analysis may be descriptive, to describe how and why the policy came to be and to describe the current state of a policy, or it may be prescriptive, to consider what could occur if a proposed policy is implemented.

Healthcare Policy Analysis Methods

Multiple approaches can be used in policy analysis depending on the impetus for conducting the analysis (i.e., qualitative or quantitative). The DNP student may decide to use one of the following models, as outlined by Porsche (2012); however, keep in mind there are other models that are not described here:

- *Eightfold path* uses a problem-solving process to clarify the problem and identify solutions.
- *Participatory policy analysis (PPA)* is used to ensure that the ideals of democracy are included in policy alternatives.
- *Logical-positivist model* uses a deductive reasoning approach to analyze a policy (hypothesis testing).
- *Process model* analyzes each of the stages associated with policy making.
- *Substantive model* focuses on the policy issue.

Other Healthcare Policy Analysis Considerations

Policy analysis can focus on micro-level issues (efficient allocation of resources) or macro-level issues (structural focus, sociocultural issues). The policy analysis process can use a variety of methods to obtain relevant data. However, conducting the analysis is only one part of the picture. Disseminating the results of the analysis to the appropriate stakeholders is a critical component of policy analysis; it is a part of the implementation and evaluation portion of the DNP project.

Program Development and Evaluation

Programs that are developed to address health and healthcare needs are of critical importance and definitely essential to the health of our nation. Gaps in healthcare access or delivery across the nation have been addressed through implementation of a variety of healthcare programs. They can be complex and multifaceted or relatively simple, such as providing health education to a community.

Program Development and Evaluation Focus

The types of programs that DNP scholars could potentially develop are vast and wide-reaching. A DNP program development and evaluation project may include an intervention that involves planning and implementing activities that will ultimately improve the health of a specific group or decrease known health problems within a community ("Program Development," 2015). The process involves identifying a gap in care, developing a program to address the need, and finally evaluating the outcome.

Program Development and Evaluation Focus Methods

Methods used for program planning and evaluation are variable but may include items such as surveys, individual interviews, and, more recently, focus groups. As mentioned, focus groups comprise individuals who represent a defined target population. These and other methods are used to gather information to determine the program needs, participant satisfaction, policy making, organizational development, and outcome evaluation. Irrespective of the method used to glean the desired information, it is imperative that the expectations are clear to the participants and the purpose well-articulated.

Other Program Development and Evaluation Focus Considerations

The DNP student embarking on a program development and evaluation project may benefit from the guidance of an expert in program development, implementation, and evaluation, especially as it relates to his or her area of interest. It may be helpful to include such an individual on the DNP project team (if applicable). It is also recommended by the AACN (2015) Implementation of the DNP Task Force to include an organizational mentor as part of the project team to be a liaison within the organization. Acting in this capacity the mentor could open doors to key personnel and inform the project from the organizational perspective.

Clearly, the potential project options for the DNP scholar are boundless. In fact, there are many more options than are listed within this chapter. When considering the options, the key is to focus on a phenomenon that meets the needs of society, is interesting, and in which the DNP scholar has sufficient expertise; to choose a project that will result in a personally meaningful outcome (because the time commitment to complete scholarly work is significant); and to develop a network of support in areas in which the DNP scholar has limited knowledge. There are many outstanding exemplars of DNP scholarly work. Consider the work by Dr. Bonnie Freeman, RN, DNP, ANP-C, ACHPN, which involved a practice innovation that resulted in the development of a tool to aid in the care of dying patients. The intent was to bridge the gap between current, evidence-based knowledge and what was being applied at the bedside. For more information about this very important work see the following article: CARES: An Acronym Organized Tool for the Care of the Dying, *Journal of Hospice & Palliative Nursing, 15*(3), 147–153. The CARES tool is available for downloading free of charge at the City of Hope Pain and Palliative Care Resource Center Web site: http://prc.coh.org.

Key Messages

- The literature review is a method used to support the value of and/or the need to study the phenomenon of interest.
- The assessment can lead to the identification of a gap in the current state of a phenomenon or help validate current perceptions.
- The problem statement encompasses a phenomenon in need of inquiry that is examined to better understand the phenomenon in order to develop a potential solution.

- When articulating the problem statement, the goal is to identify an issue, describe it clearly but succinctly, and adequately articulate why it is important that the problem be addressed.
- Key stakeholders are those individuals or groups who touch the project in some way or have an interest in the project outcome.
- Project goals describe what the student intends on delivering within the context of the project.
- The project scope includes all the work that needs to be accomplished in order to fulfill the project goals.
- The IRB oversees all research involving human subjects and ensures that studies meet all federal regulation criteria and ethical standards.

Action Plan—Next Steps

1. Conduct a literature review.
2. Conduct an assessment.
3. Write the problem statement.
4. Identify key stakeholders.
5. Define the project goals and scope.
6. Select a project theory and framework.
7. Determine the project type.
8. Submit for IRB review (if required).

REFERENCES

American Association of Colleges of Nursing. (2015). *Implementation of the DNP task force.* Retrieved from http://www.aacn.nche.edu/news/articles/2015/dnp-white-paper

Brown, S. J. (2014). *Evidence-based nursing: The research-practice connection* (3rd ed.). Burlington, MA: Jones & Bartlett Learning.

Business Source Premier. (2012). Retrieved from: http://www.ebscohost.com/academic/business-source-premier

Conceptual framework. (2015). *The Free Dictionary.* Retrieved from: http://medical-dictionary.thefreedictionary.com/conceptual+framework

Database. (2015). *Merriam-Webster.* Retrieved from: http://www.merriam-webster.com/dictionary/database

Donabedian, A. (1988). The quality of care: How can it be assessed? *Journal of the American Medical Association, 260,* 1743–1748.

EBSCO Publishing. (2011). *CINAHL databases.* Retrieved from: http://www.ebscohost.com/cinahl/

Fogarty International Center. (2013). What is implementation science? Retrieved from: http://www.fic.nih.gov/News/Events/implementation-science/Pages/faqs.aspx

Goal. 2015. *Merriam-Webster.* Retrieved from: http://www.merriam-webster.com/dictionary/goal

Health Resources and Services Administration (HRSA) (2011). Quality improvement. Retrieved from: http://www.hrsa.gov/quality/toolbox/508pdfs/qualityimprovement.pdf

Hemon, P., & Schwartz, C. (2007). What is a problem statement? *Library and Information Science Research, 29,* 307–309.

Houser, J. (2015). *Nursing research: Reading, using, and creating evidence.* Burlington, MA: Jones & Bartlett Learning.

Institute of Medicine. (2001). *Crossing the quality chasm: A new health system for the 21st century.* Retrieved from http://www.iom.edu/~/media/Files/Report%20Files/2001/Crossing-the-Quality-Chasm/Quality%20Chasm%202001%20%20report%20brief.pdf

Langley, G. L., Moen, R. D., Nolan, K. M., Nolan, T. W., Norman, C. L. & Provost, L. P. (2009). *The improvement guide: A practical approach to enhancing organizational performance* (2nd ed.). San Francisco, CA: Jossey-Bass Publishers.

Methods for conducting educational needs assessment. (2008). Retrieved from: http://www.extension.uidaho.edu/admin/needsassessment/01introduction.pdf

Moran, K., Burson, R., Critchett, J., & Olla, P. (2011). Exploring the cost and clinical outcomes of integrating the registered nurse certified diabetes educator in the patient centered medical home. *The Diabetes Educator, 37*(6), 780–793.

National Institute of Nursing Research. (2011). *Bringing science to life: NINR strategic plan.* Retrieved from: https://www.ninr.nih.gov/sites/www.ninr.nih.gov/files/ninr-strategic-plan-2011.pdf

Peerpoint. (2012). *The definition of healthcare quality and the Institute of Medicine.* Retrieved from: http://www.peerpt.com/performancequality-improvement/the-definition-of-healthcare-quality-and-the-institute-of-medicine/

Polit, D. F., & Beck, C. T. (2014). *Essentials of nursing research: Appraising evidence for nursing practice.* Philadelphia, PA: Wolters Kluwer/Lippincott Williams & Wilkins.

Porsche, D. J. (2012). *Health policy: Application for nurses and other healthcare professionals.* Burlington, MA: Jones & Bartlett Learning.

Price, B. (2009). Guidance on conducting a literature search and reviewing mixed literature. *Nursing Standard, 23*(24), 43–49.

Problem. (2015). *Merriam-Webster.* Retrieved from: http://www.merriam-webster.com/dictionary/problem

Program development. (2015). *The Free Dictionary.* Retrieved from: http://medical-dictionary.thefreedictionary.com/program+development

PubMed. (n.d.). Retrieved from: http://www.ncbi.nlm.nih.gov/pubmed/

Research. (2015). *Merriam-Webster.* Retrieved from: http://www.merriam-webster.com/dictionary/research

Timmins, F., & McCabe, C. (2005). How to conduct an effective literature search. *Nursing Standard, 20*(11), 41–47.

University of Maryland Library. (2014). *Primary, secondary, and tertiary sources.* Retrieved from: http://www.lib.umd.edu/tl/guides/primary-sources#primary

Helpful Resources

Citation Management Resources
EndNote—http://www.endnote.com/endemo.asp
RefWorks—http://www.refworks.com/

Data Resources

Agency for Healthcare Research and Quality, Clinical Guidelines and Recommendations. http://www.ahrq.gov/professionals/clinicians-providers/guidelines-recommendations/

Agency for Healthcare Research and Quality, Quality Indicators. http://www.qualityindicators.ahrq.gov/

American Nurses Association. http://www.nursingworld.org

Business Source® Premier. http://www.ebscohost.com/academic/business-source-premier

CINAHL® Plus with Full Text—http://www.ebscohost.com/academic/cinahl-plus-with-full-text/

Education Resources Information Center (ERIC). http://www.eric.ed.gov/

Emerald. http://www.emeraldinsight.com/

Health and Wellness Resource Center. http://www.gale.cengage.com/Health/HealthRC/about.htm

Joanna Briggs Institute. http://joannabriggs.org/

PsycINFO®. http://www.apa.org/pubs/databases/psycinfo/index.aspx

PubMed. http://www.ncbi.nlm.nih.gov/pubmed/

The Cochrane Collaboration. http://www.cochrane.org/

Quality Improvement Resources

Agency for Healthcare Research and Quality. http://www.ahrq.gov

American Health Quality Association. http://www.ahqa.org

FADE Model. http://patientsafetyed.duhs.duke.edu/module_a/methods/methods.html

Fogarty International Center. http://www.fic.nih.gov/News/Events/implementation-science/Pages/faqs.aspx

Institute for Healthcare Improvement. http://www.ihi.org

National Association for Healthcare Quality. http://www.nahq.org

National Quality Forum. http://www.qualityforum.org

Plan-Do-Study-Act (PDSA) Cycle. http://www.ihi.org/IHI/Topics/Improvement/ImprovementMethods/HowToImprove/testingchanges.htm

Six Sigma. http://www.isixsigma.com/new-to-six-sigma/getting-started/what-six-sigma/

Total Quality Management (TQM). http://www.thecqi.org/Knowledge-Hub/Resources/Factsheets/Total-quality-management/

CHAPTER 7

Interprofessional and Intraprofessional Collaboration in the Scholarly Project

Dianne Conrad

CHAPTER OVERVIEW

As the doctor of nursing practice (DNP) student formulates the question for the scholarly project, additional resources will be needed to assist in assessment and in planning, implementing, and evaluating the outcomes of the project. This process allows the student to practice the skills outlined in *The Essentials of Doctoral Education for Advanced Nursing Practice* (American Association of Colleges of Nursing [AACN], 2006) related to organizational and systems leadership, as well as forming and leading collaborative teams. This chapter will define collaboration with professionals within nursing and other professions, as well as populations and patients served. Nationally, nurses are called to actively collaborate within interprofessional teams to improve quality, cost-effective, and efficient care and improve outcomes (Institute of Medicine [IOM], 2003). The Implementation of the DNP Task Force (AACN, 2015) emphasized that organizational and systems leadership knowledge and skills are critical for the DNP prepared nurse to develop and evaluate new models of care delivery. The scholarly project for DNP students provides the opportunity for attaining and refining the competencies needed for collaborative team participation and leadership.

CHAPTER OBJECTIVES

After completing the chapter, the learner will be able to:
1. Discern the difference between the terms *interdisciplinary collaboration, interprofessional collaboration,* and *intraprofessional collaboration*
2. Discuss the importance and value of interprofessional and intraprofessional collaboration in the DNP project and in clinical practice settings
3. Identify the competencies needed for the DNP leader in an interprofessional team

GATHERING RESOURCES FOR THE DNP PROJECT

Developing the DNP project is a comprehensive and rigorous process. As the clinical question for inquiry develops, the DNP student may find gaps in knowledge and skill sets to carry out the project. The student will require assistance not only from DNP faculty but also from key players in the university and the organizational setting in which the clinical question is studied. Other collaborative efforts may be needed to effectively implement the project and develop an appropriate evaluation strategy. Finally, the DNP student may require assistance from appropriately qualified personnel to disseminate the results. This process will involve gathering not just one but perhaps several teams consisting of members from nursing and other disciplines.

Clearly, the DNP project is not accomplished by the DNP student without guidance, but it is an opportunity for the student to experience and, in particular, refine the skills required for DNP *Essential II: Organizational and Systems Leadership for Quality Improvement and Systems Thinking* and *Essential VI: Interprofessional Collaboration for Improving Patient and Population Health Outcomes* (AACN, 2006). DNP Essential II involves the ability of the DNP graduate to organize care to address emerging practice problems as well as collaborate with others to manage risks ethically, based on professional standards. Essential VI delineates the components of interprofessional collaboration and states that the DNP graduate should be able to:

- Effectively communicate and collaborate with others to develop and implement practice models, peer review, practice guidelines, health policy, standards of care, and/or other scholarly products
- Develop the ability to lead interprofessional teams in an organization to address complex practice issues
- Demonstrate the skills required to lead and collaborate with intraprofessional and interprofessional teams to address the change needed in health care and complex healthcare delivery systems (AACN, 2006).

Draye, Acker, and Zimmer (2006) advised that DNP education should include opportunities for students to form interprofessional teams. This experience allows students to refine skills in effective team leadership, in effective communication, and in guiding team members to the highest level of function to effectively improve health outcomes for patients and populations. The profession of nursing also benefits by the DNP student modeling to other members of the team and organization the behaviors of doctoral-level nursing leadership and collaboration in scholarly practice inquiry. The DNP graduate is equipped to serve on leadership teams with other practice doctorates in healthcare systems to address the complexities of health care.

DEFINITIONS

The origin of the word *collaborate* comes from the Latin word *collabratus*, meaning to labor together. *Collaborate* is defined as "to work jointly with others or together especially in an intellectual endeavor" ("Collaborate," 2015, para. 1). Ash and Miller (2016) noted that the concept of collaboration in successful business and management fields that includes "strategic alliances" and "interpersonal networks" can be transferred to the health sector. Collaborative partnerships that allow interaction between health professionals to share ideas and knowledge, as well as shared decision making, can improve quality and cost-effective care. The processes of collaboration involve communicating, cooperating, transferring knowledge, coordinating, problem-solving, and negotiating. Collaboration can occur within the framework of formal and informal teams that the DNP student may encounter during the scholarly project process. The DNP student may work with formally identified teams during the project, such as his or her project team or other teams of professionals within the clinical site. The student may also use the same skill set in communicating and working with informal team members such as statisticians or other experts needed for consultation on specific aspects of the project.

The concepts of *interdisciplinary* and *interprofessional* have been used interchangeably in the literature regarding collaboration in teams. Using the term *interdisciplinary* can limit the concept to knowledge ascribed to a particular discipline. The term *interprofessional* offers a broader definition than *interdisciplinary*; interprofessional collaboration refers to the interactions among individual professionals who may represent a particular discipline or branch of knowledge but who *additionally* bring their unique educational backgrounds, experiences, values, roles, and identities to the process. The collaboration with other professionals is enriched with shared or overlapping knowledge, skills, abilities, and roles (Ash & Miller, 2016).

To enhance the understanding of the phenomenon of interprofessional collaboration, D'Amour and Oandasan (2005) proposed the concept of *interprofessionality*. They defined *interprofessionality* as "the process by which professionals reflect on and develop ways of practicing that provides an integrated and cohesive answer to the needs of the client/family/population. . . [I]t involves continuous interaction and knowledge sharing between professionals, organized to solve or explore a variety of education and care issues all while seeking to optimize the patient's participation. . . Interprofessionality requires a paradigm shift, since interprofessional practice has unique characteristics in terms of values, codes of conduct, and ways of working" (p. 5). *Interprofessional collaboration* will be the term used in this text to refer to interactions with nursing and other health team members who do not belong to the nursing profession. The concept of *intraprofessional collaboration* is defined as interactions among colleagues *within the nursing profession* who share nursing professional education, values, socialization, and experience. However, the term interdisciplinary may be used at times in the discussion to accurately cite work from other authors.

COMPONENTS OF COLLABORATION IN THE DNP PROJECT: WHO, WHAT, WHERE, WHEN, AND HOW

The process of developing the DNP project will require collaboration with members of the nursing profession as well as other health professionals. Members of the team a DNP student gathers to complete a scholarly project can include, but are not limited to, nursing and other disciplinary faculty project team members, organizational leadership and healthcare workers, business and management personnel, experts in informatics, statisticians, and the patients who are part of the intervention. To explore the components of collaboration with different professionals and members of scholarly project teams, the framework of *Who, What, Where, When, and How* will be used.

Whom to Collaborate With?

When the DNP student gathers resources needed for the scholarly project, *who* will be needed to assist in assessment, planning, implementing, and evaluating the process may include members from the nursing profession as well as members from outside the profession, including patients and populations served.

> *Who* will be needed for the scholarly project team can include members from the nursing profession as well as members from outside the profession.

Intraprofessional Collaboration

The DNP student will find resources within the profession from both faculty and other nursing professionals in the clinical setting. Nursing faculty are the primary role models and resources for collaboration for the DNP student. The Implementation of the DNP Task Force recommended a doctorally prepared faculty member to help guide the student (AACN, 2015). Cronenwett and colleagues (2011) described the optimal learning environment for DNP students as "one in which doctorally-prepared faculty members are actively engaged in teaching, clinical practice, translational science and systems improvement, preferably within an environment characterized by robust interprofessional learning opportunities" (p. 14). Identifying faculty as mentors as well as content and research consultants in identified areas of the projects is important early in the scholarly project work. These faculty members may also serve as part of the DNP project team to guide the work of the student during the project. For more on the project team and their functions, see Chapter 8, The DNP Project Team.

As the practice doctorate programs in nursing continue to grow, the collaboration of PhD- and DNP-prepared nurses in contributing to evidence-based practice will be realized. DNP students collaborate with their PhD-prepared nursing faculty, and research collaboration between nursing PhD students and DNP students provides a multifaceted approach to healthcare problems. Many universities already have both nursing research and nursing practice doctorate programs.

This is an ideal setting for PhD and DNP students to collaborate in research projects from their respective viewpoints of knowledge generation and practice.

Clinton and Sperhac (2009) stated that the two doctoral degrees in nursing are complementary and overlap. The interaction between the research and practice degrees in nursing can be applied to projects in which research questions are generated by the practice doctorate from clinical questions and then tested in the practice environment for application and evaluation with the assistance of the research doctorate. The process can be reversed in that the nurse researcher coming from a particular field of interest can enlist the aid of the practice doctorate in the clinical environment to test theory. In all, the nursing profession benefits from the collaboration of the practice and research doctorates in the generation of evidence-based practice.

> The nursing profession benefits from the collaboration of the practice and research doctorates in the generation of evidence-based practice.

The opportunities for collaboration also occur with other nurses in the clinical setting where the scholarly project takes place. DNP students can model doctoral nursing leadership skills with other nurses—such as nursing administration, nursing staff, and nursing informatics experts involved in their project—and include them in their project team when appropriate. DNP students in administrative advanced practice roles can influence institutional policy with projects, such as instituting a new program to benefit a specific population. For example, the administrative DNP student might gather a team of nursing administrators, clinicians, and other departments, such as pharmacy and information technology, to inform a project aimed at serving the local uninsured population. The DNP student not only would model leadership behaviors in a project proposal for his or her university but also may present the project to the board of the institution to implement the innovative change.

The opportunity for intraprofessional collaboration can also occur with DNP students working with each other to complete different aspects of a project topic, such as diabetes care. See Chapter 4, Scholarship in Practice, for a discussion of scholar teams of DNP students working together on a scholarly project.

Interprofessional Collaboration

In the 2001 report *Crossing the Quality Chasm: A New Health System for the 21st Century*, the IOM outlined aims for healthcare improvement, which included care that is safe, effective, patient centered, timely, efficient, and equitable.

To provide that care, the IOM, in *Health Professions Education: A Bridge to Quality* (2003), called for a change in how healthcare providers are prepared to meet these challenges, which includes working in teams. Many health professional programs are now collaborating to educate students to learn by, with, and from others from outside their own profession. Interprofessional education is the interactive learning and collaboration of students from different health and social professions "for the explicit purpose of improving interprofessional collaboration or the health/well being of patients/clients (or both)" (Reeves et al., 2013, p. 4).

Educational preparation for multiple professions working in teams often begins with simulation exercises to develop interprofessional team communication skills (Wagner, Liston, & Miller, 2011) and interprofessional mentoring in the clinical setting (Lait, Suter, Arthur, & Deutschlander, 2011).

To fully operationalize the concept of interprofessional collaboration in practice, the Robert Wood Johnson Foundation (2015) states that:

> Effective interprofessional collaboration promotes the active participation of each discipline in patient care, where all disciplines are working together and fully engaging patients and those who support them, and leadership on the team adapts based on patient needs.
>
> Effective interprofessional collaboration enhances patient- and family-centered goals and values, provides mechanisms for continuous communication among caregivers, and optimizes participation in clinical decision-making within and across disciplines. It fosters respect for the disciplinary contributions of all professionals (p. 1).

Interprofessional Clinical Models

Traditionally, healthcare professionals have practiced in the silos of their perceived professional boundaries. Lack of communication and coordination of care has led to fragmentation, excess cost, and a healthcare system that is disease oriented rather than health oriented. In 1983, Bonnie Wesorick began work to address these issues, developing the Clinical Practice Model (CPM) Framework™ to create the best places to give and receive care. One goal of the CPM Framework™ was to unravel the complexity of factors impacting healthcare culture in a holistic framework with an integrated team approach rather than focusing only on individual issues in patient care (Elsevier CPM Resource Center, 2012).

Today, the Elsevier CPM Framework™ is implemented in hundreds of acute care settings in North America. Elsevier's CPM Framework™ is founded on core beliefs, healthcare related theories and principles that describe the nature of the work and the actions steps necessary to transform health care at points of care (Wesorick & Doebbeling, 2011). The patient, family, community, and caregiver are at the core of the model because they are impacted by transformational change and their stories live at the center of the healthcare experience (see **Figure 7-1**, The CPM Framework). This framework is designed to assist practitioners to focus on practice priorities, evidence-based clinical decision support, and practice expertise to ensure improved patient outcomes, compliance with national patient safety standards, and an overall improvement in interprofessional staff collaboration and satisfaction.

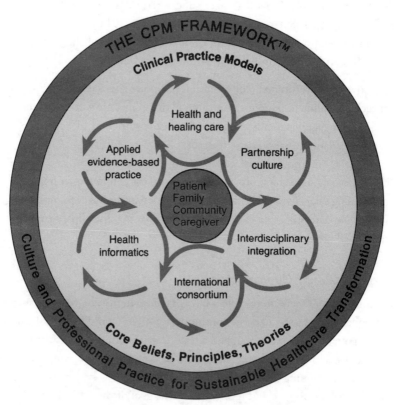

FIGURE 7-1 The CPM framework.

This figure was published in The CPM Framework™: Culture and professional practice for sustainable healthcare transformation [Brochure], Elsevier CPM Resource Center. Copyright Elsevier (2011).

Fundamental skills used in the CPM Framework ^{TM} that enhance interdisciplinary communication and influence cultural and practice transformation include dialogue, partnership, and polarity management. Because many problems plaguing health care today are considered dilemmas and contain more than one right answer, it is important to prioritize polarity management as first steps in solving healthcare issues. Polarities involve interdependent pairs of values or of view. Polarity thinking invites the various disciplines to look at a health dilemma from different points of view when there is tension between the two "sides" and the issue cannot be fixed by choosing one or the other. The technique encourages professionals to think differently and enhances communication as team members appreciate and work through these paradoxes or dilemmas (Elsevier CPM Resource Center, 2012) (see **Table 7-1**).

Many of the cultural shadows that haunt us today and prevent us from reaching a higher ground of a healthy work culture and integrated care are the result of trying to fix problems that are really polarities (Wesorick, 2002).

Table 7-1 Polarity Thinking^{TM}

Polarity Thinking *"LIFE" Polarities*

Home Life	Work Life
Activity	Rest
Self	Others
Candor	Diplomacy
Gentle Love	Tough Love
Yin	Yang

"Healthcare" Polarities

Framework-Driven Change	Project/Initiative-Driven Change
Autonomous Care	Standardized Care
Integrated Competency	Individual Competency
Mission	Margin
Hospital Interest	Physician Interest
Staff Satisfaction	Patient Satisfaction
Patient Safety	Staff Freedom

Wesorick also encourages the DNP nurse to be aware of the polarity of individual "task" versus "scope of practice," which can divide members of different health professionals trying to work together. The leader must be clear on each profession's scope of practice to effectively lead the team.

This is a challenge for the team leader but essential to break the silos of professionals trying to protect their domain, yet attain an integrated competency of working together as a team. The ultimate goal is to bring each profession's expertise together to benefit the individual patient, society, and the healthcare delivery system (B. Wesorick, personal communication, September 19, 2012).

Bonnie Wesorick is a pioneer in interprofessional nursing practice and embodies the leadership reflected in the DNP *Essentials* that enhances the nursing profession. Her work began and continues in the clinical setting and reflects the impact of scholarly practice.

The Robert Wood Johnson Foundation (2015) has identified exemplar healthcare organizations that have embraced interprofessional collaboration and published best practices in their report "Lessons from the Field: Promising Interprofessional Collaboration Practices." Key findings from the report show that successful interprofessional collaboration models include:

- Putting patients first.
- Demonstrating leadership commitment to interprofessional collaboration as an organizational priority through words and actions.
- Creating a level playing field that enables team members to work at the top of their license, know their roles, and understand the value they contribute.
- Cultivating effective team communication.
- Exploring the use of organizational structure to hardwire interprofessional practice.

DNP students can use these principles of integrated clinical models and interprofessional collaborative best practices during their immersion experiences and in implementing their scholarly projects.

WHAT TYPE OF INFORMATION IS NEEDED?

The gathering of resources includes identifying the gaps in knowledge that the student may need to inform the scholarly project. The DNP student may need to look outside the nursing profession to other disciplinary fields to inform

> What type of information is needed to complete the scholarly project? Answering this question may involve investigation and study in other disciplinary fields.

the development of the DNP project question. For example, in preparing for this author's DNP scholarly project regarding the use of standardized nursing language in the electronic health record (EHR), independent study was needed in the area of nursing standardized language, healthcare informatics, and the development and function of the EHR. This preparation involved collaborating with nursing informatics experts in an independent study class as well as working with information technology experts at a national conference of EHR vendors. Nursing informatics is a rapidly developing field, and the independent study allowed an in-depth exploration of the current status of the visibility of nursing practice reflected in electronic documentation. Learning the new technical language of information technology allowed dialogue with EHR vendors to understand how advanced practice nurses can be involved in asking for the tools, such as reference terminologies available in EHRs, to reflect nursing language and nursing care. (See Chapter 15, Disseminating the Results, Appendix A, for the *Journal of the American Academy of Nurse Practitioners* article "Identifying the Barriers to Use of Standardized Nursing Language in the Electronic Health Record by the Ambulatory Care Nurse Practitioner," by Conrad, Hanson, Hasenau, & Stocker-Schneider, 2012.)

Other types of information needed by the DNP student can be provided by business, management, and statistical professionals, as well as professionals in other healthcare disciplines. For example, to explore the feasibility of purchasing new equipment to relieve pressure ulcers in the hospitalized patient used in a safety study, the DNP student may need to gather information from equipment vendors, budget office personnel (for funding), and clinicians who may use the equipment on the clinical units. The DNP student will need a broad lens to explore his or her chosen field of study to narrow down the clinical question to be studied. Gathering the resources and interacting with other members of the identified team provide an opportunity for the DNP student to practice interprofessional competencies, including leadership and communication skills. Faculty mentors and the DNP student's project team can assist in identifying and linking the student with the appropriate resources needed to inform the project. The DNP student will continue to perfect these skills as the project matures in the context of his or her clinical immersion experiences.

WHERE AND WHEN DOES COLLABORATION TAKE PLACE?

> When and where to implement an intervention in a scholarly project may be guided by the collaborating team.

Gathering the team together, particularly in the planning and implementation phases of the project, will likely take place during the immersion experience in the facility chosen to implement the DNP project. During this time, the DNP student will use the organizational evaluation techniques learned in DNP core courses as well as implement change theory techniques if the project involves a practice intervention.

Evaluation of the culture of the organization is critical to not only identifying clinical problems but also designing and implementing a successful clinical intervention. Several tools are available for assessing organizational culture (see Chapter 12, The Scholarly Project Tool box, for organizational assessment tools). These types of tools assign a score for organizations for current and future assessments in areas such as organizational leadership, management of employees, and strategic emphases. Organizational assessments can be invaluable to the student as he or she evaluates and assesses organizational potential for change for a DNP project intervention.

Enlisting the help of key members of an organization is important to the success of a project. For example, a DNP student who is working with a home healthcare organization for implementation of a nurse practitioner on staff will need to not only evaluate the existing organizational structure for support for the new position but also assess financial viability, the collaborative resources available to the advanced practice nurse, and needs of the population to be served.

The team that the DNP student gathers can have a formal or informal structure. An example of a formal team is the DNP project team (see Chapter 8, The DNP Project Team). Informal members of the team can be people who the DNP student consults to plan and implement a project within an organization. This could be the nursing manager of a unit or a nurse informatics specialist who the student will consult to inform various aspects of project implementation.

After identifying the organizational structure and individuals who will be part of the collaborating team for the DNP project, the student then embarks on implementing the project. Change theory can guide the DNP student in planning and implementing the intervention. **Table 7-2** features just two examples of many change theories that can be used in understanding the process of change.

Table 7-2 Examples of Change Theory

Model	Components of the Change Theory
Lewin/Schein's Change Theory (Wirth, 2004)	Stage 1: Becoming motivated to change (unfreezing)
	Stage 2: Change what needs to be changed (unfrozen and moving to a new state)
	Stage 3: Making the change permanent (refreezing)
Kotter's 8-Step Change Model (Kotter, 1996)	Step 1: Create urgency
	Step 2: Form a powerful coalition
	Step 3: Create a vision for change
	Step 4: Communicate the vision
	Step 5: Remove obstacles
	Step 6: Create short-term "wins"
	Step 7: Build on the change
	Step 8: Anchor the change in corporate culture

When and where to implement the change may be influenced by the DNP student's collaborating team based on the assessment of

> The DNP project allows the DNP student to practice and refine skills on how to lead a collaborative team.

the organization. Ash and Miller (2016) cautioned that even a desirable change can meet resistance by the team members and other members of the organization. DNP prepared nurses must be change agents for successful collaboration and understand and apply various change theories to accomplish collaborative team goals.

HOW TO ACCOMPLISH A SUCCESSFUL SCHOLARLY PROJECT USING COLLABORATION

The skill set of leading successful interprofessional teams is multifaceted and involves specific competencies to be attained by the DNP student.

In response to the IOM's (2001) call for improvement by the healthcare professions in addressing the American healthcare delivery system, the National Center for Healthcare Leadership (2010) defined leadership competencies for medicine, nursing, and administration. The model consists of three domains—*transformation, execution,* and *people*—that "capture the complexity and dynamic quality of the health leader's role and reflect the dynamic realities in health leadership today" (p. 3). Each domain has specific competencies related to that domain to further outline the specific skill set needed by the healthcare leader (see **Figure 7-2**).

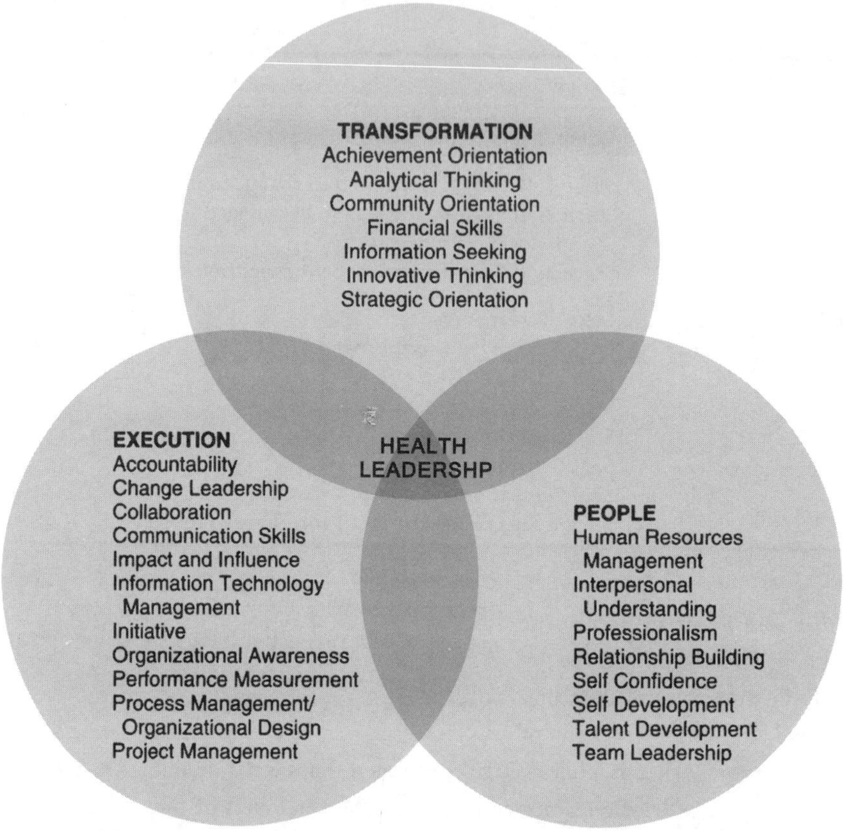

TRANSFORMATION
Achievement Orientation
Analytical Thinking
Community Orientation
Financial Skills
Information Seeking
Innovative Thinking
Strategic Orientation

EXECUTION
Accountability
Change Leadership
Collaboration
Communication Skills
Impact and Influence
Information Technology
 Management
Initiative
Organizational Awareness
Performance Measurement
Process Management/
 Organizational Design
Project Management

**HEALTH
LEADERSHP**

PEOPLE
Human Resources
 Management
Interpersonal
 Understanding
Professionalism
Relationship Building
Self Confidence
Self Development
Talent Development
Team Leadership

FIGURE 7-2 NCHL Health Leadership Competency Model™.
Reproduced with permission from the National Center for Healthcare Leadership.

In 2011, the Interprofessional Education Collaborative released *Core Competencies for Interprofessional Collaborative Practice*, a report that outlined action strategies to support implementation of the interprofessional education competencies. These competencies include working in interprofessional teams, using evidence-based practice, applying quality improvement, and using informatics in providing patient-centered care. The competencies also reflect the IOM's goals for interprofessional care delivery.

Action strategies are used to educate health professionals to work in interprofessional teams and include principles of care delivery that are:

- Patient and population oriented
- Relationship centered
- Stated in "common" language across professions
- Applicable across practice settings

- Applicable across professions
- Able to be integrated across the learning continuum
- Outcome driven (performance)
- Relevant to all the IOM's goals for improvement: patient-centered, efficient, effective, safe, timely, and equitable care.

The opportunity to practice these skills arises within the process of the DNP project. Developing a successful collaborative team requires progress through various stages of team development, according to Tuckman and Jensen (1977). The stages include teams progressing through phases of *forming, storming, norming, performing,* and *adjourning.* See Chapter 9, Creating and Developing the Project Plan, for a detailed discussion of each phase.

The DNP student can address the following factors to assist the team to achieve the DNP project goals:

- *Shared purpose, goal, and buy-in of members:* The DNP student must be clear on articulating the purpose of his or her scholarly project in relation to the benefits to the patients, members of the team, and organization.
- *Reciprocal trust in team members:* The DNP student will utilize the immersion experience in the organization to foster a culture of trust and transparency.
- *Recognition and value of the unique role or skills each team member brings:* Respect for team members and modeling this behavior by the DNP student allow for successful interaction with and among team members.
- *Functioning at the highest level of skill, ability, or practice:* The DNP student has the opportunity to utilize clinical expertise in formulating and implementing a scholarly practice innovation and can model the aim of the *Future of Nursing's* (IOM, 2010) call for nurses to practice to the full extent of their education and training.
- *Clear understanding of roles and the responsibilities of team members to meet goals:* The DNP student must use high-level communication skills throughout the project to ensure that each team member understands his or her role in completing the project. This can decrease conflict and uncertainty among team members and enhance timely completion of the project.
- *Work culture and environment that embrace the collaborative process:* The DNP student's evaluation of organizational culture and environment is necessary to identify barriers to implementing and completing the project and enlist the help of the team to overcome the barriers.

- *Collective cognitive responsibility and shared decision making:* The DNP student is the leader of his or her project team but must enlist the aid of team members for timely and appropriate decision making during all aspects of the project process.

The DNP core courses provide the opportunity to explore leadership competencies. The DNP student will refine leadership skills in clinical practice as well as in the completion of the scholarly project. Dr. Stephanie Brady outlines many of these competencies in the following description of her scholarly project.

THE IMPACT OF MINDFULNESS MEDITATION ON A CULTURE OF SAFETY ON AN INPATIENT PSYCHIATRIC UNIT
Stephanie Brady, DNP, APRN-BC

My project, "The Impact of Mindfulness Meditation on a Culture of Safety on an Inpatient Psychiatric Unit," involved the implementation of a 6-week program on mindfulness meditation for a multidisciplinary team that worked on an inpatient adult psychiatric unit. The hypothesis was that if we could teach the multidisciplinary teams how to be present for patients, we would see a decrease in the number of falls, a reduction in the number of patient incidents of aggression, and an increase in patient satisfaction. The Mindfulness Meditation class was conducted weekly for an hour along with daily homework assignments. The class size was limited to a maximum of 15 participants. Staff were required to attend every session for the 6-week time frame. The multidisciplinary team included physicians, nurses, social workers, mental health technicians, and recreational therapists. The outcome metrics were gathered for the period 6 months before the class and the 6 months post-class. I was able to demonstrate a clinically significant reduction in patient falls, a decrease in the number of patient aggressive incidents, and a significant increase in patient satisfaction.

This project required me to work closely with the nurse manager of the inpatient unit to facilitate the scheduling of the interested staff, the psychologist who was teaching the class, the nurse who is the risk manager for the facility, the recreational therapist for the room space, and the psychiatrists for their buy-in to the project. Although advice was provided by my DNP research committee, the operational perspective of the project really fell to me for implementation. In my role in behavioral health within our health system, I interact on a daily basis with the interdisciplinary team. I found that the leadership role I took as a DNP student was not really any different than that of being a leader in the system. I find that my leadership style is to influence via relationships versus power. Because this project was successful, there has been a great deal of interest in expanding this work to other units of the same hospital and other sites within the health system. There has also been a lot of positive feedback from the staff on this unit for more classes/refreshers on this topic because many felt that this class was helpful to them in their entire life, not just at work, and they appreciated the workplace for giving them this opportunity.

SUMMARY

The complexity of health care requires innovative approaches to solve the multifaceted health issues of individuals and populations. Healthcare professionals must work together to change the current linear disease-oriented care system to new models in which all disciplines are contributing specialized skills and abilities that allow them to practice to the full scope of their education and training. However, high-level communication and leadership skills are needed to form and guide the team to function at each individual professional's highest level to accomplish a goal. See **Table 7-3** for interprofessional and leadership resources. In this way, the collaborative team can contribute to high-quality, cost-effective, and safe patient-centered care (Ash & Miller, 2016). The DNP-prepared nurse begins to actualize this skill set in carrying out the DNP project in the context of interprofessional and intraprofessional collaboration.

Table 7-3 Interprofessional and Leadership Resources

Resource	Purpose	For More Information
Robert Wood Johnson Project on Interprofessional Collaboration	Identifying and Spreading Practices to Enable Effective Interprofessional Collaboration	http://www.rwjf.org/en/library/research/2015/03/lessons-from-the-field.html
Clinical Practice Model (CPM)	A clinical framework to integrate evidence-based practice with multiple disciplines to improve patient care	http://www.cpmrc.com/company/overview/
NCHL Health Leadership Competency Model	Defined health leadership competencies for multiple health disciplines	http://www.nchl.org/Documents/NavLink/Competency_Model-summary_uid31020101024281.pdf
Core Competencies for Interprofessional Collaborative Practice	Defined action strategies to support implementation of the interprofessional education competencies	http://www.aacn.nche.edu/education-resources/ipecreport.pdf

Key Messages

- The DNP student is expected to model doctoral-level leadership skills in forming and leading interprofessional and intraprofessional teams to accomplish the scholarly project.
- *Who* will be needed for the DNP project team can include members from the nursing profession and members from outside the profession.
- *What* types of information needed to complete the DNP project may involve investigation and study in other disciplinary fields.
- *When and where* to implement an intervention in a DNP project may be guided by the collaborating team.
- The DNP project allows the DNP student to practice and refine skills on *how* to lead a collaborative team.

Action Plan—Next Steps

1. In selecting the phenomenon of interest or the DNP project, identify gaps in the knowledge and skills needed to formulate the question and design, implement, and evaluate the scholarly practice inquiry.

2. Gather resources and faculty members who can assist in filling the knowledge and skill gaps, keeping in mind that consultation with other disciplines may be needed.
3. Consider professional development in other areas of study to broaden the knowledge base needed to complete the project.
4. Study and practice the leadership skill competencies needed to participate and lead interprofessional teams.
5. Formalize the relationship of faculty mentors and other team members with the formation of the DNP project team or other advising structure recommended by the university.
6. Begin relationship building with potential team members within the immersion experience organization.

REFERENCES

American Association of Colleges of Nursing. (2006). *The essentials of doctoral education for advanced nursing practice.* Washington, DC: Author.

American Association of Colleges of Nursing. (2015). The doctor of nursing practice: Current issues and clarifying recommendations. Retrieved from http://www.aacn.nche.edu/aacn-publications/white-papers/DNP-Implementation-TF-Report-8-15.pdf

Ash, L., & Miller, C. (2016). Interprofessional collaboration for improving patient and population health. In S. M. DeNisco & A. M. Barker (Eds.), *Advanced Practice Nursing* (3rd ed., pp. 123–147). Burlington, MA: Jones & Bartlett Learning.

Clinton, P., & Sperhac, A. M. (2009). The DNP and unintended consequences: An opportunity for dialogue. *Journal of Pediatric Health, 23*(5), 348–351. doi:10.1016/j.pedhc.2009.06.004

Collaborate. (2015). *Merriam-Webster's Online Dictionary.* Retrieved from http://www.merriam-webster.com/dictionary/collaborate

Conrad, D., Hanson, P. A., Hasenau, S. M., & Stocker-Schneider, J. (2012). Identifying the barriers to use of standardized nursing language in the electronic health record by the ambulatory care nurse practitioner. *Journal of the American Academy of Nurse Practitioners, 24*(7), 443–451. doi:10.1111/j.1745-7599.2012.00705x

Cronenwett, L., Dracup, K., Grey, M., McCauley, L., Melies, A., & Salmon, M. (2011). The doctor of nursing practice: A national workforce perspective. *Nursing Outlook, 59*, 9–17. doi:10.1016/j.outlook.2010.11.003

D'Amour, D., & Oandasan, I. (2005). Interprofessionality as the field of interprofessional practice and interprofessional education: An emerging concept. *Journal of Interprofessional Care, 19*(Suppl 1), 8–20.

Draye, M. A., Acker, M., & Zimmer, P. A. (2006). The practice doctorate in nursing: Approaches to transform nurse practitioner education and practice. *Nursing Outlook, 54*(3), 123–129.

Elsevier CPM Resource Center. (2012). Retrieved from http://www.cpmrc.com/company/overview/

Institute of Medicine. (2001). *Crossing the quality chasm: A new health system for the 21st century.* Retrieved from http://www.iom.edu/-/media/Files/Report%20 Files/2001/Crossing-the-Quality-Chasm/Quality%20Chasm%202001%20%20 report%20brief.pdf

Institute of Medicine. (2003). *Health professions education: A bridge to quality.* Retrieved from http://www.nap.edu/openbook.php?record_id=10681&page=45

Institute of Medicine. (2010). *The future of nursing: Leading change, advancing health.* Washington, DC: National Academies Press.

Interprofessional Education Collaborative. (2011). *Core competencies for interprofessional collaborative practice.* Retrieved from http://www.aacn.nche.edu/education-resources/ ipecreport.pdf

Kotter, J. P. (1996). *Leading change.* Boston, MA: Harvard Business School Press.

Lait, J., Suter, E., Arthur, N., & Deutschlander, S. (2011). Interprofessional mentoring: Enhancing students' clinical learning. *Nurse Education in Practice, 11*, 211–215. doi:10.1016/j.nepr.2010.10.005

National Center for Healthcare Leadership. (2010). *National Center for Healthcare Leadership competency model summary.* Retrieved from http://www.nchl.org/Documents/ NavLink/Competency_Model-summary_uid31020101024281.pdf

Reeves, S., Perrier, L., Goldman, J., Freeth, D., & Zwarenstein, M. (2013). Interprofessional education: Effects on professional practice and healthcare outcomes (update). *Cochrane Database of Systematic Reviews,* CD002213. doi: 10.1002/14651858. CD002213.pub3

Robert Wood Johnson Foundation. (2015). Lessons from the field: Promising interprofessional collaboration practices. Retrieved from http://www.rwjf.org/en/library/ research/2015/03/lessons-from-the-field.html

Tuckman, B. W., & Jensen, M. A. C. (1977). Stages of small-group development revisited. *Group & Organizational Management, 2*(4), 410–427. doi:10.1177/10596011 7700200404

Wagner, J., Liston, B., & Miller, J. (2011). Developing interprofessional communication skills. *Teaching and Learning in Nursing, 6,* 97–101. doi:10.1016/j.teln.2010.12.003

Wesorick, B. (2002). 21st Century leadership challenge: Creating and sustaining healthy healing work cultures and integrated service at the point of care. *Nursing Administration Quarterly, 26*(5), 18–32.

Wesorick, B., & Doebbeling, B. (2011). Lessons from the field: The essential elements for point-of-care transformation. *Medical Care, 49*(12, Suppl 1), S49–S58.

Wirth, R. A. (2004). *Lewin/Schein's change theory.* Retrieved from http://www.entarga .com/orgchange/lewinschein.pdf

CHAPTER 8

The DNP Project Team

Marisa L. Wilson, Shannon Reedy Idzik, and Dianne Conrad

CHAPTER OVERVIEW

Many doctor of nursing practice (DNP) programs require faculty members and other disciplinary experts to serve on a project team to guide the student through the DNP project process. According to the American Association of Colleges of Nursing (2015a), the project team should consist of a DNP student or group of DNP students with a minimum of a doctorally prepared faculty member (project faculty mentor) and a practice mentor. The project faculty mentor, along with the project team, will oversee the project, ensuring that the topic, processes, and timelines stay within school policy and procedure and that the final product is at an acceptable level of rigor for the degree and the program. This chapter outlines the purpose, roles, and function of the DNP project team. The DNP student's role in refining the leadership competencies and collaborating with members within and outside the nursing profession, beginning with the DNP project team members, is discussed. Finally, alternatives to the traditional academic committee structure are presented as outlined in the DNP Task Force recommendations (AACN, 2015a) to provide efficient use of resources and support student learning.

CHAPTER OBJECTIVES

After completing the chapter, the learner will be able to:
1. Discern the differences between a DNP project and a dissertation or thesis
2. Explore the role of the DNP project team and project faculty mentor in the project completion process
3. Formulate plans for project team and project faculty mentor interactions and management

THESIS, DISSERTATION, AND THE DNP PROJECT

A graduate student demonstrates mastery of the core essentials of a program of study in a variety of ways. Presentation, scholarly writing, and article development are just a few. The thesis, dissertation, and DNP project are usually culminating demonstrations of knowledge, competencies, and skills attained through a program of study. Some DNP students may be familiar with a master's thesis, having completed one during a previous program of study. DNP students are also usually familiar with doctoral dissertations because they probably see the rigorous process their PhD peers undergo as they pursue completion of this work. DNP students also face demonstrating proficiency and integration of required competencies in the completion of a rigorous scholarly project. Both the student and the academicians guiding these graduate students can find themselves having difficulty with differentiation between these products. What are the purposes of and differences between the thesis, dissertation, and DNP project? The detailed answers will lie in the individual university student handbook, and students are encouraged to review and discuss that information with their project faculty mentor or advisor. However, there are some basic purposes and differences.

In the context of academic studies, the definition of *thesis* and *dissertation* is a written, formal document that supports the student's candidacy for a degree. The *thesis* may be the term used for this product at the master's level in some universities, whereas the term *dissertation* often refers to a written document produced in the framework of doctoral studies, advancing a new point of view resulting from research (Thesistown.com, 2012). The Doctor of Nursing Practice *scholarly project* is the deliverable that demonstrates the student's achievement of the eight

DNP *Essentials* of Doctoral Education for advanced nursing practice,
as outlined by the American Association of Colleges of Nursing. The
final DNP project should demon-

> The products of a program of study
> move the frontiers of knowledge
> and answer a contestable question.

strate "synthesis of the student's work" and lay the groundwork for future scholarship (2006, p. 20). The common theme is that the main purpose of the thesis,
dissertation, and DNP project is to serve as a tangible demonstration of skills and
competencies that integrates each through a culminating experience.

The competencies to be demonstrated in the final work are different between
the nursing practice doctorate and the research doctorate. Gardenier and Stanik-
Hutt (2010) state that

> DNP programs prepare nurses to transform health care through leadership
> and evidence-based practice within a transdisciplinary environment. To
> accomplish this, students need to be able to evaluate and apply available
> evidence, fully use clinical information systems, analyze and influence health
> policy, and lead interdisciplinary teams—all with the goal of improving
> care quality in the broader healthcare system. In contrast, research doctoral
> programs are designed to prepare nurse scientists to expand nursing
> knowledge through independent research. These students need advanced
> preparation in theory construction, qualitative and quantitative research
> methodology, sampling, measurement, and an in-depth understanding of
> descriptive and inferential statistics (p. 364).

Therefore, the purpose and content of a product to demonstrate the competencies of a research versus a practice doctorate can be different but equally
rigorous.

The thesis, dissertation, and DNP project are also used as a means for faculty
to judge whether a student has mastered a body of knowledge. Each is meant to
provide novel intellectual contributions to a field. Each of these products of a
program of study moves the frontiers of knowledge further and answers a con-
testable question.

A major difference between a thesis, a dissertation, and a DNP project in some
cases lies in the method of inquiry. In a thesis or dissertation, graduate students propose a research study in which data are collected, analyzed, and reported in the final
product. With a dissertation, one is engaged in original research work, whereas a
thesis can require an analysis of secondary information (perhaps faculty provided).
The dissertation is based on the student's own background research about a topic,

whereas a thesis provides arguments to defend a standpoint or hypothesis. The thesis or dissertation will often have a broader scope than a DNP project. The DNP project may have a more narrow area or topic because of its practice and translation nature. The thesis and dissertation are also solo activities, whereas the DNP project may be accomplished in a group. See Chapter 4, Scholarship in Practice, for an in-depth discussion of what qualifies as a scholarly project.

The DNP project starts with a thorough literature review that addresses a problem or issue. This literature synthesis is followed by a discussion describing the unique contribution that the student intends to make in addressing the problem or issue in his or her professional endeavors. The student then describes a translational process meant to address the problem or issue (the project plan), implements the plan, and follows this with an evaluation of the implementation and a plan for disseminating the findings. See Chapter 9, Creating and Developing the Project Plan. Often the scholarly project includes specific recommendations or offers materials that can be used in implementing the proposed method of addressing the problem or issue. The average length of time required to complete the DNP project will vary, but it may take a year or longer to complete. However, the DNP student must note that some universities require the scholarly project to be completed in a prescribed number of semesters. The DNP student should carefully ascertain his or her university's requirements for scholarly project completion.

CHOOSING THE DNP PROJECT FACULTY MENTOR AND PROJECT TEAM MEMBERS

It is important that any doctoral student be mentored through this rigorous process by experienced faculty. For some students, this mentoring will be formalized through a committee structure and process that may be regulated by the school of nursing or the graduate school, depending on which school awards the degree. Not all schools use a committee structure, and the student will be guided by the individual policies of the institution. However, for those that do, the size, requirements, and constituency of this committee are outlined in the doctoral student handbook and will vary slightly from one school or university to another. According to AACN (2015a), "the DNP Project team should consist of a student or a group of students with a minimum of a doctoral prepared faculty member and a practice mentor who may be from outside the university" (p. 5). Often the practice mentor is from the organization where the project will be implemented, to provide organizational context to the project.

Forming a cohesive and collegial team whose members will work together, however, is vital to the success of the student. The first step is selecting the appropriate DNP project faculty mentor, who, as mentioned, should be a doctorally prepared member of the graduate faculty of the school of nursing. The student should consult the DNP project guidelines for all requirements related to timing and selection criteria for the project faculty mentor and project team members. However, one of the first considerations, aside from the expertise of the faculty mentor, is that the student and the faculty mentor should have mutual respect for one another and should have positive regard toward each other (Magnan, 2016). Magnan indicated that the faculty member fulfilling this role must possess an interest in the topic; theoretical, methodological, or content expertise; and the wherewithal to get the student through the final project on time (p. 132).

The next step is for the student and the project faculty mentor to determine the skills and expertise needed within the project team to complete the DNP project and ensure success. The specific talents that will be needed are directly determined by the nature of the student's proposed work. Some questions to consider are:

1. Will this work be done in a specific organization?
2. Will a specific population be affected by the project?
3. Will the student need to implement certain tools, technologies, or guidelines?
4. Will there be a methodological or analytical process that requires certain expertise?

The student will want a well-rounded team whose members have complementary areas of expertise. Choosing team members carefully will ensure that the student has the depth of knowledge available for a successful completion. The project faculty mentor and the student should also be familiar with the school policies regarding faculty affiliation when choosing members.

> Forming a cohesive and collegial project team whose members will work together is vital to the success of the student.

Often schools will impose a maximum number of team members whose primary affiliation is outside the school or university. Other schools may require a member of the organization where the project will be implemented to be part of the project team to assist the student in navigating the facilitators/barriers of project implementation.

"How does one find project team members?" a doctoral student may ask. Many schools have a list of faculty and their stated areas of expertise available for students to review. The doctoral student should review this list and then do some further investigation by looking at publications, presentations, and the teaching expertise of the potential team members. When inviting new team members, it is important for students to take a professional approach. The invitation should be a formal email or letter introducing themselves, describing their proposed project, and identifying other members serving on the project team. The request should include how the potential project team member's expertise would benefit the team.

ROLES AND EXPECTATIONS OF PROJECT TEAM MEMBERS

The role of the project faculty mentor is to act primarily as the scholarly advisor to the student. The project faculty mentor must be prepared to evaluate the process and progress of the project. In addition, the project faculty mentor is usually responsible for evaluation of all written work, ensuring that the project and process come to completion in a timely manner. The project faculty mentor must also be a member of the school's graduate faculty. The specific university expectations of the project team are often described in the doctoral student handbook.

The project team members, on the other hand, have the primary roles of lending their expertise to help develop the ideas, to direct specific aspects of the work, to serve as mentors through the DNP process, and to evaluate the project as a whole. The DNP project team members will be responsible for helping to craft and approve the project, for participating in the completion of a defense or comprehensive examination testing overall student knowledge of the domain, and for approving the final product. Because the DNP student is pursuing a practice doctorate, one member of the team should serve as a practice mentor who will guide and advise the student through the DNP project process at a particular site. As mentioned, the practice mentor should be from within the organization where the project will be implemented, giving the student access to organizational leaders with whom he or she might not otherwise engage in the translation process.

In addition, when putting together the project team, it is important that the student and the project faculty mentor look outside the discipline of nursing. Creating an interprofessional committee with representation from medicine, business, public health, law, the allied health sciences, and research can help to shape a very rich scholarly project. This interprofessional team has the potential to influence other members of the healthcare team and can assist the DNP student in developing leadership skills and competencies as outlined in Essential VI. Chapter 7, Interprofessional and Intraprofessional Collaboration in the Scholarly Project, provides additional information and guidance in forming quality interprofessional and intraprofessional collaborations that can be manifested through the DNP project.

An important role in the project team is that of the student. This is not a passive role. In many universities, it is expected that the student will take an active role in selecting a project faculty mentor (i.e., based on expertise, in vetting team members, and in managing the team activities). However, in some universities, the project faculty mentor is assigned by the college of nursing. Therefore, it is important for the DNP student to check with the DNP handbook or advisor before seeking a DNP project faculty mentor. The DNP student must use communication and leadership skills to keep all activities moving toward completion of the final scholarly project. Moreover, it is the responsibility of the student to stay in close contact with the project faculty mentor to apprise him or her of progress.

DEFINING THE TIMELINE FOR THE DNP PROJECT

A very important role of the project faculty mentor and the project team is to assist the DNP student in developing a project that can be completed within the time frames outlined by the school or university. It is not uncommon for doctoral students to propose a grandiose project that would take much longer than time permits. Team members and the project faculty mentor often must help the student to narrow the focus to meet a reasonable time frame while maintaining a level of rigor and scholarly outcome.

> The project team members and the project faculty mentor must help the student to narrow the focus of the project to meet a reasonable time frame while maintaining a level of rigor and scholarly outcome.

The student and the project faculty mentor must be aware of any constraints placed on the timeline by the plan of study, and together they must formulate a schedule to meet those targets. See Chapter 12, The Scholarly Project Toolbox, for scheduling tools such as the project timeline. Meetings should be set up in advance between the student and the project faculty mentor, and subsequently between the project faculty mentor and other team members, at regular intervals so that adequate control and appraisal of progress may be maintained. Doctoral students must be aware that most project faculty mentors and team members will require 2 weeks or longer to review work and provide feedback, so the student must build this time into the plan.

ENHANCING TEAM PRODUCTIVITY

Leadership skills, including the ability to facilitate effective and productive meetings, are an essential attribute of DNP graduates. Learning meeting productivity and facilitation skills starts during the educational process. Doctoral students should prepare for and lead their own project team meetings as a demonstration of this competency. In many ways, doctoral project team meetings are no different from most other meetings. Sometimes early in this process, doctoral students feel that they are being shuttled back and forth by the opinions and experiences of the project faculty mentor and the project team members. As doctoral students become confident in their skills and knowledge, it is incumbent on them to step up and lead their project with the project faculty mentor and project team members providing guidance.

> Leadership skills, including the ability to facilitate effective and productive meetings, are an essential attribute of DNP graduates.

Preparation is essential. Key components in preparing for a project team meeting are meeting necessity, purpose, and outcomes; inviting the right people; agenda; logistics, including room and equipment; and proper lead time.

The first step in preparation is determining whether a meeting is actually necessary. Meetings should not just be automatic events. What are the purpose and outcome of the project team meeting? If the meeting is only scheduled to share information, could an email suffice? Meetings may need to be held at various times throughout the DNP project. Meetings held during the formative stages of the project and those held during summative stages may have very different purposes and outcomes. For example, a formative meeting may be necessary to discuss a major change in the student's implementation plan. However, a summative meeting may be held for the student to present the final proposal of his or her implementation plan for approval. As the number of doctoral students increases, the toll on faculty workload will become evident. Not all meetings require all members to be present, and it is important to invite only relevant members. Initial meetings may include only the student and the project faculty mentor, whereas meetings in which project approval is needed may require all members.

Keep in mind that there are alternative technologies available that allow for team members to attend by conference call or virtual meeting computer applications, when necessary. There may also be times when ad hoc members are needed for problem solving, or the student may be working directly with one team member who possesses expertise that is needed for a certain section.

Key Components of a Project Team Meeting

- Meeting necessity, purpose, and outcomes
- Inviting the right people
- Agenda
- Logistics
- Proper lead time

Once it has been determined that a meeting is needed, a purpose and outcome have been identified, and participants have been selected, an agenda should be created. The agenda should be detailed and include the outcome expected for each topic, the person responsible for each topic, and the amount of time allotted to each. See Chapter 12 for tools such as a meeting agenda template. The agenda should be distributed in advance of the meeting to allow the participants to prepare. The project faculty mentor and the student should be familiar with the school policies on reserving rooms and equipment. Although this is a seemingly simple step, being caught without a room or proper equipment can be disastrous for a meeting.

Facilitating a meeting is a learned skill and can be difficult even for expert leaders. Early in the project, the project faculty mentor may need to assist the DNP student. Janice Francisco (2007), a change facilitator, suggested four steps to facilitating a meeting:

1. Get everyone on the same page.
2. Strike a balance between creative and critical thinking to productively support discussion and decisions.
3. Document the meeting and its accomplishments by capturing meeting minutes and actions.
4. Evaluate the effectiveness of the meeting.

A formal approach to meetings sets the stage for an effective meeting. All meetings should start with ground rules for how the meeting will be conducted.

A brief introduction of new members and the role of each and a review of the agenda should follow.

Project team members are often chosen because of their diversity and variety of expertise. Although this leads to an improved product, conflict can result from differences. The best way to resolve conflict within the committee is to prevent it (Mind Tools Limited, 2015), and the best way to prevent conflict is to be prepared for the meeting and reduce the opportunity for conflict. Spotting potential conflicts early and managing them can prevent them from becoming problematic. If a conflict does arise, conflict management skills are essential. Depersonalizing, questioning, removing/reducing the perceived threat, and taking issues offline are all conflict management skills to use. Depersonalizing involves making the conflict about the issue rather than about the person raising the issue. Questioning involves asking the members with the conflict for specific details about the concern and suggestions for resolution. Conflict in meetings can arise when a member perceives a threat to his or her reputation or success. For example, if a team member disagrees with the path that the project faculty mentor has recommended for the student, the project faculty mentor may feel that his or her reputation is being threatened. Removing/reducing the perceived threat by supplying the correct information or clearing up unknowns may help to resolve the conflict. The DNP student must realize that it is the duty of the project faculty mentor to manage these high-level conflicts with team members, and the project faculty mentor may need to have a one-on-one discussion with the team member or replace a team member who is blocking progress. This can be a difficult discussion, particularly for a doctoral student. It is very important for the student to have a mentor as a member of the project team who can guide him or her through this process. It may be difficult for the doctoral student to take an active role in negotiating disagreements to consensus, but it is necessary. This process prepares students for their eventual responsibilities as a doctorally prepared nurse, which will require them to be tactful but direct with those they may view as having more experience or authority. However, most team interactions are productive in moving the student toward the goal of completing the project. See Chapter 10, Driving the Practicum to Impact the Scholarly Project, for a discussion of the importance of developing the emotional competence that enables a leader to manage the relationships between individuals and groups.

Once the meeting is over, the real work often begins. The most important component of a meeting is the follow-up and follow-through. All members who attended the meeting should understand the action plan at the end of the meeting. Additionally, meeting minutes and action items should be sent out right away to the appropriate people. See Chapter 12 for tools to help in managing and communicating your project, as well as Chapter 9, Creating and Developing the Project Plan. If possible, the action plan items should be addressed before the next meeting to ensure timely progression of the scholarly project.

ALTERNATIVE APPROACHES TO A TRADITIONAL COMMITTEE FOR PROJECT SUPERVISION

Many schools began DNP programs as post-master's programs and implemented committee structures similar to the traditional PhD programs. Although that structure is the standard for traditional PhD programs, the structure for DNP programs is evolving. For example, some schools have implemented alternatives to the committee structure. As the number of students in DNP programs grows exponentially and faculty resources to supervise projects become stretched, it will become necessary for schools to investigate and implement alternative structures. Recognizing this mounting concern, the Implementation of the DNP Task Force (AACN, 2015a) has recommended that the traditional committee designations and structures be replaced with the concept of the DNP project team to minimize confusion between the PhD dissertation committee and the faculty and mentors who oversee the final DNP project.

Managing the practice doctoral student versus the research doctoral student presents several challenges. The sheer number of students seeking practice doctorates is challenging. Over three times as many students are enrolled in DNP programs (18,352) as are enrolled in PhD programs (5,290) (AACN, 2015b). In addition, research can often be done without community partnerships. For example, PhD students have opportunities to do bench research or secondary data analyses within the confines of the school. Most DNP practice projects require community partners. Finding and forging these relationships can be a challenge for some practice doctoral students, although many DNP students may have practice connections that will overcome these difficulties. Another challenge is that DNP students are more likely to be practicing full-time and are less likely to be full-time students. In many schools, the admission criteria are less likely to require that the student be matched exactly with a faculty member's area of scholarship. This is an advantage for the admission process but has led to DNP cohorts with diverse practice interests that are more difficult to match to the skills of the current faculty.

Membership also varies between DNP project teams and PhD committees. PhD committees almost always require the expertise of a statistician. Although some DNP projects require statisticians, it is less likely that they will be formal members of the DNP project team. If needed, a statistician may be an ad hoc member or a consultant. However, it is important to have current practice experts on DNP project teams, which may not be necessary on PhD committees. Because many DNP projects involve community partners, it is often necessary to have members outside the school of nursing on DNP project teams.

Alternative approaches to the traditional committee structure are becoming more prevalent. The committee structure may vary depending on school project requirements. One variation from the traditional approach is to assign each student (or a team of students) to a single project advisor and develop one overseeing project team to review all proposed and completed projects. This scholarly project process is being used particularly in schools where students progress from a bachelor of science in nursing (BSN) to DNP. It is not uncommon to see students working on projects in teams in these programs. Because the sheer number of DNP students in a post-BSN-to-DNP program and their relative lack of clinical experience as they approach the scholarly project can quickly create a faculty workload issue, new ways of managing the process are being tested.

> Alternative approaches to traditional committee structure are evolving.

Another alternative approach in well-established programs is using a faculty member as the primary advisor and DNP alumni as project team members and community partners. The various approaches to creating project teams to guide the student through the DNP project have pros and cons. The traditional approach of assembling a chair and several members provides a team with a strong understanding of the student's project, but the faculty workload for this type of structure is significant. Because of the amount of interaction with team members and the significance of their input, students can sometimes be pulled in many directions. Having a sole advisor and then having the project go out to a project review team decreases the faculty workload but decreases the amount of input from experts in the student's project. Having only one faculty member responsible up to the point of proposal could result in wide variability in projects as well as the student needing to make significant revisions once the project is reviewed by the project team. Using DNP alumni as part of the project team structure is a promising avenue because DNP alumni are often excited to share their knowledge and practice expertise. This method again decreases the number of faculty on project teams but may increase the amount of work for the project faculty mentor because the alumni may need to be coached along the process.

Brown and Crabtree (2011) have proposed a seminar course series approach for group mentoring of DNP projects. This approach has eased faculty workload connected to the increasing numbers of DNP students and project team responsibilities. Core DNP courses are the prerequisites to the seminar course series. One faculty member is responsible for the same cohort of DNP students for an academic year. The faculty member establishes an ongoing relationship with the students working in groups on projects on a similar topic. It is important that the cohort be a manageable size, usually fewer than 10 students. The goals of the seminar course series are to develop, implement, and evaluate the DNP project in a group format in a quality, cost-effective way. This is an innovative approach to addressing the concern expressed regarding faculty workload and the length of time required to complete the DNP project. As mentioned in Chapter 3, Defining the Doctor of Nursing Practice: Current Trends, the Implementation of the DNP Task Force recommendations (AACN, 2015a) related to designing DNP programs with attention to program efficiency include the following:

- Consider new models and processes for implementing DNP project teams that provide efficient use of resources and support student learning.
- Adopt a process that allows for oversight and evaluation of DNP projects that ensures quality and equity of resources.
- Provide faculty development to ensure quality student learning outcomes to include:
  - Curricular design of DNP programs
  - Development of new, innovative teaching strategies
  - Development of innovative, new practice opportunities to support achievement of the DNP *Essentials* learning outcomes
  - Strategies to support and evaluate the DNP project
  - Implementation of quality improvement processes
  - Interprofessional education and practice experiences

CREDITING THE PROJECT TEAM

After completion of the project, the deliverables for communicating the results may include scholarly project submissions to the university, a manuscript submitted for publication, public presentations of the result of projects, or practice portfolios. See Chapter 15, Disseminating the Results. Because the committee has provided substantial guidance regarding process and content for the DNP project, crediting the project faculty mentor and/or project team members in the publications and presentations is a way to recognize their contributions.

The DNP student should seek guidance from his or her doctoral student handbook and/or the project faculty mentor for the university's policy or usual procedure on crediting the project team and other acknowledgments of significant contributors to the DNP project when communicating results.

SUMMARY

Schools and universities operationalize their DNP project oversight teams in various ways. Many schools began by modeling the traditional PhD dissertation committee structure of one chair and committee for each doctoral student but are finding that they have to develop new ways to manage clinically based scholarly projects because of different complex clinical issues, student demand, and faculty workload. The prudent DNP student should investigate the practice doctorate requirements at the beginning of the program of study or while making decisions about programs.

The DNP student must also be aware of and familiar with policies, directions, and procedures that guide and impact the doctoral student in his or her school or university. The DNP student handbook for each school must be reviewed frequently and followed to ensure successful completion of the DNP project. All DNP students (or team of students) should understand that they will be guided in their scholarly project work by more experienced faculty and clinical mentors. Their purpose is not to do the work for the student or to impede progress, but to ensure that the product and demonstrations of work of the DNP student truly represent the synthesis of all required competencies and that the student is prepared to confidently and capably move forward to doctoral-level scholarly practice after completion.

The following excerpt by Dr. Katie Alfredson highlights the value of the DNP project team and the impact on the overall project quality.

My Experience with the DNP Project Team
Katie Alfredson, DNP, RN

Throughout my DNP project, the support and contributions of my committee members were vital to its success. My project examined the structures and processes used at a private, primary care practice identified as a Patient-Centered Medical Home (PCMH) that enabled successful outcomes, particularly the success realized in the Meaningful Use Incentive Program. This practice had successfully attested for Meaningful Use Stage 2 during the first quarter of 2014 while the rest of the nation continues to struggle to meet Stage 2 requirements. I wanted to know what enabled this practice to be so successful in this program so I could recommend a framework for others to replicate and potentially experience similar benefits.

As my project developed, it was clear the nursing staff, as members of the interdisciplinary team, played a pertinent role in conducting the processes that were required to meet the Meaningful Use objectives. I struggled, however, in determining how their essential roles could be quantified. This is where my committee proved to be invaluable.

I originally thought I could quantify the value of nurses in the primary care setting by, literally, timing their productivity as they completed tasks requiring the nursing skillset versus the skill set of a medical assistant or other unlicensed personnel. I thought I would then quantify the reimbursement realized as a result of these tasks and determine the return on investment for incorporating nurses in the primary care setting. This turned out to be a laborious and impossible feat.

Upon this realization, I consulted with my committee, which was composed of a DNP-prepared nurse practitioner, a physician, a business doctorate, and a PhD-prepared nurse. It was because of breakthrough conversations with these committee members that I realized one component of the interdisciplinary team could not be separated from the rest. Each team member was needed for the others to be successful. Placing a price-tag value on an individual team member was not possible or desirable as it breaks down the system to a non-beneficial level.

Project development and evolution occurred as a result of conversations with committee members. These conversations led to the success of the final project. Once I realized that the project could not be broken down to the individual team member level, I changed the project methodology and began tracing processes that were vital to Meaningful Use Stage 2 attainment. Contributions from various members of the interdisciplinary team were identified as they were required for each process. In doing so, processes enabling the success of the practice in the Meaningful Use program were described and a case was made for the inclusion of key team members used for the completion of these processes.

Collaborating with committee members not only helped guide the direction of my project but also provided me with a broader understanding of what is needed to conduct a successful project. It was through this collaboration that I developed an understanding regarding the fluidity of a project. A project cannot be approached with a concrete plan. There must be flexibility to adapt and alter original plans and perspectives.

I also came to the first-hand realization that so much more can be accomplished through the use of an interdisciplinary project team. Each committee member brought their unique experience and background to the table. This created an environment rich in creativity for project development. My project ended up being so much more than it ever could have been if I had completed it independently or from the perspective of a single discipline. Collaboration with committee members enriched the entire experience.

Key Messages

- The DNP project differs from a master's thesis and PhD dissertation in scope as well as method of inquiry and has a practice focus. The final product should reflect the mastery of the practice doctorate competencies within a rigorous and scholarly process.
- Forming a cohesive and collegial team whose members will work together is vital to the success of the student.

- The project faculty mentor and project team members guide the DNP student during the scholarly project and provide expertise needed to help develop the ideas, to direct specific aspects of the work, to serve as mentors through the DNP process, and to evaluate the project as a whole.
- Leadership skills, including the ability to facilitate effective and productive meetings, are an essential attribute of DNP graduates.
- As DNP programs mature, alternative approaches to the traditional committee structure for project supervision are evolving.
- DNP students must familiarize themselves with their institution's DNP student handbook to ensure that they understand the particulars about the project team structure, function, and timing; this will greatly impact successful completion.

Action Plan—Next Steps

1. Review your university's requirements for the DNP project team, if any, including composition requirements (i.e., for the project faculty mentor and other team members).
2. Check the timeline for completion of the DNP project according to university policies.
3. Choose the project faculty mentor and other team members who will provide the expertise, guidance, and mentoring needed to complete the project (if part of the process in your program).
4. Practice the leadership skills required of doctoral students in working with the project team members and other collaborators during the DNP project.
5. Make sure all interactions between you and the oversight committee are executed in an efficient and effective way; be prepared.

REFERENCES

American Association of Colleges of Nursing. (2006). *The essentials of doctoral education for advanced nursing practice.* Retrieved from http://www.aacn.nche.edu/DNP/pdf/Essentials.pdf

American Association of Colleges of Nursing. (2015a). The doctor of nursing practice: Current issues and clarifying recommendations. Retrieved from http://www.aacn.nche.edu/aacn-publications/white-papers/DNP-Implementation-TF-Report-8-15.pdf

American Association of Colleges of Nursing. (2015b). *Custom report on doctoral program enrollments, 1997–2014.* Washington, DC: AACN Research and Data Services.

Brown, M. A., & Crabtree, K. (2011, November 15). *Maturational issues in DNP practice inquiry/improvement projects* [Webinar]. National Organization of Nurse Practitioner Faculties. Retrieved from http://www.nonpf.org/displaycommon .cfm?an=1&subarticlenbr=64

Francisco, J. (2007, November–December). How to create and facilitate meetings that matter: Learn how to plan and run a successful meeting using crucial checklists. *Information Management Journal, 54–58.*

Gardenier, D., & Stanik-Hutt, J. (2010). Should DNP students conduct original research as their capstone projects? *The Journal for Nurse Practitioners, 6*(5), 364–365.

Magnan, M. A. (2016). The DNP: Expectations for theory, research, and scholarship. In L. A. Chism (Ed.), *The doctor of nursing practice: A guidebook for role development and professional issues* (pp. 117–148). Sudbury, MA: Jones and Bartlett.

Mind Tools Limited. (2015). *Mind tools: Essential skills for an excellent career* (6th ed.). Retrieved from http://www.mindtools.com

Thesistown.com. (2012). *What is the definition of thesis?* Retrieved from http:// thesistown.com/writing/basics/definition-of-thesis/

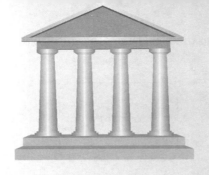

CHAPTER 9

Creating and Developing the Project Plan

Rosanne Burson and Katherine Moran

CHAPTER OVERVIEW

It is important for the doctor of nursing practice (DNP) student to have an appreciation of doctoral work, which is not linear but rather more circular or spiral in nature. Much of the cognitive work that occurs as the student explores an area of interest will be reworked through the process of developing the DNP project. The phenomenon will continue to be ruminated on, the proposal will develop, literature will continue to be reviewed, and the methodology for the design will develop.

If one considers the DNP project development process holistically, it is very similar to the nursing process—assess, diagnose/determine the problem, plan how to manage the problem and measure the outcomes, implement the plan, then evaluate (see **Figure 9-1**). All DNP projects should have a planning, implementation, and evaluation phase (AACN, 2015). The DNP student will select a phenomenon of interest, identify a problem or opportunity for improvement, develop a clinical question, develop a project plan, implement the plan, monitor the implementation to ensure that the process is working as intended, and then evaluate the outcome to determine if the goal has been met. Indeed, the DNP project is the ultimate nursing *practice* activity because it utilizes the nursing process at the doctoral level.

> The DNP project is the ultimate nursing practice activity because it uses the nursing process at the doctoral level.

189

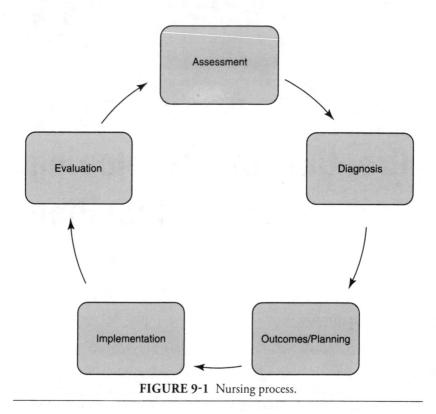

FIGURE 9-1 Nursing process.

The DNP project plan is a formal document used to plan and design the scholarly project in preparation for implementation. Successful project implementation depends on a carefully considered plan, with attention to detail. This process is just as important as planning the initial proposal, because if significant problems occur during implementation, it can lead to unsuccessful outcomes. The intent of this chapter is to present a broad overview of points to consider in creating an innovative project and developing a plan to successfully prepare for project implementation.

CHAPTER OBJECTIVES

After completing the chapter, the learner will be able to:

1. Create alternate strategies for potential innovation implementation
2. Choose a best solution based on a cost-benefit analysis

3. Develop an understanding of the various components of a project plan for use in planning project implementation

4. Analyze which components may be helpful for the individual project

5. Consider aspects of the institutional review board (IRB) approval process that will impact the timeline of the project

CREATION OF INNOVATION

Once the phenomenon of interest has evolved, the student will have a deep understanding of the topic of interest. The literature review will build on the understanding of the phenomenon, which leads to new ideas and innovations that could improve care or make a contribution to nursing. As mentioned in Chapter 6, Developing the Scholarly Project, it will be important to commit to a general concept that will continue to evolve and mature as the student encounters additional coursework and applies new knowledge to the understanding of the phenomenon. Through this process, the student will also develop new skills that can be applied to the development of a project.

Within each phase of the project development process, the DNP is able to use more concepts to expand the process to incorporate health systems and populations of patients. For instance, in the *assessment* phase, the DNP student explored the information at hand. Factors included in this phase are the necessity that goals and outcomes of the project are aligned with the organization's strategic plan, development of project specifications, financial analysis, and the identification of the team that will be able to move the project forward (Waxman, 2013). An assessment was critical and helped define the issues that will now guide decisions in the project planning phase (see Chapter 6). Tools to help the student with the assessment phase can be found in Chapter 12, The Scholarly Project Toolbox.

The *diagnosis* phase of the nursing process translates to the development of a problem statement based on all the information that was pulled together when the student identified the issues surrounding the problem. Here is where framing the problem occurs. In Chapter 6, the DNP student chose the appropriate data that highlighted the specific issues surrounding the problem and presented this information in a problem statement.

Table 9-1 Developing Project Innovations

Phase	Tools
Assessment	SWOT analysis
	Force field analysis
	Community analysis
	Needs assessment
	Organizational data
Diagnosis	Framing the problem
	Problem statement
Planning	Potential alternative solutions
	Cost-benefit comparisons
	Identify optimal solution
	Plan for implementation (project plan)
	Metric/outcome development
Implementation	Project plan in process
Evaluation	Metrics
	Satisfaction (patient/staff/provider)
	Clinical outcomes
	Cost outcomes
	Other measures

The *planning* phase includes the determination of potential alternative solutions with pros and cons. The student must describe how each solution will address the identified need and consider the feasibility and impact potential of each solution. Creative thinking and innovative ideas are a part of this phase.

Identify the optimal solutions based on analysis of the costs and benefits; then follow through with the decisions and begin developing a project plan. Remember, part of the planning phase will also include planning for *implementation*—developing the project plan and determining outcome measures and metrics for the project.

Evaluation incorporates the measurement of all metrics/identified outcomes. **Table 9-1** identifies the various components in each phase. See Chapter 12, The Scholarly Project Toolbox, for a closer look at items that can assist in each phase.

THE DNP PROJECT PLAN

Once a basic project concept has developed, the focus moves to preparing for the specifics of the project. There is extensive environmental planning required

> The DNP student will need to select the most appropriate items to use for his or her project planning—*not every item is needed for every project.*

that includes identifying the setting, collaborating with a content expert, and interfacing with the DNP project team and/or faculty mentor. In addition, written work is required for developing the proposal, obtaining IRB approval (if needed), submitting a grant proposal to support the project (if applicable), and, finally, developing the scholarly project plan. The DNP student will need to select the most appropriate items to use for his or her project planning—*not every item is needed for every project.*

Identifying the Setting

As the project plan takes shape, identifying the setting is an important aspect that must be considered early in the plan development. Will this project be applied in the acute care, primary care, community, or another environment? The student will need to investigate options and secure a location to move forward in the project plan development process. For students who are interested in implementing their project in a setting outside their work environment, it is important to schedule extra time for the approval process. This is especially true in the corporate setting, where multiple levels of approval may be required.

Once the setting is secured, it is time to begin the development of the project plan. To help the student through this process, the following information is presented using an example of an actual project plan template in an annotated format. The student should keep in mind that this is just one of many project plan formats available. It is best to check with the DNP project team or project faculty mentor to determine the format used by the university prior to beginning the planning process. Although a multitude of topics are presented here, the DNP student will want to *choose* the aspects *specific* to his or her scholarly project.

When reading this section, note that each part of the plan includes section descriptions, and some sections point out additional documents that may be needed to complete the plan. See Chapter 12, The Scholarly Project Toolbox, for a project plan template. This plan is designed to address most project sizes; however, smaller projects may not require completion of the entire plan. What follows is the plan example.

(Project Name)

Project Plan

(Student Name)

(University)

(Date)

Table of Contents

1. Introduction
    1.1 Purpose of the Project Plan
2. Executive Summary
3. Project Goals and Objectives
4. Scope
5. Project Administration
    5.1 Structure
    5.2 Boundaries
    5.3 Roles and Responsibilities
6. Project Management
    6.1 Assumptions and Risks/Constraints
    6.2 Risk Management Plan
    6.3 Monitoring Plan
    6.4 Staffing Plan
    6.5 Communication Management Plan
7. Software and Hardware Requirements
    7.1 Security
8. Work Breakdown Structure
    8.1 Work Structure
    8.2 Relationships
    8.3 Resources
    8.4 Cost Management
    8.5 Schedule/Time Management
9. Quality Management
    9.1 Milestones
    9.2 Quality Indicators
10. Project Initiation Plan
11. Training Plan
12. Procurement Plan
13. Appendices

1. Introduction

1.1 Purpose of Project Plan

In this section, describe the purpose of the project. When a project charter is used to gain organizational approval for the project, the description of the purpose from the project charter can be used in this section. See Chapter 12, The Scholarly Project Toolbox, for a description of the project charter. It is helpful to identify the intended audience of the project in this section as well.

2. Executive Summary

This section is used to give a quick preview of the project plan. It is a high-level overview of the project that should include a brief description of the project scope, deliverables, required resources, scheduling requirements, budget, and any reference material necessary to fully understand the project. The goal is to grab the attention of readers by providing them with enough information to gain a reasonable understanding of the project but not bore them with the specific details. It is best to limit the summary to one page. Again, if the student already developed a project charter, include a reference to the approved project charter.

3. Project Goals and Objectives

In this section, describe the overall project goals, and then describe in detail the objectives that will be used to reach the goals. See

Chapter 6 for more information regarding the development of goals and objectives.

4. Scope

The project scope describes the breadth of the project—that is, what is relevant and what is not relevant to the project. As indicated in Chapter 6, it should include all the work that needs to be accomplished to successfully complete the project. Budgetary requirements and the time required to complete the work should be considered in the scope.

5. Project Administration

The project administration section is used to describe the overall project structure, how the project is organized in relation to team member responsibilities, and how the project interfaces with the organization and potentially other organizations—especially related to organizational boundaries.

5.1 Structure

An organizational chart can be used to describe the management structure of the project, including lines of authority (where applicable) and responsibility. See Appendix A.

5.2 Boundaries

When the project includes more than one organization or team, the boundaries of each are identified in this section. This helps everyone understand the organizational/team expectations right from the beginning.

5.3 Roles and Responsibilities

The roles and responsibilities of each team member are briefly described in this section.

6. Project Management

The management process section includes the project assumptions, risks/constraints, risk management plan, monitoring plan, and staffing and communication management plan.

6.1 Assumptions and Risks/Constraints

Assumptions

Project assumptions include those items that are assumed to be provided so that the project will move forward, for example, access to the setting, access to participants where applicable, use of equipment, etc.

Risks/Constraints

Project constraints include any event that could potentially have a negative impact on the project objectives, for example, lack of staff, subjects, or material resources.

6.2 Risk Management Plan

To successfully manage any potential project risks/constraints, a risk management plan should be developed. This section should describe the identification and potential impact of the risks and how they will be mitigated. The improvements made can be documented as lessons learned. If a project charter was developed, a reference to the project charter is appropriate. See Chapter 12 for an example of a risk assessment tool.

6.3 Monitoring Plan

The monitoring plan should include those tools that will be used for monitoring or tracking adherence to the project plan. This section should also include a description of how information will flow, how change will be approved and implemented (if warranted), and how progress is reported. See Chapter 12 for examples of project management tools.

6.4 Staffing Plan

In this section, indicate the total number of people who will be required to complete the project objectives; it is helpful to also include the schedule (see Chapter 12).

6.5 Communication Management Plan

The purpose of the communication plan is to describe how communication will occur during the project. This plan includes how and when information will be communicated (i.e., meetings, email, memorandums, etc.), who communicates the message (based on roles), and what is communicated. See examples of a communication plan, project agenda/minutes, status report, and issues log template in Chapter 12.

7. Software and Hardware Requirements

Describe any software and hardware requirements for the project. For example, describe the computer software system that will be used (if applicable), what it will be used for (e.g., documentation), and who will have access to the software. Any policy or procedure required to implement or utilize this software should be described in this section as well.

7.1 Security

Specify security requirements that will be needed to both support the project and access the specific software (where applicable). For example, perhaps only a few key team members will have access to all the software features, whereas others may have only limited access based on what is needed for their role.

8. Work Breakdown Structure

This section of the project plan will specify the work structure, identify the relationships among them, state the project resource requirements, provide a cost management plan, and establish a project schedule.

8.1 Work Structure

A description of the work breakdown structure (WBS) for all activities is required to complete this section. An example of a WBS is provided in Chapter 12.

8.2 Relationships

This section should describe the relationships between various aspects of the work needed to complete the project. It should include any dependencies or interdependencies among the various tasks, as well as any external dependencies or interdependencies.

8.3 Resources

A list of all the resources required to complete the project is included in this section. Included are all material resources, such as computers and computer software and hardware, training time, travel, and maintenance requirements.

8.4 Cost Management

In this section, clearly describe the project budget and how the project costs will be managed. The project budget should include specific information on the financing required to complete the project from start to finish. This section identifies the person responsible for the budget plan, discloses how changes are made to the budget and who has responsibility for those changes, describes how cost variances will be managed and who has responsibility for those variances, and discusses how and when costs will be reported. An example of a project budget is provided in Chapter 12.

8.5 Schedule/Time Management

This section describes the project schedule, including all activities, milestones, and team member roles and responsibilities in relation to time to complete. An example of a project schedule is provided in Chapter 12.

9. Quality Management

The quality management section describes the project milestones/key deliverables and quality indicators.

9.1 Milestones

*Milestones are important events or key deliverables that are completed during the life cycle of the project. A table can easily be utilized to describe and track the estimated time of completion for each milestone (see **Table 9-2**).*

9.2 Quality Indicators

Quality indicators are those items that are considered desirable and promote project success. Examples include staying within the projected budget and meeting project milestones. It is helpful to indicate the desired quality baseline in this section to use as a point of reference throughout the project and to describe measures that will be

Table 9-2 Project Milestones

Milestones	Description	Estimated Completion Date

taken to ensure that the desired quality is met and maintained (e.g., audits, inspections) (see Chapter 6 for more information on quality indicators).

10. Project Initiation Plan

In this section, describe how the project will be rolled out. Provide a detailed description of each step in the process, from securing the setting to delivering the end project.

11. Training Plan

Most projects will require some type of training. When considering the training plan, it is important to describe the training process in as much detail as possible. Include information on who will provide the training, who will be trained, when the training will occur, the tools that will be used in the training process, the time required to provide the training, and where the training will be held.

12. Procurement Plan

This section describes how the resources for the project will be acquired, that is, hardware, software, licenses, and any other resources needed to successfully complete the project.

13. Appendices

Include any appendices to the project in this section. Items to consider for this section include those that add meaning or that may help one understand the project plan.

13.1 Appendix A—Organizational Structure

13.2 Appendix B—Definition of Key Terms

Any terms or acronyms used in the plan or by the organization are listed in this appendix.

13.3 Appendix C—References

List any documents referenced in the plan and where they are located.

APPENDIX A

Organizational structure

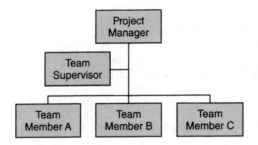

APPENDIX B

Definitions

The following table provides definitions for terms and acronyms that may be used throughout the project plan.

Term/Acronym	Definition
Budget	An itemized summary of planned income and expenditures over time.
Customer	The individual or group for which a project is designed.

APPENDIX C

References

The following table includes all the documents referenced within the project plan.

Name	Description	Location

This plan (pp. 194–208) was adapted from the Centers for Disease Control (n.d.), North Carolina Enterprise (2004), and Project Management Docs (n.d.).

COLLABORATING WITH CONTENT EXPERTS

As the project plan becomes clearer, it will be important to collaborate with content experts and begin interfacing with the identified DNP project faculty mentor (see Chapter 8, The DNP Project Team). The DNP student should assess the areas in which he or she has expertise and the areas in which a content expert may be required. It may be helpful to consider the multiple aspects of the general plan in the assessment. For example, in a health policy project, the DNP student may be a content expert on the impact of the advanced practice nurse (APN) in reducing costs in transitional care. In addition, the DNP student may have considerable expertise in the area of interacting with legislators on this same topic. However, the DNP student may need assistance in the area of policy development. If this is the case, the DNP student could seek out a policy expert to further explore the content required for the project and its success. An important part of doctoral work is collaboration, which assists the student in growth and adds to the richness of the project (see Chapter 7, Interprofessional and Intraprofessional Collaboration in the Scholarly Project).

> An important part of doctoral work is *collaboration*, which assists the student in growth and adds to the richness of the project.

INSTITUTIONAL REVIEW BOARD APPROVAL

As part of the project development, consideration should be given to human subject approval. The student should note that acceptance of the proposal by the DNP project team must occur prior to IRB application submission. Therefore, thinking about the IRB process in the project development stage is important. It is imperative that the student ascertains the policy of the university regarding DNP projects and the IRB.

However, when the IRB application is required, the process can be daunting for doctoral students. Incomplete or flawed submissions have the potential to slow down the progress of the project. This can be a problem because of the short time frame the DNP student may have to complete the program. Understanding the IRB process and addressing potential areas of concern will help ensure a smooth, efficient, and more predictable outcome.

All projects may need to be reviewed by the IRB. Typically, the proposal will initially be reviewed by the IRB chair to determine the type of review required. There are three categories of review: (1) exempt, (2) expedited, and (3) full review. If an IRB application is exempt, no formal IRB review is required because there is no risk for human subjects. Typically this is reserved for projects that use surveys, noninvasive procedures, secondary documents, or methods in which the data are deidentified (Houser, 2015). Expedited review occurs when there is minimal risk to human subjects, described as discomfort or risk that is not greater than that encountered in daily life. The expedited review is usually completed by one or two members of the committee. A full review is completed by the entire committee and is done for projects that do not qualify for exempt or expedited review (Houser, 2015). The type of review that is determined by the IRB will affect the timeline. Often, committees meet at predetermined monthly times, so if a full review is required, the time from application to approval could be lengthy.

In previous years, quality improvement (QI) projects did not require IRB review. However, today, QI projects may be included in an IRB review. Over the past decade, there have been discussions regarding when to consider a project a research study, as opposed to a QI project. QI did not use research methods and always aimed to directly benefit participants, and the work was not published. Today, the distinction between research and QI has become more blurred, with many projects being published. In addition, QI projects now may use research methods (Weiserbs, Lyutic, & Weinberg, 2009). As a result, some IRBs have instituted IRB-QI subgroups to fast-track QI projects. Defining QI projects and policies regarding protection of human subjects can be reviewed at http://www .hhs.gov/ohrp/policy/qualityfaqsmar2011.pdf.

Understanding IRB-related requirements ahead of time will help prepare the DNP student for the process. For instance, in addition to IRB approval at the site of the project, approval through the university IRB may be required. In addition, in preparation for IRB application, accrediting processes ensure the understanding of human subject protection. The student can complete these certifications ahead of time. Typically, a module review, test, and printed certifications are included in the IRB application packet.

Identifying which IRBs will be needed and the requirements of each can smooth the process. "One of the most important steps that a new investigator can take regarding the IRB process is to schedule a meeting with an IRB representative to learn about the institution's IRB processes" (Weber & Cobaugh, 2008, p. 2062).
Some of the questions to consider include:

1. Is there a contact person who may be helpful for answering questions?
2. What is the process of application?

3. Is there a template to be used for the application?
4. What are the educational/certification requirements? Can these be completed ahead of time?
5. How will the completed application be forwarded to the committee?
6. Will the university IRB work with the format of any other IRB committees, or is a separate application process required?
7. What is the usual time frame for IRB approval in each institution?

Remember that the IRB is not there to block research or QI, but to "help researchers by looking for risks in a research proposal that the investigator may have overlooked or underemphasized, thereby protecting the researcher, the institution, and all potential research subjects" (Colt & Mulnard, 2006, p. 1607). Federal regulations require that any research on human subjects be approved by an IRB. The IRB committee must complete a very detailed review to accept the proposal. Understanding the components of the review will assist the DNP student in preparing for the application.

Pech, Cob, and Cejka (2007) outlined the areas that the IRB committee must review:

1. Ensure that risks to the subjects are minimized.
2. Risks are reasonable in relation to anticipated benefits.
3. There is equitable selection of subjects.
4. There is informed consent.
5. There is monitoring of data to ensure safety of subjects.
6. Protection of subject privacy and data confidentiality is ensured.

The role of the investigator is to "explain in simple terms the reason for the research and its risk to human subjects, and to clearly demonstrate how those subjects will be protected" (Colt & Mulnard, 2006, p. 1605). There are many types of people on IRB committees, so simplicity and clarity are of particular importance. The student will need to describe each of the preceding areas of concern in the IRB application.

Typically, the format of the application process will include an institution-specific application and a narrative proposal that incorporates the purpose, clinical question, and procedures that will be utilized for the project. All forms are submitted, such as consent, surveys, tools, and questionnaires. Because many IRB applications are now web based, they can be accessed and developed over time. The goal for the student when preparing the IRB submission is to submit a thorough application to reduce approval delay and to maintain subject protection.

Here are some tips to prepare well for IRB submission:

1. Avoid an incomplete or flawed submission. This includes:
   - Proofreading for content and grammatical errors
   - Being sure that all elements of the form are completed
   - Ensuring that all signatures are completed
   - Providing complete information in all required documents.
2. Be consistent in all documents—ensure that the information provided is the same across all documents.
3. Provide all survey tools that will be used.
4. Be in contact with your assigned IRB member—identify potential areas of concern and usual questions prior to the submission.
5. Consider the audience—use simplified, easy-to-understand language.
6. Prepare a thorough application to reduce time to approval.
7. Keep requirements in mind to justify the project.
   - Provide rationale for the study and the design.
   - Describe the risk to subjects.
   - Describe how subjects are protected throughout the research.
8. Allow for a realistic time frame (Colt & Mulnard, 2006; Greaney et al., 2012).

The IRB committee will review the application and make a decision. There may be full or conditional approval. In the case of conditional approval, revisions may need to be made prior to initiating the project. There is also the possibility of the committee denying approval, in which case the student should work carefully with the IRB representative to identify the changes that need to be made prior to resubmission. Of course, the project cannot be implemented prior to approval (see the Helpful Resource section at the end of this chapter for IRB resources).

SUBMITTING FOR GRANT SUPPORT

An additional area of consideration is submitting a grant proposal. Small grants can provide financial assistance for the project. The process of applying for a grant can encourage the writer to work on clarity of the project problem statement, goals, and objectives. Look for available small grants in areas of one's specialty, such as perianesthesia nursing, or within nursing organizations, such as local chapters of Sigma Theta Tau. Also consider grants available for novice researchers or students, such as the Blue Cross Blue Shield of Michigan Foundation Student Award. Walsh and Bowen (2012) have provided the following suggestions for writing a grant:

1. Tailor the grant to the funding agency's mission.
2. Showcase your expertise and the environment.
3. Minimize the reviewer's work by having a clear, concise, and well-organized application.
4. Follow instructions exactly.
5. Take advantages of any resources for preparing and submitting the grant.
6. Contact the funding agency's program officer with any questions.
7. Be sure the application tells an interesting story (p. 22).

Obtaining a grant can lend credibility to the project, assist with the budget, and build experience for future grant opportunities.

PREPARING FOR IMPLEMENTATION OF THE DNP PROJECT

Once the project plan has been finalized with your project team, the proposal has been defended and approved, and IRB status has been approved (if needed), the implementation process will commence. The following items should be considered prior to the initiation of the project.

Earlier in this chapter, the student learned about key points to consider when developing a project plan. Although the project plan provides the framework for success, what actually constitutes a successful project is dependent on several variables: (1) completing the project on time, (2) completing the project within budget, (3) achieving the intended goals, and (4) achieving stakeholder satisfaction (Pinto & Slevin, 1987). Therefore, careful attention will be needed when implementing the plan.

Clearly, project implementation will involve more than simply dropping the project in place. The implementation phase of the project is complex and may require "simultaneous attention to a wide variety of human, budgetary, and technical variables" (Pinto & Slevin, 1987, p. 167). The student will need to consider the environment where the project will be implemented, as well as the processes involved for training. "If you think through implementation from a holistic approach and communicate well, there is a much greater likelihood that your project will end as a win" (Mochal, 2003, para. 5). It is clear that the implementation of the project will require not only project management but also change management. These are two distinct disciplines that are integrated for the purposes of achieving a project goal.

Project management involves planning, organizing, acquiring, managing, leading, and controlling resources to achieve the overall project goal(s) ("Project Management," 2012). Generally, project management focuses on the activities one will need to complete to accomplish a goal and is achieved through the use of project management processes (Creasey, 2012). Therefore, project management begins long before the implementation of the project; it begins with the planning and designing of the project.

> The implementation phase of the project is complex and may require "simultaneous attention to a wide variety of human, budgetary, and technical variables" (Pinto & Slevin, 1987, p. 167).

As discussed earlier in the chapter, first the project goals are determined, objectives are outlined, specific activities to achieve the objectives are developed, and so forth.

Change management, on the other hand, focuses on helping the people involved in the process make the changes required effectively and efficiently. For example, change management begins with gaining buy-in from stakeholders but also includes training of individuals involved in the project implementation phase. As one can imagine, much of the

> Change management focuses on helping the people involved in the process make the changes required effectively and efficiently.

work involved in change management includes effective communication. See Chapter 7 for information regarding how change theory can be used to guide the DNP student in planning and implementing the project.

Both project management and change management techniques and processes are useful and help the student implement the project successfully. Another important point to consider when implementing a project is that it is often a circular process. For example, as is the case with most projects, the process will involve continued monitoring that may result in further project refinement and/or adjustments to the plan. **Figure 9-2** illustrates the project implementation process.

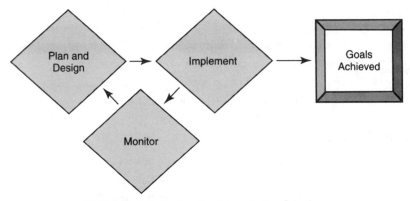

FIGURE 9-2 Project implementation flowchart.

Project Structure

Now that the process is understood and the tools are in place to help ensure a positive outcome, it is time to look at the project structure. This includes finalizing project implementation details with the project setting, which encompasses coordinating with the organizations that are involved in the project, preparing the infrastructure for implementation, identifying the participants and covariables, and, finally, implementing the training (if applicable).

Coordinating with Organizations

Regardless of the type of project being implemented, successful implementation will require activities such as coordinating schedules and resources with organizations involved in implementation. This may require simple one-time communication efforts to confirm that the affiliation agreement is in place, or it may involve several meetings to ensure that everyone involved is on the same page. The goal is to coordinate efforts with everyone or every group with a role in the project. For example, for information technology solutions, there may be an operations group and several infrastructure groups that will need

> . . .failure to plan ahead and coordinate efforts with those involved leads to increasing levels of frustration and roadblocks and may lead to a lack of commitment to completing the project.

to be communicated with prior to implementing the project (Mochal, 2003). The student should recognize that failure to plan ahead and coordinate efforts with those involved leads to increasing levels of frustration and roadblocks and may lead to a lack of commitment to completing the project.

The following focus questions will help the student coordinate organizations:

Focus Questions

- Who are the people or groups that touch the project in some way or form?
- Have all the required relationships been established?
- Has the project implementation plan been communicated effectively?
- Do the stakeholders all understand and agree on the project goals and objectives?
- Is there top management support?
- Have all their questions or concerns been addressed?
- Are there any hidden barriers that have not been uncovered?

Preparing the Infrastructure

It is essential that the characteristics of the DNP project environment be considered and that the project infrastructure be in place prior to implementation. In other words, successful project implementation requires the student to gather the support he or she will need, including resources (i.e., people, technological resources, materials, and supplies). Although in many cases, the project will be implemented in an organization that is familiar to the student, it is still important to carefully review the resources that are available to support the project. For example, the student may need to conduct a review of computer hardware or software, or review the documentation and communication tools to confirm that the information technology infrastructure (databases) will support the project as intended. In doing so, the student is able to identify potential issues and problem solve before it becomes a barrier to implementation. Chapter 10, Driving the Practicum to Impact the Scholarly Project, discusses how to evaluate and prepare the environment for the DNP project.

A few questions to consider include:

Focus Questions

- Are the needed documentation tools in place?
- Does the documentation system capture the data needed for the project?

- Are there any security or access issues that have not been addressed?
- Are the data secured?

Forming the Team

Building a successful organizational project team is critical to a successful project outcome. All of those within the organization that will impact the implementation of the DNP project should be considered as project team members. The DNP student should identify all stakeholders as potential team members dependent on the specific project. Examples of team members may include providers, clinical and administrative staff, management, and patients. To ensure that all members of the team are appropriately invested and to improve the likelihood of the project's success, the manager should be cognizant of the team's development stages. This information will help the manager resolve problems early and keep the project moving forward. Typical group development stages include *forming, storming, norming,* and, finally, *performing* (Tuckman & Jensen, 1977).

The *forming* stage occurs when the team comes together before project implementation. There may be several opportunities for forming to occur: during the initial meeting when the project is introduced, during project implementation planning meetings, during project training meetings, and during other meetings designed to help ensure the project's success. During this stage, some team members meet other team members for the first time; people start to understand the project's objectives, become engaged in the process, and come to understand their role in the process; team member relationships are developed; and members' strengths, weaknesses, and authority are recognized. The DNP student project manager will direct the team at this stage of team orientation.

The next group development stage is *storming*. During this stage, team members may compete for specific roles or responsibilities, there may be disagreements over how to get things done, and individual hidden agendas may become more evident. The DNP student project manager will need to lead the group by example, keep on top of issues between members, and implement problem-solving strategies and conflict management techniques to keep the project moving forward.

The *norming* stage of team development is characterized by congruent team behavior. During this stage, specific rules are developed (either formally or informally), and each team member's role and responsibility are established. The team becomes more efficient and productive. There is a sense of comradery. The DNP student project manager should focus on facilitating group meetings and including everyone's perspective when possible.

The *performing* stage occurs when the team is working well together and objectives are being met. Team members rely on each other to perform their roles and responsibilities to the standard established by the group and help each other where possible. At this stage of team development, the team is cohesive, and there is a sense of unity. The DNP student project manager focuses on meeting the project objectives.

Training the Team

Most projects will require some form of team member training or coaching prior to implementation. This training should occur close to the time the project is ready to start. If a significant amount of time passes between the initial training and the project implementation, there is a risk that the critical elements required for implementation may be forgotten.

The focus of the training is on key functions of each team member. During training, team members should be provided with a document that summarizes the project training key elements and identifies a contact person for questions or problem-solving during implementation. By the end of the training, members should have an understanding of what will be required to implement the project as a whole and be comfortable performing their roles.

In some cases, a dress rehearsal may be feasible. This can be a very valuable exercise because modifications to the plan can be incorporated that address problems identified in this process. Rehearsing the project prior to implementation also serves to decrease team member performance anxiety and builds confidence.

Once the training is complete the student should ask:

Focus Questions

- Are the members of the team clear on the purpose of the project?
- Are they clear on the project goals and initiatives?
- Do the team members understand the objectives and how they will be measured?
- Were team members' questions answered sufficiently?

In summary, as the DNP student progresses through coursework, the project plan and proposal will continue to develop. Expect to continue to work through more details of the project plan as time progresses. The practicum is an opportunity to work some elements of the DNP project into place and will be discussed in Chapter 10.

The following excerpt from Michele Corker, DNP, FNP-BC, AN/Maj, highlights the planning experience for the DNP Project:

Evaluation of an Army Regulation Electronic Contingency Notebook as a Process Improvement Tool During Soldier Readiness Process at Fort Hood Soldier Readiness Center
Michele Corker, DNP, FNP-BC, AN/Maj

My DNP QI project was to evaluate and analyze the effectiveness and ease of use of a technological electronic database repository. The database repository would be used as a tool to improve the Soldier Readiness Process (SRP) at a large military multiforce installation. Planning the evaluation included identification of all stakeholders, review of deployment medicine and military fit for duty standards, and an evaluation of consistency in practice and provider accountability. Development of an interview tool, that involved collaboration between military and civilian providers, was included in the plan.

The student must have an awareness of all required processes for approval in the environment where the project will be implemented. In this case, applications and approvals from multiple sources such as the SRC Medical Officer in Charge (OIC), Deployment of Medicine Chief Officer, university IRB, and the Army Medical Center IRB were obtained.

Following the Institute for Health Improvement (IHI) model, planning the "how" of the evaluation was initiated by using Process Mapping and the Logic Model as a planning tool-framework to show clarity of purpose and organization of actions and outcomes of the project and to obtain the support of leadership. Process mapping provided a visual display or outline of the project focus, helped keep the ultimate mission in mind, and was used to track progress. The Logic Model is a visual outline to display inputs (what is needed to perform the project), outputs (activities to perform QI, participation of stakeholders), and outcomes (short, medium, and long: goal of QI). An interview tool for evaluation of the project was authored to determine if the outcomes were met.

Finally, planning also included the Plan-Do-Study-Act (PDSA) model to test effectiveness of the electronic database (notebook) through comparison of the expected and actual outcomes and continuous evaluation of rapid cycle change. Modifications were made through observation and experiences from the team as they used the notebook. The PDSA model allowed for continuous flexibility, improvements, and reevaluations during the evaluation process. The notebook continues to be revised, which contributes to the relevance and sustainability of the project.

Key Messages

- Use the nursing process at a doctoral level to refine your innovation and project plan based on assessment data.
- Successful project implementation depends on a carefully thought-out plan, with attention to detail.
- Multiple tools are available to assist in the development of the innovation idea and the project plan.
- Collaborate with content experts to build a team for the project.
- Understand all the specific requirements of the university and the organization where the project will be implemented.

Action Plan—Next Steps

1. Create alternative solutions to the identified problem.
2. Choose the best solution as the innovation.
3. Prepare for implementation using appropriate components of the project plan document.
4. Be aware of all requirements within the university and the organization.
5. Consider using the practicum as a stepping stone for project implementation.

REFERENCES

American Association of Colleges of Nursing. (2015). The doctor of nursing practice: Current issues and clarifying recommendations. Retrieved from http://www.aacn.nche .edu/aacn-publications/white-papers/DNP-Implementation-TF-Report-8-15.pdf

Centers for Disease Control. (n.d.). *Project management plan*. Retrieved from http://www .google.com/url?sa=t&rct=j&q=project%20management%20plan%20template& source=web&cd=1&ved=0CLIBEBYwAA&url=http%3A%2F%2Fwww2.cdc.gov %2Fcdcup%2Flibrary%2Ftemplates%2FCDC_UP_Project_Management_Plan_ Template.doc&ei=VOPYT7zFMYG26gG54cn-Ag&usg=AFQjCNHjbv1ppJiJlixqH 3gH2BBofxGGHA

Colt, H. G., & Mulnard, R. A. (2006). Writing an application for a human subjects institutional review board. *Chest, 130*, 1605–1607.

Creasey, T. (2012). *Definition of change management*. Retrieved from http://www .change-management.com/tutorial-defining-change-management.htm

Greaney, A. M., Sheehy, A., Heffernan, C., Murphy, J., Mhaolrunaigh, S. N., Heffernan, E., & Brown, G. (2012). Research ethics application: A guide for the novice researcher. *British Journal of Nursing, 21*(1), 38–43.

Houser, J. (2015). *Nursing research: Reading, using and creating evidence*. Burlington, MA: Jones & Bartlett Learning.

Mochal, K. (2003). *Project implementation: Eight steps to success*. Retrieved from http://www .techrepublic.com/article/project-implementation-eight-steps-to-success/1054399

North Carolina Enterprise. (2004). *Project management plan template*. Retrieved from http://www.google.com/url?sa=t&rct=j&q=project%20management%20plan%20 template&source=web&cd=7&ved=0CLsBEBYwBg&url=http%3A%2F%2Fwww .epmo.scio.nc.gov%2Flibrary%2Fdocs%2FSPMPLAN.doc&ei=VOPYT7zFMYG 26gG54cn-Ag&usg=AFQjCNGuGKiwZjr3YxU-Cbv1Lbyfz0dT-g

Pech, C., Cob, N., & Cejka, J. T. (2007). Understanding institutional review boards: Practical guidance to the IRB review process. *Nutrition in Clinical Practice, 22*, 618. doi:10.1177/0115426507022006618

Pinto, J. K., & Slevin, D. P. (1987). *Critical success factors in effective project implementation*. Retrieved from http://gspa.grade.nida.ac.th/pdf/PA%20780%20(Pakorn)/8 .Critical%20Success%20Factors%20in%20Effective%20Project%20Implementati.pdf

Project management. (2012). *Wikipedia*. Retrieved from http://en.wikipedia.org/wiki/ Project_management

Project Management Docs. (n.d.). *PM docs*. Retrieved from http://www.google.com/ url?sa=t&rct=j&q=project%20management%20plan%20template&source=web& cd=3&ved=0CJgBEBYwAg&url=http%3A%2F%2Fwww.projectmanagementdocs .com%2Ftemplates%2FProject%2520Management%2520Plan.doc&ei=J__ YT-qJL42I8QSgu_DOAw&usg=AFQjCNFinqXApwAKgBSS9d-j_a2MHZRRIA

Tuckman, B. W., & Jensen, M. A. C. (1977). Stages of small-group development revisited. *Group & Organizational Management, 2*(4), 410–427. doi:10.1177/ 105960117700200404

Walsh, M. M., & Bowen, D. M. (2012). An introduction to grant writing: De-mystifying the process. *Canadian Journal of Dental Hygiene, 461*(1), 17–48.

Waxman, K. T. (2013). *Financial and Business Management for the Doctor of Nursing Practice*. New York, NY: Springer.

Weber, R. J., & Cobaugh, D. J. (2008). Developing and executing an effective research plan. *American Journal of Health-Systems Pharmacy, 65*, 2058–2065.

Weiserbs, K. F., Lyutic, L., & Weinberg, J. (2009). Should QI projects require IRB approval? *Academic Medicine, 84*(2), 153. doi:10.1097/ACM.0b013e3181939881

Helpful Resources
Grant Resources

Blue Cross Blue Shield of Michigan Student Award. Available at http://www.bcbsm.com/foundation/pdf/student_award_program.pdf

Fastweb. Scholarships. Available at http://www.fastweb.com/content/featured_scholarships

Institutional Review Board Resources

Collaborative Institutional Training Initiative. Available at https://www.citiprogram.org/Default.asp

National Institute of Health Office of Extramural Research. Protecting human research participants. Available at http://phrp.nihtraining.com/users/login.php

Protection of Human Subjects in Non-Biomedical Research: A tutorial. Available at http://mypage.iu.edu/~pimple/hspt-nbm.pdf

U.S. Department of Energy. Human subjects protection resource book. Available at http://humansubjects.energy.gov/doe-resources/files/HumSubjProtect-Resource-Book.pdf

U.S. Department of Health and Human Services, Health Resources and Services Administration. Protecting human subjects training. Available at http://www.hrsa.gov/publichealth/guidelines/HumanSubjects/

http://www.hhs.gov/ohrp/policy/qualityfaqsmar2011.pdf

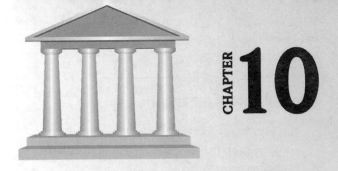

CHAPTER 10

Driving the Practicum to Impact the Scholarly Project

Rosanne Burson

CHAPTER OVERVIEW

The practicum is a unique opportunity to plan field experiences that support the development of doctor of nursing practice (DNP) competencies and professional scholarly growth. Immersion experiences provide an opportunity to apply, integrate, and synthesize the DNP *Essentials* necessary to demonstrate achievement of desired outcomes in an area of advanced nursing practice (American Association of Colleges of Nursing [AACN], 2015). There is also the potential to use the practicum in preparation for implementation of the DNP project. This chapter reviews a process to focus and organize plans for an effective practicum with the designed outcomes. The practicum plan is driven by the DNP student's identified needs in collaboration with faculty and mentors.

CHAPTER OBJECTIVES

After completing the chapter, the learner will be able to:

1. Assess professional growth needs in relation to the DNP *Essentials* and the project needs
2. Develop objectives for the practicum to successfully attain goals for professional development
3. Identify an appropriate site and effective mentor for the practicum in collaboration with the faculty
4. Use the opportunities within the practicum for professional growth and to prepare for DNP project implementation

PRACTICUM PURPOSE

As the time for the practicum course approaches, DNP students may be at very different points in their preparation for the scholarly project. The DNP student may have developed a keen view of the phenomenon and reviewed many aspects of the literature surrounding the phenomenon. There may be an understanding of the clinical question and the process that will be used for outcome improvement. Some of the integral structural parts of the plan may be in place, such as potential nursing theories that will support the project, or there may be some early thoughts on the methodology that will be utilized in the DNP project.

At this point in the curriculum, the student may have completed the DNP program coursework, which undoubtedly strengthened the student's skill set related to the DNP *Essentials*. The student should also be deciding on a project type and should begin thinking about all the components that will be required to complete the project successfully. It is important that the student understand that the DNP project team members and faculty support is available for assistance. (See Chapter 8, The DNP Project Team, for specific information related to relationships with the project team members.)

The practicum is another opportunity for the student to hone skills within the DNP *Essentials*. However, this course can also be used to further networking relationships and assess the organizational climate as a precursor to the implementation

> The practicum is an ideal location to build the required skill set of the student and develop the setting for the project.

of the DNP project. The practicum is an ideal location to build the required skill set of the student and develop the setting for the project.

This field time is also an opportunity to showcase the abilities of the DNP student and market the potential of DNP education to assist organizations in transition driven by data.

IDENTIFYING THE SETTING

The DNP student should consider the potential setting of the DNP project as he or she plans for the practicum. For instance, a project that will improve the quality of care delivered to ventilated patients in the intensive care unit will require an acute care setting. Does the student have access to an acute care organization? The student may be working within an acute care organization, or he or she may have a professional contact within another organization.

It is important for the student to have a full understanding of the university requirements of the practicum. Some universities do not allow practicum hours within the organization of their place of work; others require that the student not work within the confines of his or her current role in the organization.

> It is important for the student to have a full understanding of the university requirements of the practicum.

Each practicum setting choice has distinct positives and negatives. A practicum in an organization of which the student is not a member or employee offers a new lens that can broaden understanding of the project topic. The DNP student may identify issues within the practicum organization that are similar to the student's experience, or issues may be considerably different. The organization may benefit from a fresh pair of eyes viewing areas in which the organization has an interest, as well as expert hours offered to work on these specific aspects of the organization.

If the student is completing a practicum within his or her organization, one can assume that a relationship and a level of trust have developed. A good reputation can take one far. The student may have knowledge of different departments that he or she will need to work with to complete practicum and project objectives. The student may be knowledgeable about the organization and the current environment. Although this knowledge is helpful, it is important for students to separate themselves from their usual workday competencies. The student should keep in mind that it may be difficult for others whom the student works with on a daily basis to relate to him or her in another capacity.

Regardless of employment status, the bulk of the practicum can be positioned in the organization where the DNP project will be implemented. In this way, understanding the organization and developing relationships and trust, which are critical features that have already been established, will help the student successfully implement the project. Caution should be exercised, however, because the organization and the student may have competing goals. Further, the practicum design should incorporate specific experiences and deliverables that will give the student the opportunity to demonstrate the development of relationships and networks to facilitate the DNP project. For instance, as discussed in Chapter 9, Creating and Developing the Project Plan, identifying the institutional review board (IRB) representative and spending time asking specific questions related to the organization's IRB application process will develop a collaborative relationship and smooth the way for this part of the process. Practice experiences may include direct patient care but should also include indirect care practices in healthcare environments (AACN, 2015) to attain DNP competencies.

> The student is demonstrating the DNP *Essentials* to the organization and so may be "sowing seeds" for potential roles suitable for the DNP.

Finally, the student must remember several items. The student is demonstrating the DNP *Essentials* to the organization and so may be "sowing seeds" for potential suitable roles for the DNP prepared nurses. The student is marketing not only himself or herself but also the value-added benefits of the DNP prepared nurse. Expect many opportunities within the practicum to discuss what the DNP prepared nurse is all about and why the student has chosen this path.

Sometimes a student will identify the need for an independent study to become further immersed in a specific topic. An example is the DNP student who completed an informatics independent study to become more fully informed regarding available software and information technology (IT) issues, to implement a project. As the DNP student considered the project scope, his or her realization of the need for additional understanding of informatics evolved. Many university programs have elective courses built into the curriculum and encourage independent studies that will strengthen the project.

MATCHING STUDENT COMPETENCY WITH PROJECT NEEDS

> An assessment of the student's current skill set prior to the onset of the practicum is essential in developing a practicum plan that will address strengthening core skills.

An assessment of the student's current skill set prior to the onset of the practicum is essential in developing a practicum plan that will address strengthening core competencies. A recommended approach is to review each of the DNP *Essentials* competencies (AACN, 2006). The DNP student will identify specific areas for one's professional growth. For example, consider Essential IV: Information Systems/Technology and Patient Care Technology for the Improvement and Transformation of Health Care. One of the identified competencies is to demonstrate the conceptual ability and technical skills to develop and execute an evaluation plan involving data extraction from practice information systems and databases. The student may choose to design a plan for the practicum hours that will incorporate experiences to strengthen this core competency by spending time within the IT department or with the informatics nurse.

In addition to identifying learning needs for the student, an assessment of the competencies that will be needed specifically for the DNP project is in order. For example, the student may determine that outcome data for a population will need to be extracted as a step in the project. So, within the practicum, the student will want to identify a specific outcome or deliverable that will assist him or her in the project. Examples of deliverables may include defining data sets that are applicable for the DNP project, or it may be identifying and working with the data or IT department within the organization. Both of these outcomes will assist in moving the project forward through the practicum.

The student should move through each of the DNP *Essentials* competencies and determine what additional experiences will be needed for the project, differentiating current student strengths from competency areas that will be attained in the practicum (see **Table 10-1**).

In this table, column 1 describes the specific competencies for this Essential. Column 2 is a self-rating by the student of his or her current

> Move through each of the DNP *Essentials* competencies and determine what additional experiences will be needed for the project—differentiating areas of student strength with what will need to be pursued in the practicum.

Table 10-1 Competency Assessment for Practicum Design

Essential II: *Organizational and Systems Leadership for Quality Improvement and Systems Thinking* **Competencies**	DNP Student Competency Rating (Low, Moderate, High)	Needed for Project	Needed for Practicum
Use advanced communication skills/ processes to lead quality improvement and patient safety initiatives in healthcare systems.	High	*	*
Employ principles of business, finance, economics, and health policy to develop and implement effective plans for practice-level and/or systemwide practice initiatives that will improve the quality of care delivery.	Moderate	*	* *
Develop and/or monitor budgets for practice initiatives.	Low		^

Key: **Assessment**	**Explanation**
Low-Moderate-High	Student self-rated competency
*	Competencies needed for the scholarly project
* *	Identified professional growth need for the project
^	Additional identified professional growth need

Reprinted with permission from the American Association of Colleges of Nursing. (2006). The essentials of doctoral education for advanced nursing practice. Retrieved from http://www.aacn .nche.edu/publications/position/DNPEssentials.pdf

competency on a scale of low, moderate, or high competency level. An asterisk (*) in column 3 indicates that this particular skill set is needed for the project. All competencies needed for the project, regardless of level of student competency, should be planned for in the practicum and identified by an *. If the student identified a professional growth need that is also needed for the project, column 4 will identify the need for practicum time in this area, identified by an additional *.

The practicum can also be used to strengthen a student's skill set that may not be required for the DNP project. The ^ sign will map this out as well.

In the preceding competency assessment example, the DNP student is reviewing competencies within *Essential* II. The student has identified that he or she has advanced communication skills, as evidenced by the rating of high competency.

This is a skill set needed for the project (as indicated in column 3*). Even though the student has a high competency in this area, practicum time will need to be incorporated to move the project forward. The networking and collaboration accomplished during the practicum will assist the student in completing the project within that specific organizational environment. For this reason, column 4 identifies an *, indicating that it is needed for the practicum.

In the second competency, the student identifies a growth need in the area of business and finance to implement a practice initiative (self-rating moderate). This is also identified as a component needed for the project. For this reason, column 4 posts **. In this case, practicum time is needed for both professional development and the project. The student will need to incorporate the cost initiatives as part of the project, so he or she will need to understand specific costs. In addition, the practicum time can be used to develop networks within the financial teams of the organization. For example, time spent with the chief financial officer (CFO), the business manager, or the finance team will build relationships for use during the project as well as an understanding of the cost factors that drive the organization.

In the final competency, the student again identifies a growth need in the area of budget monitoring. However, it is determined that this specific skill is not needed for the project. Here, the DNP student uses the opportunity within the practicum to improve on the budget monitoring skill set even though it is not specifically needed as a skill in the project. This time is identified with the ^ sign. The *competency assessment for practicum design* tool template is available in Chapter 12, The Scholarly Project Toolbox, Appendix A. It includes all the DNP *Essentials* and related competencies.

Once the student has worked through all the DNP *Essentials* and competencies in relation to the self-identified learning needs and project needs, he or she will be able to design an individualized plan for experiences within the practicum. The student will also be required to

> Once the student has worked through all the DNP *Essentials* and competencies in relation to the self-identified learning needs and project needs, he or she will be able to design an individualized plan for experiences within the practicum.

develop objectives and measurable outcomes for the practicum that address the self-identified assessment plan. The student collaborates with faculty in the assessment of learning needs and designing practice experiences to assure attention to all of the DNP *Essentials* (AACN, 2015). Also see Chapter 16 for use of the tool to identify competencies.

SITE AGREEMENTS

It is important for the DNP student to understand that a site agreement may need to be in place prior to beginning the practicum. More information regarding the university-specific process may be available in the DNP program policies. This is important to note because it can take time for the university to negotiate a new site agreement. Work closely with faculty and the DNP program director to be sure that the site agreements are in place prior to initiating field time within the institution. In addition, organizations may have varied requirements that must be met prior to the practicum. The university will most likely have requirements as well. These may include basic life support certification, tuberculosis test results, as well as proof of immunization or titers for varicella, MMR, hepatitis B, malpractice insurance, and others. These items may take time to procure, so be sure to allow for this time when planning your practicum.

> Work closely with faculty and the DNP program coordinator to be sure that site agreements are in place prior to initiating field time within the institution.

Practicum site decisions are a very important part of completing the *Essentials* competencies for the DNP student and for prepping for the scholarly project. Students should consider their personal needs assessment, their professional contacts, and the objectives for their practicum in making this decision. For some students, there may be multiple practicum sites to accomplish the determined objectives. Therefore, it is wise to check with an advisor early in the process to determine if the university will be making the contacts or if the student is expected to initiate contact with potential sites.

PRACTICUM HOURS

DNP programs are accredited through a certification process administered by the Commission on Collegiate Nursing Education. The practicum requirement is based on AACN DNP *Essentials*, which require 1,000 hours of postbaccalaureate clinical hours in a practice setting. For post-master's DNP programs, each institution determines the number of relevant graduate hours required to have been attained per enrollee and how many additional hours are needed. A typical scenario is 500 hours post-MSN to be completed within the doctoral program. Advanced nursing practice hours are assessed individually by the program to determine the amount of required additional hours to develop DNP competencies

(AACN, 2015). The DNP student should be well acquainted with all written descriptions and policies related to the practicum within one's university. Planning for these hours in one's life is very important. Therefore, the student should consider his or her fixed responsibilities (work, other courses, family, etc.) and the potential for reorganizing his or her life to commit to and complete the practicum and the scholarly project. As rigorous as the process is, the student will want to be prepared to become immersed in the experience, grow as much as possible, and even enjoy it!

> Consider reorganizing your life to commit to and complete the practicum and the scholarly project.

CHOOSING A MENTOR

Choosing a mentor is a critical feature of preparing for a successful practicum. "Mentoring is a developmental partnership through which one person shares knowledge, skills, information and perspective to foster the personal and professional growth of someone else. The power of mentoring is that it creates a one-of-a-kind opportunity for collaboration, goal achievement and problem-solving" (Stone, n.d., para. 1).

In a qualitative analysis of the characteristics of outstanding mentors, Cho, Ramanan, and Feldman (2011) identified the following attributes:

- Exhibits enthusiasm, compassion, and selflessness
- Acts as a career guide, tailored to the mentee
- Is able to make a time commitment
- Supports personal/professional balance
- Has effective communication skills
- Is respected in the workplace by peers and senior administrators
- Is politically astute
- Is highly knowledgeable in the field.

When considering a mentor, the student should be sure to have an understanding of the requirements of the mentor in the specific DNP program. Many programs identify formal and professional experience as a requirement for the professional role, preferring a graduate degree in a specialty area of practice. For example, if the DNP student is working with the CFO, it is expected that the CFO has a graduate degree in finance.

Often, the written descriptions of the practicum and the mentor–mentee relationship will set the stage for a successful practicum. This may include clearly defined roles and expectations of the mentor. Mentor–mentee expectations are particularly important because the DNP student may be rather new to the healthcare scene and unlikely to have an in-depth understanding of the DNP degree and the potential associated roles. Taking the time to review the expectations of both the mentor and mentee will lay the groundwork for a mutually respectful relationship.

> Taking the time to review the expectations of both the mentor and the mentee will lay the groundwork for a mutually respectful relationship.

As the student considers potential mentors, he or she should think about the expertise the mentor possesses as well as the opportunity to think differently and achieve the next stage of growth. The following characteristics of the mentor should be considered in relation to the specific needs of the student. The mentor should:

- Understand the nuances of the organization
- Hold a position in the organization that matches the student need
- Be able to network with multiple departments and high-level executives
- Have expertise in an area that the DNP student requires
- Be willing to share time and knowledge with the student.

In considering mentors, review the primary areas that have been identified for professional growth and project requirements. For instance, a DNP student who is a primary care nurse practitioner may be expert in the management and care of patients with asthma. The identified goals of professional growth may include informatics, the use of technology to reach patients, data mining, and the budgetary process for office management. The DNP may consider a mentor who is in the finance or informatics area to develop a deeper understanding of these areas. The DNP will also use the skills learned to apply to the project. In addition, if the project is completed within this organization, the DNP student will have developed relationships in these areas to assist with data or finance issues specific to the project.

Sometimes it may be difficult for the DNP student to identify an appropriate mentor. Discussing one's specific goals and objectives for the practicum with faculty, student peers, and work colleagues may elicit a potential list of mentor candidates for consideration.

While working with the mentor, the DNP student may require additional contacts to fulfill all the defined objectives. A mentor who is well respected within the organization, networks well, and has a good understanding of the corporate dynamics will be able to advise the student on additional experiences and follow-up contacts. The DNP student in this example may wish to spend time with the director of the primary care practices or the IT department that works directly with the primary care office. Because the practicum plan is driven by the objectives, the additional contacts and experiences are unique and individualized to each student's identified needs.

Grossman (2007) described a *multiple mentoring model* whereby "the mentee can seek out advice from more than one mentor as well as use the most qualified mentor for each need" (p. 9). The DNP student may very well seek out multiple mentors to achieve the identified goals of the practicum. Various mentors will offer very different perspectives and be able to coach with different skill sets. In addition, at this time, many DNP students are being mentored by people who are not DNP prepared nurses. Because of the lack of DNP mentors, the student may choose to seek out multiple mentors with various specific characteristics and skill sets. This is evolving as more DNP prepared nurses become a part of organizations and offer the specific skill sets that the student is seeking. Even as the DNP mentor becomes a reality, the student will selectively choose additional mentors to focus on areas they wish to develop.

> The DNP student may very well seek out multiple mentors to achieve the identified goals of the practicum.

Reverse mentoring is defined as the mentee mentoring the mentor (Grossman, 2007). Sometimes the student will be able to offer expertise and mentoring in an area the mentee would appreciate. Of course, this varies based on the expertise of both mentor and mentee. For instance, the DNP student may bring a wealth of clinical background that can be used by the mentor. Mentoring is often thought of as a synergistic relationship in which all concerned learn, develop, and share.

As the DNP student considers the practicum experience in the mentee role, it is advantageous to reflect on the *Essentials* competencies of the mentee.

- Internal locus of control
- Interest in learning
- Emotional competence
- Achievement focused

For the practicum to yield maximum results, the DNP student needs to drive the experience, seeking out people and situations that

> For the practicum to yield maximum results, the DNP student needs to drive the experience, seeking out people and situations that will serve to meet the identified objectives.

will serve to meet the identified objectives. These characteristics exemplify internal locus of control and achievement focus. Further, an attitude that exemplifies an interest in learning will encourage the mentor and others that one comes in contact with to develop new relationships and share pearls from their experience. In essence, the DNP student must showcase emotional competence.

Emotional competence is defined as a "collection of perceptions, behaviors, knowledge, and values that . . . enable a leader to manage meaning between individuals and groups within an organization" (Porter-O'Grady & Malloch, 2015, p. 396). Emotional competence is critical in a new environment, where having a sense of appropriate behavior within the setting can make or break the experience. Some of the attributes of emotional competence include self-awareness, mindfulness, openness, appreciation of ambiguity and paradox, appreciation of knowledge, compassion, passionate optimism, and resilience (Porter-O'Grady & Malloch, 2015).

> Emotional competence is critical in a new environment, where having a sense of appropriate behavior within the setting can make or break the experience.

The following excerpt by Dr. Lisa Zajac demonstrates all these attributes as she describes her practicum experience:

DNP Practicum Reflection
Lisa M. Zajac, DNP, RN, ANP-BC, OCN

In my DNP program, our first practicum experience was in the policy course. Looking back, I remember how uninterested I was with policy in general. I always associated policy with lobbying and knew that I was not the type to march on Capitol Hill or influence legislators; I was fully content letting others speak on my behalf. However, after being immersed in the course content, spending 2 days at our state capitol meeting legislators, and meeting with my city councilwoman at a local town hall meeting, I learned that I did have a voice. I shared my concerns regarding community health issues and made suggestions for improvements; and they wanted to hear it. I realized that I could positively impact the health of my community and that motivated me to do more.

The momentum continued in my epidemiology and population health course. My practicum experience in this course included conducting a windshield survey, which I chose to conduct in several ZIP codes in Detroit. Through this first-hand experience I was able to see the great aspects of the community, but also the incivilities and lack of healthcare resources in some of the neighborhoods. After researching the literacy, employment, crime, and healthcare statistics for the city, I realized that the residents could benefit from healthcare education as well as other resources. I took advantage of an opportunity that presented to talk to the residents in the community about their health concerns. They were open and honest and willing to share; and at the top of their list was the need to improve the safety of their neighborhoods.

This led me to attend a public "Conversations with the Councilwoman" forum focusing on public lighting. Approximately 150 residents attended the session. Representatives from the regional electric company were asked to attend the meeting to inform the residents of their plan to update all of the residential street lighting. While the residents were pleased to hear that residential street lights would be replaced, they were concerned because alley lighting was not included in the plan; which would be needed to deter crime. After hearing their concerns, the representatives from the electric company agreed to replace the alley lights for free; however, the cost of maintaining the alley lights would fall on the resident where the light was located. The representatives estimated that the cost would be about $15 a month to maintain one alley light. The residents were visibly disturbed by this. In a district where more than half of the residents are living in poverty, it was clear that this would be difficult for residents to sustain.

After the meeting, I introduced myself to the councilwoman, told her I was a DNP student and asked if she would be willing to meet with me to discuss the data I had collected that related to the health and welfare of the district that she represented. She agreed. While I was pleased to gain the interest of the councilwoman, I knew that I needed to come up with a feasible alternative that would address the residents' concerns about safety. This was the beginning of my community healthcare recommendation focusing on safety and security: the most basic health care need. A couple of weeks later, I walked into the city council office and presented my "Adopt an Alley" lighting initiative. She was impressed with my plan and offered her full support. The councilwoman quickly arranged a meeting with the executives from the electric company and asked me to present the "Adopt an Alley" lighting initiative. While they were initially resistant to the plan, after I addressed their concerns and presented a proposed operationalized plan, they agreed to support the initiative.

My final practicum course began the following term, which allowed me the opportunity to continue to work on my policy initiative. I was able to secure my practicum placement with the director of the Office of Nursing Policy for the state of Michigan. When I met with my mentor the first time, I shared my "Adopt an Alley" initiative and briefed her on what had transpired to date. She quickly connected me with key stakeholders in Michigan who she thought would have interest in my work, and the potential for dissemination began.

While the initiative began as a recommendation in my population health course, it was during my final practicum experience that I was able to see how all of the *DNP Essentials* (AACN, 2006) were incorporated and how all of my previous practicum experiences had laid the foundation to move this initiative forward. For example, early in the process my advanced nursing skills were used to assess the needs of the community, develop a plan to address the identified needs, and guide individuals and groups through the transition (Essential VIII). To accomplish this, I first analyzed both nursing and public health research to determine the nature and significance of the health problem. Since nearly all policy directly or indirectly impacts health, it was clear that a policy change was needed that would address the community's concern about safety and their overall well-being. As a result, an innovation was designed to meet the community's needs that was mindful of the ethical principles of justice and fidelity (Essentials I, III, and V). Throughout my doctoral coursework, I took advantage of opportunities to enhance my skill sets in leadership, advocacy, and principles of negotiation. As a result of these advanced skills, I was able to capitalize on my capacity to facilitate interprofessional collaboration in order to address the needs of the community. Even though I was initially met with resistance, I was eventually able to convince the executives from the electric company of the merit of my recommendation (Essentials II, VI, and VII). While I already possessed advanced informatics skills, it was because of my ability to translate the potential use of technology from a conceptual to an operationalized plan that the executives from the electric company were even willing to listen (Essential IV).

To close, as future DNP students look toward planning their practicum, I urge them to fully embrace each hour, for had I not, I would not have had the experience I did in Detroit. For my final practicum, I looked for opportunities where I could strengthen my skill set as a DNP student; I did not seek experiences where I felt most comfortable. Because of this, I am fully confident as a nursing leader who can truly make a difference in both policy and population health.

Prior to meeting with the identified mentor, the DNP student must have a complete understanding of the practicum requirements, mentor–mentee expectations, and objectives for the practicum, from both a program perspective and a professional development perspective. This will serve to increase the DNP student's confidence and will start the experience off in the right direction, with all participants on the same page. Dye and Garman (2006) have suggested a few expert tips in relation to approaching a mentor:

- Convey that one is grateful for the help
- Be well prepared
- Honor the meeting arrangements
- Use time efficiently
- Make it a two-way relationship.

In that first meeting with the mentor, using the preceding tips will help the DNP student get off to a great start. For example, a "thank you for the opportunity" can be a good introduction and lead-in for the meeting. When the student is well prepared, is on time, and uses the meeting time efficiently, a message of respect, professionalism, and time well spent is conveyed. Finally, by asking questions, listening attentively, and being engaged in the conversation, the student demonstrates true interest in the mentor's perspective, which will help develop the relationship. All these behaviors demonstrate emotional competence, an important characteristic of a successful mentee in laying the groundwork for the practicum.

DEVELOPING OBJECTIVES FOR THE PRACTICUM

After identifying the specific professional growth and project needs, the DNP student is responsible for developing objectives that will drive the experiences within the practicum. By way of review, the final outcome of the practicum experiences is the achievement of a goal (Bastable, 2014). Goals are typically broad and difficult to directly measure. To begin, the student should consider the overall goal that he or she would like to reach. For example, perhaps the student's goal is to develop an innovation that will improve asthma care in the primary care setting. In this case, the DNP student will require a working knowledge of the asthma database within the health system to obtain preliminary data. After the overall goal is identified, the student needs to determine related objectives that are more specific to help him or her reach the overall goal. In other words, the objectives will describe the steps needed to reach the goal. In this example, a few of the objectives might be to (1) meet with the informatics specialists to review the data system and to identify key aspects of asthma reports and (2) identify potential clinical areas that receive asthma reports and would be amenable to working on their current processes related to asthma care.

Mager (1997) identified three parts to the objective:

1. A measurable verb (what the learner should be able to do)
2. A condition that the performance will occur within (under what conditions the learner should be able to do it)
3. Criteria for acceptable performance (how well the learner should be able to do it).

Writing objectives provides the learner with a way to organize activities in order to reach a goal, communicates to the mentor/faculty the activities for the design of the practicum, and provides deliverables that indicate when the objectives have been accomplished. The process of developing and communicating objectives will ensure that the practicum time is well designed and goals are met.

The process of developing and communicating objectives will ensure that the practicum time is well designed and goals are met.

For the DNP student, writing of objectives allows one to focus on self-assessment and to design activities that will allow attainment of objectives. Reviewing the DNP program objectives, the DNP *Essentials*, and the practicum course objectives will assist the student in maintaining congruence in expectations of doctoral study. Objectives are the measurable actions that result in goal achievement. They are the first step in designing an organized plan to ensure that the student will use time effectively in the field. For the faculty and the mentor, objectives describe the steps that the student will take to reach professional growth needs and to lay the groundwork for the practicum evaluation.

Higher level objectives typical of doctoral study are in the area of application, analysis, evaluation, and creation. **Table 10-2** identifies verbs for each level objective based on the Iowa State University's model of learning objectives. The model was defined by Heer (updated in 2012) using Anderson and Krathwohl's 2001 revision of the original Bloom taxonomy. Compare the table's objective levels with the program objectives of one's DNP program. As one develops objectives, use verbs that are consistent with an appropriate level, such as analysis, evaluation, and creation.

Table 10-2 Level Objective Verbs

Level Objective	Verb				
I. Remember	Recall	Retrieve	Recognize	Identify	
II. Understand	Illustrate	Categorize	Summarize	Explain	Describe
III. Apply*	Execute	Implement	Demonstrate	Employ	
IV. Analyze*	Distinguish	Discriminate	Calculate		
	Organize	Differentiate	Critique		
	Compare	Appraise	Contrast		
V. Evaluate*	Judge	Monitor	Critique	Detect	Test
	Appraise				
VI. Create*	Hypothesize	Design	Construct		

*DNP Level.

Data from Rex Heer, Iowa State University, Center for Excellence in Learning and Teaching, updated 2012.

A common format in developing objectives is the acronym SMART, which specifies that objectives should be:

- Specific—Be as concrete as possible, use action verbs to communicate effectively
- Measurable—How will one know that the objective has been attained?
- Achievable—Within the allowed time frame
- Realistic—The resources and the time allowed set one up for success
- Timely—When will the objective be achieved?

Here is a sample for review:

1. Identify the overall goal related to the *Essentials,* professional growth, and the project:
   Advance the use of information, IT, communication networks, or patient care technology in a particular patient practice setting.
2. Identify specific objectives (steps) that will move toward goal achievement:
   a. *Analyze (verb—analysis level) current IT used in this practice setting (the setting this will occur) by field time with IT and the practice manager to observe practice specifics and compare with current literature (how this will occur).*
   b. In SMART format, the objective would read as: *Analyze current technology utilized in this practice* (specific) *by field time with IT and the practice manager to observe practice specifics in comparison with current literature* (measurable *and* achievable *based on time frame, with appropriate* resources) *by the fifth week of the practicum* (timely).
3. The student may determine that a practicum deliverable will assist in meeting the identified goal.

PRACTICUM DELIVERABLES

In determining the practicum deliverables, one must identify which of the developed objectives will have a concrete item to be delivered to the faculty/mentor or organization. The student will need to determine which items will be helpful in connecting the objectives and outcomes to the *Essentials* and the project. Here are some examples of practicum deliverables related to the objectives discussed in the previous paragraph:

Analyze the current state of this practice's use of the electronic health record, database, and patient portal in comparison with the current IT availability and report to the practice, mentor, and faculty in a one-page summary by week 6 of the practicum.

Sometimes a practicum deliverable will expand beyond the immediate site to incorporate next steps that will develop the DNP student in preparation for the scholarly project. Here are a few examples:

Organize and complete a poster presentation on the exclusion of advanced practice nurses for the HITECH Act incentives. Present the poster at the Summer Institute of Nursing Informatics on July 23, XXXX, in Baltimore, Maryland.

Design an independent study proposal that will contribute to an understanding of the full scope of the scholarly project, which is an exploration, analysis, and synthesis of the current state of standardized language of advanced nursing practice in electronic health records. The independent study elective application will be developed with faculty in nursing informatics by fall XXXX.

The next example relates to implementing a change process within a clinical area. In this case, an organizational assessment may be a concrete deliverable. By performing the assessment, the DNP student demonstrates the ability to operationalize this skill in order to determine feasibility for the project success. In addition, strengths and weaknesses can be determined prior to project implementation and plans developed based on the results. The process of being involved with the staff will also begin to solidify relationships prior to implementation. Following is an example of an objective related to these skills:

Explore with key stakeholders within the system the status of the organizational culture in relation to transforming primary care offices, specifically two employed physician practices. The results will be submitted in the form of SWOT (strengths/weaknesses/opportunities/threats) analyses specific to the overall system and to each of the two practices to faculty by 7/1/XX.

Note that in the next examples, the objective is also tied to course practicum objectives, DNP *Essentials*, and competencies:

Meet with key stakeholders within the organization to discuss the organizational structure and culture within the primary care setting. Effective communication skills will be utilized in these meetings, articulating the purpose of the project and collaborating where appropriate to meet the needs of the specific care settings where the pilot will take place. A summary paper will be submitted to faculty by June 28, XXXX, as evidence of meeting practicum objective numbers 4 and 8 and DNP Essentials II-2a and e; VI-1; VII-2, 3; and VIII-1, 3, and 7.

In exploring business and finance aspects of the environment the following objectives have been defined:

> *Examine budgets utilized within the organization specific to two identified offices. The purpose of the examination is to identify line items to consider in implementing new programs within primary care offices. The knowledge will be used to develop a budget proposal to sustain the nurse certified diabetes educator (CDE) within the patient-centered medical home (PCMH). The budget will be submitted for review to faculty and the business mentor by 7/23/xx (Essential II-1, 2a, b, c).*
>
> *Examine the cost-effectiveness and financial sustainability of integrating the RN CDE in the primary care setting by evaluating current reimbursement for education and specific care management within a sample of primary care practices. This will be accomplished by evaluating the patient education reimbursement, evaluation and management codes used, billing charges submitted, and reimbursement received within a sample of these practices. A budget that summarizes the costs for integrating a CDE in this setting and the potential reimbursement will be submitted to faculty by July 24, XXXX, as evidence of meeting practicum objective numbers 2 and 3 and DNP Essentials II-2b, c, and d; IV-3; and VIII-7.*

The key aspects of the practicum objectives are that they are driven by the needs of the DNP student, are designed to incorporate growth in doctoral essential competencies, and prepare the student for implementation of the DNP project.

PRESENTING THE PRACTICUM PLAN

The DNP student will present the objectives and deliverable plan to faculty and mentor(s) prior to initiation of the practicum. Input from faculty and/or mentor(s) may identify additional networking opportunities with departments or key players within the organization. Concurrently, the student will plan with the faculty/mentor regarding how, when, and where time will be spent to achieve the objectives within the practicum time frame. Practicum experiences should be tied back to student-developed professional objectives, practicum course objectives, and DNP *Essentials*. Practice experiences should prepare

> Input from faculty and/or mentor(s) may identify additional networking opportunities with departments or key players within the organization.

Table 10-3 Practicum Tracking

Date/Topic	Description	Course Objective	DNP Essential	Hours

Modified from Madonna University, Livonia, MI.

the student with outcomes delineated in all of the DNP *Essentials* and should be integrated into the student's practice (AACN, 2015). **Table 10-3** suggests a format for tracking the practicum hours.

IMPLEMENTING THE PRACTICUM

As the practicum is implemented, evaluate the progress toward goals and be ready to adjust the plan as needed. Take advantage of opportunities that develop that were not originally discussed. The richer the practicum experience, the more informed the student will be regarding the phenomenon of interest and the organization as a potential project site.

Multiple areas within the practicum can make for a smoother transition to the DNP project. Exploring specifics to the environment, such as the organizational structure, can prepare the DNP student for the scholarly project. Conducting a SWOT analysis of the environment in preparation for the project and developing relationships with the key stakeholders in order to understand the structure is time well spent (see Chapter 6).

Potential barriers to the scholarly project may be identified during the practicum experience as well. Recognizing real or potential barriers early on will give the student the opportunity to develop action plans to either remove the barriers or to alter the plan. This again can smooth the project implementation experience and save valuable time.

Learning the IRB process within the organization during the practicum can also help move the project forward. Understanding the process and making contacts with the key players in the process will smooth the transition for the project and save time. Review Chapter 9 for more detailed information on the IRB process.

PRACTICUM EVALUATION— WERE THE OBJECTIVES MET?

At the completion of the practicum, an evaluation of the objectives should be undertaken. The evaluation is completed by both mentor and student. Completion is validated by the deliverables that were identified in the planning phase of the practicum. If an objective was not met, barriers to achieving the outcome should be identified.

SETTING THE STAGE FOR THE DNP PROJECT

By using the practicum well, the student will be able to (a) identify a project site that is well prepared for implementation of the scholarly work; (b) develop key relationships that will assist him or her in working within the system; (c) assess the organizational culture to determine probability of successful implementation; (d) consider potential barriers so that a plan to move forward can be realized prior to the implementation of the project; and (e) learn aspects of the organizational system, such as formal and informal reporting and the IRB process, for use during the project implementation.

The site of the practicum may continue as the site for implementation of the DNP project depending on university requirements for the project. Utilizing one's mentor for a smooth transition to the project is essential for credibility and consistent messaging. The mentor may also continue to be a valuable resource during the project implementation.

CLOSING OUT THE PRACTICUM

As the practicum comes to a close, the DNP student will want to tie up loose ends by communicating with all key stakeholders. The method of communication should mirror the organization's preferred methods—verbal, email, or formal report.

Showing appreciation to the mentor for time spent and knowledge shared is part of the closure of the practicum. The DNP student will want to choose a way to thank the mentor and may also want to keep the lines of communication open for future networking opportunities.

Key Messages

- The practicum is an ideal location to build the student's required skill set and develop the setting for the project.
- It is important for the student to have a full understanding of the university requirements of the practicum.
- The student is demonstrating the DNP *Essentials* to the organization and so may be "sowing seeds" for potential suitable DNP roles.
- An assessment of the student's current skill set prior to the onset of the practicum is essential in developing a practicum plan that will address strengthening core skills.
- Taking the time to review the expectations of both the mentor and mentee will lay the groundwork for a mutually respectful relationship.
- For the practicum to yield maximum results, the DNP student needs to drive the experience, seeking out people and situations that will serve to meet the identified objectives.
- The process of developing and communicating objectives will ensure that the practicum time is well designed and goals are met.

Action Plan—Next Steps

1. Assess professional growth needs based on the DNP *Essentials* and practicum course objectives.
2. Assess specific skill set needs for the DNP project.
3. Develop overall goals for the practicum.
4. Identify SMART objectives to reach the goals.
5. Plan practicum experiences and deliverables around the objectives.
6. Choose the site and mentor for the practicum.
7. Present practicum plan to faculty and mentor, integrating additional suggestions and refining based on input.

REFERENCES

American Association of Colleges of Nursing. (2006). *The essentials of doctoral education for advanced nursing practice.* Retrieved from http://www.aacn.nche.edu/publications/position/DNPEssentials.pdf

American Association of Colleges of Nursing. (2015). *The doctor of nursing practice: Current issues and clarifying recommendations.* Retrieved from http://www.aacn.nche.edu/aacn-publications/white-papers/DNP-Implementation-TF-Report-8-15.pdf

Anderson, L. W., & Krathwohl, D. R. (Eds.). (2001). *A taxonomy for learning, teaching and assessing: A revision of Bloom's taxonomy of educational objectives.* New York, NY: Addison Wesley Longman.

Bastable, S. B. (2014). *Nurse as educator: Principles of teaching and learning for nursing practice.* Sudbury, MA: Jones and Bartlett.

Cho, C. S., Ramanan, R. A., & Feldman, M. D. (2011). Defining the ideal qualities of mentorship: A qualitative analysis of the characteristics of outstanding mentors. *American Journal of Medicine, 124*(5), 453–458. Retrieved from http://www.ncbi.nlm.nih.gov/pubmed/21531235

Dye, C. F., & Garman, A. N. (2006). Mentors: How to identify, approach and use them for maximal impact. In C. F. Dye & A. N. Garman (Eds.), *Exceptional leadership: 16 critical competencies for healthcare executives* (pp. 207–212). Chicago, IL: Health Administration Press.

Grossman, S. C. (2007). *Mentoring in nursing: A collaborative and dynamic process.* New York, NY: Springer.

Heer, R. (2012). *A model of learning objectives.* Iowa State University, Center for Excellence in Learning and Teaching. Retrieved from http://www.celt.iastate.edu/pdfs-docs/teaching/RevisedBloomsHandout.pdf

Mager, R. F. (1997). *Preparing instructional objectives* (3rd ed.). Atlanta, GA: Center for Effective Performance.

Porter-O'Grady, T., & Malloch, K. (2015). *Quantum leadership: Building better partnerships for sustainable health* (4th ed.). Sudbury, MA: Jones & Bartlett Learning.

Stone, A. (n.d.). *University of South Carolina College of Mass Communication and Information Studies, USC CMIS Alumni Society Mentoring Program handbook.* Retrieved from http://cmcismentorprogram.wordpress.com/mentoring-program-manual/definition-of-mentoring/

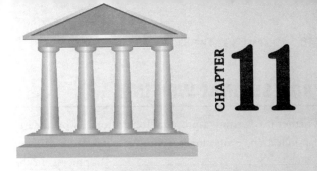

CHAPTER 11

The Proposal

Katherine Moran

CHAPTER OVERVIEW

Students enter the doctor of nursing practice (DNP) program with different levels of exposure to academic writing. As a result, writing proficiency can vary from student to student. For those students with limited writing experience, just the thought of writing a formal project proposal can be intimidating. To support the student in the project proposal writing process, this chapter (a) helps the student recognize early in the process when he or she may need some additional writing support, (b) introduces the student to the components included in a project proposal, and (c) provides a template for the student to refer to when beginning the process of writing the DNP project proposal.

CHAPTER OBJECTIVES

After completing the chapter, the learner will be able to:

1. Evaluate his or her writing skills
2. Develop a proposal outline
3. Recognize the potential components of a proposal
4. Write a project proposal according to institutional guidelines

PROFESSIONAL WRITING

Whether it is writing a proposal for doctorate work or writing for the purpose of publication, professional writing is part of the dissemination-of-knowledge process. In the case of the doctoral proposal, it represents the student's intellectual ability, knowledge in the subject area, and contributions to nursing. As a doctorally prepared nurse, there is an expectation from the profession that nursing knowledge will be distributed either in written form or through oral presentation; it is considered part of one's professional responsibility. In some ways, it can be equated to being accountable to nursing research, theory, and practice.

> The doctoral proposal represents the student's intellectual ability, knowledge in the subject area, and contributions to nursing.

Evaluating Your Writing Skill Set

Writing is a foundational skill that involves application, analysis, and synthesis (Giddens & Lobo, 2008). However, if the student is not experienced in the writing process, basic writing skills should be evaluated. For example, novice writers may inadvertently use improper sentence structure or grammar, cite secondary versus primary sources, neglect foundational literature, or simply have difficulty writing succinctly (Moos & Hawkins, 2009). As a result of these insufficiencies, some advanced writing skills, such as organization, synthesizing research, and writing evidence-based literature, may also be lacking (Moos & Hawkins, 2009). A study by Morse (2009) of academic chairs and deans ($n = 704$) that looked at academic writing (undergraduate and graduate level) revealed that formatting issues (punctuation, spelling, capitalization, and paragraph formatting) were of *moderate* concern; formatting of citations and references received a ranking of *very concerned*; and writing style (presentation of ideas, precision, and clarity) received a ranking of *moderately* to *very concerned*, indicating a need for improvement in these areas.

These concerns, however, can be overcome with faculty and institutional support. For example, most universities have a writing center to help the student with basic writing skills, grammar, formatting, and use of Microsoft Office Word software. Using simple writing strategies can make the process less arduous and help the student write more effectively. For instance, expert writers have long preferred strong use of nouns and verbs when composing a meaningful manuscript; nouns let the reader see whom the student is writing about, and the verbs show the reader the action taken (Leddy, 2011). Adverbs should be used only to add significant meaning.

> The student should seek feedback from colleagues early in the writing process.

The student should also seek guidance from his or her advisor and DNP project team members and feedback on his or her work from colleagues early in the process. Gaining this insight from the collegial perspective is invaluable. Even though it may be difficult for the student to receive constructive criticism, he or she should take it willingly because the intent is to help improve the final product. For example, some students become frustrated when revisions are made based on the feedback, only to be reversed at a later date. The student should keep in mind that this is *a process* for everyone involved—the student and the reviewers alike. Remember, as the proposal develops, it changes and evolves; and as this occurs, the true meaning of the proposal becomes more evident. An added bonus is that through this process, the student's writing skills become more refined. Generally, the more one writes, especially when completing doctoral work, the easier the process becomes. Although it may be a labor-intensive process, it will be worth it in the end.

Another writing strategy that may be helpful is to look at the situation from different perspectives. Roy Peter Clark, a renowned master writer, refers to this as writing *cinematically* (Leddy, 2011). The concept of writing cinematically is vital when describing the totality of the phenomenon of interest. Stop to think about what the main message is and how to say it effectively without using clichés or jargon. Resist the temptation to replace conversational language with complex, long-winded dialogue because of the perception that it sounds more academic (Lee, 2010). Even complex material should be presented in a straightforward and simple manner. Using appropriately labeled headings and bulleted points (where appropriate) will help with clarity and make the proposal easier to read and understand.

Another key factor to successful writing is allowing sufficient time for the writing process. Insufficient time for creative thinking, analysis and synthesis of the literature, or even careful consideration of the

> Insufficient time for creative thinking and analysis and synthesis of the literature . . . can lead to fragmented thoughts that are difficult to follow.

main message can lead to fragmented thoughts that are difficult to follow at best. Starting the proposal early is advantageous because it leaves time for revisions and final polishing (Leddy, 2011). The student should factor in enough time to deal with unexpected changes recommended by those critiquing the work prior to submission, that is, the advisor, project team members, or peers. After all, a substantial amount of the work occurs after the content of the manuscript has been established: the editing. The student should plan on the editing process constituting about 70% of the total time it takes to write a manuscript (Heyman & Cronin, 2005).

Another point worth mentioning relates to the need to properly cite sources. The student must have a clear understanding of how to reference another author's work, both parenthetically and in the reference section. Many schools of nursing in the university setting follow the *Publication Manual of the American Psychological Association* (APA) for communicating scholarly work in written form. The student should be familiar with the APA format before beginning the writing process.

The student should also understand the difference between primary and secondary sources and the importance of avoiding plagiarism. Primary sources are work from the original author; it comes from the source. For example, when a researcher conducts a study and then publishes the results, the researcher is the primary source; he or she conducted and interpreted the research. Secondary sources, on the other hand, discuss work from primary sources, offering interpretation and discussion. The problem with using secondary source material stems from the fact that one author is analyzing, synthesizing, interpreting, and then discussing another author's work. If he or she interprets the results inaccurately and the student then cites the work from this secondary source, the information provided by the student is inaccurate as well. The takeaway message here is to cite primary sources whenever possible.

> *Plagiarism* occurs when one person uses another person or group's work, idea, or words without citing the source ("Plagiarize," 2015).

Plagiarism, simply defined, occurs when one person uses another person or group's work, idea, or words as his or her own without citing the source ("Plagiarize," 2015). Some refer to this as literary theft. Certainly, this can occur inadvertently if the student is not familiar with the rules for citing sources or does not take the time to organize and document referenced material. To avoid plagiarism, the student should familiarize himself or herself with what constitutes plagiarism. For example, if the student used words from a journal article verbatim without using quotation marks and without citing the source, this would constitute plagiarism. Using quotation marks but failing to cite the source also is considered plagiarism because the source is not cited. Another example includes paraphrasing another person's work without citing the source.

Self-plagiarism is also considered as a form of plagiarism. The process of self-plagiarism involves "presenting one's own previously published work as if it were new" (APA, 2010, p. 170). Even though one may not be using another person's work, the concern centers on the potential of copyright infringement. According to APA (2010), "the core of the new document must constitute an original contribution to knowledge, and only the amount of previously published material necessary to understand that contribution should be included" (p. 16).

Remember, plagiarism occurs when one person uses another person or group's work, idea, or words without giving credit to the source, and self-plagiarism occurs when one presents his or her own previously published work as if it were new. The only exception to this is if the information being used is considered common knowledge—that is, information the average person already knows. The student can avoid plagiarism by consistently documenting sources used to substantiate or inform his or her work. For students who wish to learn more about plagiarism, Indiana University offers an online plagiarism module that may be helpful (Frick et al., 2014). This resource is available at https://www.indiana.edu/~istd/plagiarism_test.html. See Chapter 15, Disseminating the Results, for a discussion of plagiarism detecting programs.

One final thought that the student should keep in mind: his or her writing style may not be refined at the beginning of the process, but over time, it should become clearer and more fluent (Heyman & Cronin, 2005). Multiple approaches can be used to manage writing the proposal for a scholarly project. For example, some writers choose to follow a systematic approach to writing, that is, starting at the beginning with the completion of the abstract (allowing the writer to plan the manuscript content), followed by the introduction/background, literature review, and so on. Others choose to start in the middle of the manuscript. In this case, the focus is on capturing the key points on paper and then substantiating the work with the literature review, followed by the approach used, the intervention or proposed improvement process, analysis, significance and/or implications, and ending with the abstract. The DNP student will need to identify the process that works best for him or her.

WRITING THE PROPOSAL

The lessons from Stephen Covey (1989) are applicable when embarking on any significant project or major undertaking (such as writing a doctoral proposal): *to begin with the end in mind.* Simply

> Begin with the end in mind. . .

stated, this means that the writer should plan ahead. First, review the university's requirements for the DNP project, which will vary from university to university. For example, some universities use a dissertation format, while others use an executive summary format or a quality improvement process format. Second, know what it is you want to write (your message), for whom (the audience), and why (ultimate goal).

The importance of a well-written proposal cannot be overstated. This document is essentially a vehicle by which the student *makes the case* for his or her project. He or she must express why his or her project is important, that it will be valued by society (the stakeholders), and that it can be done.

Developing an Outline

Developing an outline is a great way to organize thoughts and to ensure that the key points of the manuscript are captured. However, to develop the outline, the student will need to know the expectations of the university regarding the doctoral proposal format. The student should schedule time to meet with his or her advisor or DNP project mentor to review how the manuscript should be organized, what the reviewers will be looking for, and what format should be used, including the required length, typeface, font size, word spacing, and margin size.

How to Approach the First Draft

Just start writing! It is helpful for writers, regardless of their preferred writing style, to write a rough draft as soon as possible (Happe, 2005). As the name implies, the rough draft is not the final draft. Therefore, focusing on every little detail is not the purpose of this stage in the writing process. The rough draft should be viewed as simply getting the ideas on paper; otherwise, the ability to write freely is lost (Happe, 2005). The student should allocate a certain amount of time each day or week to writing. This time should be spent *only* on those activities relevant to the proposal writing process. Do not allow other competing priorities to take precedence, even if that means sitting quietly gathering thoughts.

Once the first draft is complete, time can be spent perfecting the manuscript— adding references, checking the structure and content for accuracy, and ensuring that the message is clear and the flow is appropriate. Remember that the goal in writing the proposal is to transfer information from the writer to the reader in a manner that is easily understood. At this point, in addition to having an advisor or project faculty mentor review the manuscript it is helpful to have the manuscript reviewed by a peer with experience in the content area to ensure that the presentation of the material is both accurate and easy to follow (Happe, 2005).

Writing Resources

As mentioned, most nursing programs and professional nursing journals use APA as the preferred editorial style guide. Further, many universities offer some type of writing support for students to help them with APA style and with general writing skills. These services may be offered either on campus, such as through an academic writing center or writing labs, or via online tutorials available through the university's library and/or electronic database. A few helpful writing tips are included at the end of this chapter.

COMPONENTS OF THE PROPOSAL

Although the requirements for a doctoral proposal may vary from institution to institution, many include an informative title, an abstract or executive summary, and an introduction that includes the background, the clinical question, a statement of the problem, the project aim or purpose, and the literature review. This is typically followed by the methodology, including the intervention or proposed improvement process, analysis, and significance and/or implications. In an effort to address the broad and varying needs of DNP students across the United States, the following hypothetical pilot study is used to illustrate a comprehensive project proposal that evaluates a healthcare program and the potential to impact outcomes in a specific population. The student should follow his or her university's proposal requirements when developing the project proposal. Other resources that may be helpful when developing the project proposal include the Standards for Quality Improvement Reporting Excellence (SQUIRE) guidelines, which were developed to assist those reporting quality improvement in health care; the Consolidated Standards of Reporting Trials (CONSORT), which are useful for improvement projects or effectiveness studies that use a randomized controlled trial design; or the Strengthening the Reporting of Observational studies in Epidemiology (STROBE) guidelines for projects that use observational or qualitative techniques (Davidoff et al., 2008).

The Title

The title of the proposal is very important. It is the student's first opportunity to gain a reader's interest in his or her work. The title should briefly articulate what the project is about. Avoid using a long, descriptive title but make sure enough information is provided for the reader to understand the overall purpose of the proposal. To illustrate this, consider a hypothetical project that involves

African American women who suffer caregiver stress when caring for sick family members at home. The proposed program is provided by a parish nurse who is able to positively affect stress levels through the introduction of stress reduction techniques using a caring approach. A title using this same information would be too wordy and may disengage the reader. A succinct title that includes the necessary information would be: *Introducing a Stress Reduction Program to African American Women Suffering from Caregiver Stress.*

The Abstract

The abstract should be concise, ranging from 150 to 250 words, but should be sufficient to arouse the reader's interest. In other words, the abstract should include a succinct summary of the proposal yet give enough information to be informative. Some find writing an abstract difficult because of the need to condense the main points of the manuscript into a few short sentences. It may be helpful for the student to review abstracts from peer-reviewed journals to get a sense of how published authors accomplish this task. The abstract typically includes the statement of the problem, a description of the purpose of the project, methods or approach, data analytical procedures, and significance.

Problem Statement: African American women caring for loved ones over time are experiencing high levels of caregiver stress that negatively impact their health, increase medical costs, and result in loss of work productivity.

Purpose: Determine if a stress reduction program introduced by a parish nurse using a caring approach that focuses on the patient relationship is a cost effective method to decrease stress scores, the number of lost workdays, and increase self-rated health in African American women experiencing caregiver stress.

Methods: A two-group pretest-posttest design will be used. Participants will be recruited from three community churches. Inclusion criteria: English speaking, African American women, between 20 and 60 years of age, with no comorbid conditions, who have provided caregiving services for a loved one ≥ 6 months, with a self-rated stress score ≥ 5, who are not practicing stress reduction techniques. The intervention includes an assessment and introduction of stress reduction strategies by the parish nurse that will be practiced by the participants over a period of 6 months. All participants will be asked to complete a self-rated stress level questionnaire, a survey of workdays over the past 6 months, and self-rated perception of health survey. Analysis: Paired sample t-tests will be used to evaluate whether the participants experienced reduction in stress levels, fewer lost workdays, and higher levels of perceived health after participating in the program. A cost analysis will be conducted to determine the sustainability of the program and potential to replicate the initiative throughout local parishes.

Significance: Reducing caregiver stress may lead to a decrease in stress-related health issues, lost days of work, and an improvement in perception of health.

The Introduction

The introduction tells the reader why the topic is important; it sets the stage for what is to come. When describing the background to the project, the student should spend time describing the impetus to the project, the relevance of the topic, and the prevalence and scope of the potential problem. Why is it important for this work to be completed? What are the problems that have been identified, and what are the implications? Why should the reader be interested in this project or topic? This section should give the reader an idea of what the problem is and the characteristics of the organizations in which it occurs; it is a lead-in to the problem statement.

Using the previous example of African American women experiencing caregiver stress, the student may want to begin by giving the statistics regarding the prevalence of caregiver stress among this group. The student may want to talk about the type of problems these women experience when caring for their loved ones, perhaps describing the family members who are receiving care and the type of care the women are providing. It may also be helpful to discuss the obstacles these women have to overcome to provide care for their family members; how providing this care is affecting their physical, psychological, or emotional health; the financial cost to individuals, families, and society of providing this care; and what is likely to occur if this care is not provided (implications).

The Problem Statement

The statement of the problem should be concise but clearly articulate the breadth and depth of the problem, why it is a concern, and why it should be evaluated (i.e., the nature and the severity of the specific problem). Given that the introduction section provided the background for the problem (the lead-in), the student should spend time justifying the need for embarking on this project. Substantiating the problem with factual information or personal opinion is helpful (Nolinske, 1996). Finally, the student may want to conclude this section with a statement indicating why this is a problem for society (based on what was stated previously) and that it should be evaluated. For example,

African American women are experiencing high levels of caregiver stress that negatively impact their health, increase medical costs, and result in loss of work productivity. This is a trend that has increased >30% over the past 10 years and is not expected to change in the near future. If this trend is allowed to continue, the health status of these women is likely to continue to decline, and medical costs will increase, which will negatively impact individuals, families, and communities; therefore, this phenomenon should be evaluated.

The Purpose of the Project

The project aim or purpose should be limited to one or two key areas that are clearly articulated. It should describe what the project will involve and what it will accomplish. Those reading your proposal should have a clear understanding of what the proposal is about just from reading the project aim or purpose.

Using the previous example, the purpose may be:

This project attempts to determine if a stress reduction program introduced by a parish nurse using a caring approach that focuses on the patient relationship is a cost effective method to decrease stress scores and the number of lost workdays and increase self-rated health in African American women experiencing caregiver stress.

The Clinical Question

The clinical question helps the student describe the phenomenon of interest, informs the reader about an issue, and clarifies previous research, or it can add to the body of knowledge already available (Nolinske, 1996). One clinical question for caregiver stress could be:

Do African American women who participate in stress reduction activities rate their level of self-rated health higher after participating in the program?

As mentioned in Chapter 6, Developing the Scholarly Project, the *PICO approach* is an effective method to use to develop a good clinical question. PICO stands for Population, Intervention, Comparison, and Outcomes. In the clinical question example, the population is African American women, the intervention is stress reduction activities, the comparison includes preintervention and postintervention self-rated health data, and the outcome is how women who participate in stress reduction activities rate their level of health.

The information presented here is specific to a pilot project; however, it is useful information that is applicable to many types of DNP projects. For example, the formation of a clinical question could be used to help guide the student who is embarking on a program evaluation project, a quality improvement project, or a project with a focus on contributing to health policy. Using the example above, a program evaluation question could be: Is a stress reduction program for African American women in a parish setting beneficial, sustainable, and replicable? More information regarding scholarly project methods is available in Chapter 14, Aligning Design, Method, and Evaluation with the Clinical Question.

The Literature Review

Exploring the current literature is helpful because it gives the student an opportunity to see what has been done around his or her phenomenon of interest, to synthesize the information, and to come to a conclusion about what is available. A comprehensive literature review provides the evidence to defend a *logical argument* supporting the need for and value of the proposed scholarly project, such as:

- *African American women are experiencing high levels of caregiver stress.*
- *Caregiver stress can result in health issues and loss of work productivity.*
- *Stress reduction techniques are not being used by this population.*
- *If stress reduction techniques are introduced by a parish nurse using a caring approach, women may practice the techniques.*
- *If stress reduction techniques are being used, stress levels may decrease.*
- *If stress levels decrease, there may be a subsequent decrease in stress-related health issues, an improvement in perception of health, and a decrease in lost days of work.*

The literature review is used to present data that support the need for the project—such as a gap in knowledge or flaws within the current literature—and how the scholarly project is needed to address the findings (Schmelzer, 2006). The content of the literature review should come from peer-reviewed journals or other academic sources. The results of the search should then be discussed and appraised. The literature review is not a summarized list of literature available on the phenomenon of interest. The goal of a literature review is to obtain a representative sample of the literature that describes the concepts related to the phenomenon of interest and the results of research applicable to

> The goal of a literature review is to obtain a representative sample of the literature that describes the concepts related to the phenomenon of interest and the results of research applicable to the topic, and perhaps to identify where further clinical inquiry is needed.

the topic, and perhaps to identify where further clinical inquiry is needed. All perspectives regarding the topic should be presented, even if the perspective is not favorable. A good proposal represents all viewpoints and should articulate how the student's project is unique and separate from previous work described in the literature. A description of the process used to conduct a literature search and to write a literature review is provided in Chapter 6.

The following is the initial portion of a hypothetical literature review, with hypothetical references, using the caregiver stress phenomenon as an example.

Literature Review

African American women are more likely to experience caregiver stress than Hispanic, Asian, or Caucasian women of the same age and socioeconomic background (Jones, 2011; Peters, 2009; Smith, 2012). Many healthcare professionals caring for these women contend that this population is also developing hypertension, diabetes, and symptoms of chronic fatigue more frequently than women of Hispanic or Asian descent (Gunthre, 2012; Sindler, 2008; Vanhouser, 2009).

Paterson and Swender (2006) found that more than 40% of African American women in the United States who are caring for loved ones on a regular basis (a minimum of 5 days per week) experience at least 4 lost workdays per month. Another study by Johnson (2009) that followed 598 women over a period of 3 consecutive years confirmed this finding, with an average of 5 (25%) lost workdays experienced per month.

The literature suggests that this population is not utilizing stress reduction strategies on a regular basis (Bender, 2011; Ebstein, 2008; Marks, 2009; Paul, 2012). Further, there is a paucity of information available in the literature that looks at using stress reduction techniques in this population to improve health or reduce lost workdays. . .

The Conceptual and Theoretical Framework

A conceptual framework is similar to a map. The conceptual framework can be used to connect all the important aspects of the project. DNP students are expected to utilize a conceptual framework to guide the study as outlined in DNP Essential I: Scientific Underpinnings for Practice. As mentioned in Chapter 6, one example of a conceptual framework is the Donabedian model, which focuses on three main categories: structure, process, and outcome (Donabedian, 1988). Using this framework, the student is able to identify all the concepts that affect the project structure (the setting the project will be implemented in and who will be involved in the project), the process (what will be done and how it will be delivered), and, finally, the outcome (what will be measured, reviewed, or assessed). Using the previous example, a project could be developed and implemented in a community setting, such as community churches within the inner city.

The intervention could include a presentation given by one parish nurse introducing stress reduction techniques to the target population that will be practiced over a 6-month period. The variables measured could include preintervention and post-intervention levels of perceived stress, self-rated health, number of days of work missed over the same period, and use of stress management techniques, which would be assessed postintervention. A postintervention cost analysis could be used to determine program sustainability and the potential to spread the program to other local parishes (see **Table 11-1**).

A theoretical framework, on the other hand, helps guide and inform the project. For example, Jean Watson's theory of human caring focuses on human caring processes and experiences and makes the assumption that effective caring will promote health and individual or family growth (Watson, 2012). Therefore, using this theory as a guide, the student could illustrate how the parish registered nurse, using a caring approach, establishes a relationship with the patient and guides the patient through a stress reduction intervention to help her learn how to reduce stress levels.

Table 11-1 Project Conceptual Framework

Structure	Process	Outcome
St. Charles Church, St. Michael's Parish, and St. Bartholomew Church of Christ	Group intervention —concentrating on stress reduction techniques	Perceived stress Self-rated health
The expertise of the parish registered nurse—how the utilization of this care provider affects outcomes	The nurse–patient relationship—may help the participant integrate the stress reduction strategies	Use of stress management techniques
Inclusion criterion for participant selection—used to identify appropriate participants		Days of missed work Cost analysis

PROJECT DESIGN

The project design will be determined based on the type of project being implemented. Any proposed project should have a project design plan, which includes anything from a quality improvement project to a pilot study; and the design should be discussed in detail. For example, a pilot study could use either an *experimental design* (used to show cause and effect, such as an intervention that manipulates the variables) or a *nonexperimental design* (data are collected based on observation, without manipulating the variables), whereas a project improvement project may use rapid improvement cycles (Plan-Do-Study-Act) or Six Sigma to affect a change. The DNP student should consult with his or her advisor or partner with an experienced mentor to help guide him or her through the process.

The Methodology

This section is used to describe how the project will be done, connecting it to the project purpose. The project plan is described in detail, including ethical aspects in implementing the improvement, human subjects considerations, and a description of the participants (if applicable), the setting, the tools used to evaluate the phenomenon of interest, the data collection or process improvement/ intervention (if an intervention is included), and how the work will be evaluated. The methodology section provides an opportunity for the DNP student to describe how the clinical question will be answered.

This section may also include a financial analysis, which may be needed to demonstrate the feasibility and cost-effectiveness of a project, as well as the potential impact. Because there is an increasing need for and focus on both clinically effective and cost-effective care, a cost analysis is important to consider. The student should make a list of what would be included in the total costs of implementing the project if someone was to replicate it. These costs should include direct costs (those costs that are easily assigned to the project, for example, salary/wages of those individuals implementing the project, project supplies, and subject costs) and indirect costs (those costs that are used for more than the project alone, for example, utilities, office

> Because there is an increasing need for and focus on both clinically effective and cost-effective care, a cost analysis is important to consider.

supplies, and postage). An example of a project budget is provided in Chapter 12, The Scholarly Project Toolbox.

The Participants

When the project includes participants, it is important to discuss how the participants will be chosen, the actual description of the participants, as well as the total number of participants who will be included in the project. Accurate description of the sample population is useful to the reader because it helps him or her understand the composition of the sample and the degree to which the results of the project can be generalized to other settings.

The process for choosing participants can be accomplished using any number of sampling procedures, such as a convenience sample or a randomized sample. The description of this process becomes especially important when the project involves a pilot study. Finally, the actual description of the participants should include attributes such as gender, age, racial or ethnic group, marital status, socioeconomic status, and level of education.

The DNP student should also discuss the inclusion and exclusion criteria that will be used to identify participants. For example, the project described earlier may include only English-speaking African American female participants who are between the ages of 21 and 60 years; have no comorbid conditions; have provided ongoing caregiving services for a loved one for least 6 months; have a self-rated stress score of 5 or higher; and are not practicing any stress reduction techniques. Therefore, all males would be excluded, as would females who are not African American; African American females younger than 21 or older than 60; those who do not speak English; those who have comorbid conditions; and those who are not providing caregiving services, who have not provided caregiving services for at least 6 months, or who have a stress score lower than 5.

When conducting a pilot study, the student should also confirm that an appropriate sample size is obtained to ensure the validity of the project. A number of methods are available to assist in determining an adequate sample size. As mentioned, the DNP student should ensure that he or she is working with an experienced mentor who can guide him or her through this process.

Authorization from the institutional review board (IRB) should also be obtained (when applicable) and the results included in the proposal. It is vital that the ethical concerns related to the safety of the participants be addressed. In this section, the DNP student should describe how much information the participants will receive regarding the project's purpose, whether they will need to sign a consent form, whether a stipend for participation will be provided, and a detailed plan of how the student will maintain participant confidentiality. See Chapter 9, Creating and Developing the Project Plan, for more information regarding the IRB process.

The Setting

In this section, the student has the opportunity to describe the environment where the project will take place. This provides a clear picture of the setting for those who may want to replicate the project in the future.

The caregiver stress scenario setting could be described as follows:

> *Data will be collected in three local community churches serving Wayne County in Southeast Michigan. The population within these three churches consists of primarily African American families with a mean age of 46.2 years. More than 800 families worship at these three churches; of that number, approximately 25% have one or more family members in need of caregiver support.*

Tools

This section should include a description of the tools that will be used to evaluate the phenomenon of interest (when applicable). This would include any questionnaires given to the participants, evaluation forms, or any other tools used to measure the variables of interest. If an established tool will be used as part of the project, a description of the tool is needed as well as a description of the validity and reliability of the tool. This last point is particularly noteworthy; validity of an instrument is important because it describes how well the instrument (questionnaire, evaluation, or survey) will measure what it is *intended* to measure. In the caregiver stress scenario, the DNP student would want to choose an instrument that accurately captures the essence of *stress*. On the other hand, the *reliability* of the instrument is important because it describes how well the instrument consistently produces the same results on repeated tests. Simply stated, the DNP student will want to choose an instrument that captures the essence of the phenomenon and produces consistent, stable results over time.

> The DNP student will want to choose a tool that captures the essence of the phenomenon and produces consistent, stable results over time.

The reliability of an instrument also includes interrater and/or intrarater reliability. Interrater reliability refers to consistency of measurements from rater to rater, whereas intrarater reliability specifically involves the reliability of measurements obtained from a single rater. For instance, in the caregiver stress scenario, if several raters will be used to administer a perceived stress questionnaire, the student will want to ensure that the questionnaires are implemented consistently by all raters, that is, that all raters use the same questionnaire, that the instructions for completing the questionnaire are the same from group to group, that each rater scores the questionnaire using the same scale, and so forth. This speaks to the value of having a well-defined data collection plan in which the steps involved in implementing the project, especially measuring the variables of interest, are described in detail.

Many data collection tools are referred to in the literature. A simple search of the literature for the tool in question should produce at least one tool that would be appropriate for the project. In some instances, however, the student will need to develop his or her own tool to accurately measure the variables of interest. In this case, the student should note how it will be developed and any evidence that supports its development. Remember that the DNP student will need to work with his or her advisor or project faculty mentor to ensure that the reliability and validity of tools used in the project are maintained. Finally, a copy of the tools that the student plans on using in the project should be provided in the appendix.

The Intervention and Data Collection

When the DNP project includes an intervention, this section will be used to describe the process step by step, from start to finish. It includes the rationale for the intervention, a broad overview of the description of the intervention, and an operational plan. The intervention will be guided by the conceptual and theoretical framework of the project. Again, the purpose of this section is to describe what will be done (including the collection of data and the purpose), how it will be done (the approach or process that is appropriate for the project design), where it will occur, who will be responsible for implementing the process (including background and credentials), how many people are involved in the process, and the expected timeline. Think of this section as a plan that can be used to train the members of the project team.

Next are a few points to consider. When using a questionnaire, remember to identify the response rate that will be considered acceptable (count on an average fall-off rate of 10–20%). When describing the procedure or intervention, remember to use future tense (because the project has not yet been completed) and to clearly describe the project variables. It is also helpful to consider what will be done to increase the response rate and how nonresponders will be tracked (Saunderlin, 1994).

In the caregiver stress scenario, the following may be included:

An educational program will be implemented to impact the stress levels of the participants, reduce lost workdays, and improve perception of health. Participants will be recruited from three Southeast Michigan community churches located in Wayne County. A letter will be sent to all parishioners describing the program and the inclusion criteria. A telephone number will be included for those who are interested; individuals who meet the initial inclusion criteria will be asked to meet with the parish nurse individually. These individuals will be given a stress level questionnaire to determine continued eligibility. One bachelor's-prepared registered nurse (parish nurse) will provide the intervention across the three sites.

Each participant with a stress score of 5 or higher will be provided with a comprehensive description of the program, including the program purpose, what to expect as a participant, including potential risks, and the project lead's contact information if she has questions or concerns. Those who desire to participate will be asked to sign an informed consent.

Each participant will be directed to return to the parish on a predetermined day for a 1-hour appointment, at which time they will receive an individual assessment with the parish nurse, a survey that evaluates the participant's work history over the past 6 months, and a perception-of-health survey. The participants will be asked to return to the parish 1 week later for a 1-hour group educational intervention with the parish nurse that includes an introduction to comprehensive stress reduction strategies and a teach-back opportunity to verify understanding. Participants will be asked to follow up with the parish nurse every 2 weeks for 6 months via telephone, email, or in person to assess barriers to implementation, answer questions, and provide support. All participants will receive the parish nurse contact information for follow-up as needed between visits. A caring approach will be used by the parish nurse during all interactions to foster the development of a relationship with each participant. The parish nurse will contact any participant who does not attend the group intervention via telephone 1 week after the event and attempt a one-time makeup session.

After the completion of the 6-month intervention period, the participants will be asked to meet with the parish nurse one final time in person to complete the stress level questionnaire, the perception-of-health survey, the participant's use of mental stress management techniques questionnaire, and a work history survey for the prior 6-month period. In the event that a participant does not complete the post-intervention session, the parish nurse will make one attempt via telephone to reschedule the session.

Analysis

This section of the proposal focuses on how the student plans to evaluate the results of the project and/or analyze the data. The evaluation plan identifies the criteria that will be used to evaluate what worked and what may not have worked in the project and serves as a mechanism to help the student determine needed next steps or recommendations (i.e., what needs to occur after completion of the project). The project evaluation plan or approach may include key individuals who will be involved in the process, the overall goals of the project and/or the outcomes-based performance measures that will be used to assess change, the description of how the goal will be evaluated, and the reason for using the chosen evaluation method.

For projects involving a pilot study, the level of statistical significance must be stated, the test used for analysis described, and the statistical software identified. It is imperative that an appropriate test be chosen to measure the variable of interest, which is also influenced by the clinical question. Again, describing the rationale for using specific analytical methods is beneficial. It is also wise to consult with a statistician at this point in the project because he or she has the expertise to ensure that the appropriate test(s) is selected for analyzing the clinical question.

Following are just a few points to consider. Descriptive results, such as the number of men and women in the study, should be included to describe the population. When statistics are used to predict an outcome or to determine differences or a relationship, the student should plan on reporting the results using conventional terminology (see **Table 11-2**). Some clinical questions, on the other hand, may require methods of analysis other than traditional statistics. For example, program evaluation projects may include budget analysis and data related to potential for program replication.

The analysis section, in essence, organizes the data in a way that answers the clinical question; in other words, it addresses the problem statement (Saunderlin, 1994). An effective analysis section presents a *summary* of how the results will be interpreted in logical succession.

Table 11-2 Sample of Statistical Terminology

Test	Purpose	Statistical Symbol	Expression
p value	Tells you how likely you are to get the same results if the null hypothesis is true; the significance.	p	Report the significance (.01 or .05 are typically used). $p \le .05$
t statistic	Determines if there is a statistically significant difference in mean values between two groups.	t	Report degrees of freedom (df), the t value, and p value. $t(30) = 5.29$, $p = .000$
Pearson's product-moment correlation	Measures two variables at the interval or ratio level to determine if there is a relationship.	r	Report the df (always N – 2), the r value, and p value. $r(55) = .49, p < .01.$
Chi square	Used to analyze nominal and ordinal data to determine if there are any differences.	χ^2	Report df and sample size in parentheses, the chi square value, and the p value. $\chi^2(1, N = 80) = 0.89, p = .25$

Significance and/or Implications

Before writing this section, think about how the results of the project may impact practice, patient outcomes, and so forth. Describe how the project will provide new insight into the existing knowledge where there is currently a gap regarding the phenomenon of interest or regarding the clinical significance and cost-effectiveness implications of the project. For the DNP student it is particularly important to include information regarding the clinical significance when describing the implications of the project. Clinical significance refers to whether or not the intervention has an impact on everyday life, etc. In other words, what does it mean for the patient population that you are trying to impact or the clinical environment? How important is it clinically? Sometimes interventions can have statistical significance, but are not practical for the clinical environment and therefore are not clinically important.

The DNP student should also address the cost-effectiveness of the project whenever possible. In today's healthcare environment all costs are scrutinized. As a result, most administrators will assess projects to determine if there is a potential for a return on investment before authorizing project implementation. To this point, it is wise to also include information on how you plan on sustaining and spreading improvements; as this will invariably impact return on investment. According to the Institute for Healthcare Improvement (IHI) (2015), *sustainability* refers to locking in the progress made by an improvement initiative and *spread* [replication] occurs when best practices and knowledge about successful interventions are actively disseminated to every available care setting. Finally, it is also appropriate to discuss the potential for subsequent clinical inquiry, how the project could influence current programs, or perhaps even healthcare policy.

CITING REFERENCES

> Only the material referenced in the body of the proposal should be cited in the reference section.

Only the material referenced in the body of the proposal should be cited in the reference section. As mentioned previously, APA style of writing is used by many schools of nursing in universities across the United States. Other styles include the *American Medical Association (AMA) Manual of Style,* which is often used to present scientific data in biomedical journals. The *Uniform Requirements* for manuscripts submitted to biomedical journals is yet another example; this style focuses on both ethical and technical aspects of publishing. Again, the DNP student should consult with his or her advisor or project faculty mentor to determine the appropriate style manual. Refer to the reference section of this chapter for an example of APA-formatted references. Other styles are available in the Helpful Resources section of this chapter.

APPENDICES

When additional information is needed to support the presented work but is too cumbersome to include in the body of the work (e.g., a tool used to evaluate outcomes), the information can be presented in the appendix section. In other words, appendices are used for reference to additional documentation necessary to complete the project. The type of documents included in the appendices section will vary based on the project. The following materials may be appropriate for this section (note that it is best to confirm the requirements with an advisor or committee chair prior to submitting the final product):

- Participant invitation letter
- Tools used to measure variables

- Informed consent form
- Participant instructions
- Letters to stakeholders
- Transcripts of interviews
- Budget
- Needs assessment report
- SWOT analysis report

A proposal template is provided as a reference at the end of this chapter (see the appendix). As mentioned, the requirements for the doctoral proposal will vary from institution to institution. Therefore, the student should check with his or her advisor or project faculty mentor for specific information regarding the proposal requirements.

WRITING TIPS

The following writing tips from Venolia (2001) may help the DNP student when writing the DNP proposal.

1. Use a comma to
   a. Separate independent clauses that are joined by coordinating conjunctions—*and, but, or, for, yet,* and *so.*
   b. Separate three or more items in a series—*popcorn, peanuts, and pretzels.*
   c. Between consecutive adjectives that modify the same noun—*an inexpensive, worthwhile program.*
   d. Where needed for clarity—*whatever you decide to do, do it right (Venolia, 2001).*
2. Use a semicolon or period preceding the conjunctive adverb, not a comma—*The dean will be late for the recognition ceremony; however, she does plan to attend. Also use a semicolon to join two independent clauses that are not joined by a conjunction – The dean will not attend the recognition ceremony; she will be missed.*
3. Avoid misplaced modifiers (may alter the intended meaning)—*She told him that she wanted to move to a new location frequently.*
   a. Right: *She frequently told him that she wanted to move to a new location.*
4. And, avoid dangling modifiers—*Hidden in the armoire, Aunt Suzy found her missing sweater.*
   a. Right: *Aunt Suzy found her missing sweater hidden in the armoire.*

5. Tricky words
    a. *Affect* is most often used as a verb (to influence)—*The physician hopes to affect the patient's decision.*
    And *effect* as a noun (consequence)—*The effect of the policy change was to reduce falls on the unit.*
    b. Use *that* to introduce restrictive or defining clauses—*The sweater that needs to be washed is on my bed.* In this case, the sweater is one of several and thus must be further identified.
    And use *which* to introduce nonrestrictive clauses—*The sweater, which needs to be washed, is on my bed.* In this case, there is only one sweater that needs to be washed (*which* adds further meaning and could be dropped from the sentence without changing the meaning). Tip: A *which* clause should be separated with a comma.
    c. Who or Whom? The best guide is to substitute a personal pronoun for who or whom. If he, she, or they fits, use *who*; if him, her, or them fits, use *whom*—*The woman who entered the store* (*she* entered the store). *To whom shall I send the check?* (I shall send the check to *him, her*, or *them*).
6. Write in active voice. In the active voice, the subject acts (*Kathy passed the medications for the unit*) instead of being acted upon (*the medications for the unit were passed by Kathy*).
    Tip: Write in active voice unless the thing acted upon is more important than the person performing the action—*the game was canceled.*
7. Plural vs. singular nouns or pronouns. Check that there is agreement between the pronoun and the antecedent. For example, "Each patient took their medication . . ." is incorrect because one patient cannot be a "they" (Venolia, 2001).
8. Literature review vs. annotated bibliography
    a. A literature review is both a *product* and a *process*. The process involves collecting and reading the relevant literature, coming to some understanding (comprehension) based on what has been read, making connections/applying what is learned to your project, analyzing it (to determine how it fits together), evaluating the strengths and weaknesses of your findings, then coming to a conclusion (what you think the scientific literature says about the topic. For example, you may identify a gap in the literature). The literature review as a product is a written *synthesis* of your findings.
    b. Annotated bibliography—a list of sources used to research a topic with notes that describe and/or evaluate your findings.

9. Avoid writing in first person (i.e., using pronouns "I" or "me").

10. Introduce new topics or ideas with a transitional statement (to connect separate thoughts or ideas together for the reader).

11. The body of the work should be written in a logically succession (do not skip around) and there should be a connection between the introduction, body of the work, and the conclusion.

12. Remember: The author/researcher studied a phenomenon . . . not the article or journal.

APA Format

1. Include a running head (maximum of 50 characters, spaces, and punctuation) in the upper left-hand side of the first page (the words "running head" are on the first page only) and a page number in the upper right-hand side of every page. To create a header using Microsoft Office Word click on the "insert" tab → choose "header" and select format → check "different first page" box → click on "page number" → choose option for the page number flush right → to the left of the page number type the words "Running head:" followed by your title in UPPERCASE → then press the tab key until the title is flush-left. On the next page click on the header section and type your title next to the page number (in UPPERCASE), then press the tab key until the title is flush-left.

2. Title page: The title should be a maximum of 12 words, centered in the upper half of the page, followed by your name (omit title/degree), then your affiliation (university, organization, etc.).

3. Times New Roman 12-point typeface is the APA typeface preference, although other serif typefaces with 12-point font are also acceptable.

4. Use at least 1-inch margins all around (top, bottom, left, and right) on standard-sized paper (8.5 × 11 inches) and double-space between lines. Margins should only be left justified.

5. Abstract: This is a concise summary of your manuscript. It should be approximately 150 to 250 words. Do not indent the paragraph.

6. Introduction: starts on page 3 of a manuscript. Do not use "introduction" as a heading; the title of the manuscript is used (centered) instead.

7. In text quotations:
   a. By two authors: Research by Williams and Jones (2014) supports . . . The latest research indicates . . . (Williams & Jones, 2014)

b. By three to five authors: (Williams, Jones, Sun, Berry, & Harlow, 2014). In subsequent citations (Williams et al., 2014)

c. Six or more authors: (Williams et al., 2014)

d. Two or more works in the same paragraph: (Williams et al., 2014; Wolker & Peamont, 2012)

8. References page: the heading "References" should be centered at the top of the page; double-space reference entries; the first line of every entry should be flush left then all lines that follow are indented. To use "hanging" indent feature in Microsoft Office Word, click on the—Page Layout—tab, then click on "Paragraph" option and then use the down arrow to select "Hanging" in the "Special" box.

9. All entries in the references should be ordered alphabetically by the author's surnames (last name followed by initials, i.e., Moran, K. J.). If you have a source that is anonymous, then the title of the work is used (instead of the author's surname).

10. The author name should be inverted (last name first, then initials: "Williams, J. Q.")

11. Only the first word of a title and subtitle are capitalized. Or, if a colon is used in the title then the first word after a colon is capitalized. The same is true following a dash in a title. Of course, all proper nouns should be capitalized. When hyphenated compound words are in the title do not capitalize the second word.

12. *Block quotations* (any quotation of 40 words or more) do not use quotation marks to enclose the block. Block quotes are indented one-half inch on the left margin for the whole quote, but not on the right margin. Here's an example:

With regard to plagiarism, the *Publication Manual of the American Psychological Association* (2010) makes the following statement:

> Quotation marks should be used to indicate the exact work of another. Each time you paraphrase another author (i.e., summarize a passage or rearrange the order of a sentence and change some of the words), you will need to credit the source in the text. . . . The key element of this principle is that authors do not present the work of another as if it were their own work. This can extend to ideas as well as written words (pp. 15–16).

Key Messages

- The doctoral proposal represents the student's intellectual ability, knowledge in the subject area, and contributions to nursing.
- When writing a project proposal, insufficient time for creative thinking and analysis and synthesis of the literature can lead to fragmented thoughts that are difficult to follow.
- When starting the proposal writing process, begin with the end in mind.
- The student can avoid plagiarism by consistently documenting sources used to substantiate or inform his or her work.
- Only the material referenced in the body of the proposal should be cited in the reference section.

Action Plan—Next Steps

1. Evaluate your writing skill set.
2. Check with your advisor or project faculty mentor regarding the institutional proposal format requirements.
3. Develop an outline.
4. Choose an appropriate project title.
5. Start writing!
6. Seek feedback from colleagues early in the writing process.

REFERENCES

American Psychological Association. (2010). *Publication Manual of the American Psychological Association* (6th ed.). Washington, DC: Author.

Covey, S. R. (1989). *The 7 habits of highly effective people: Powerful lessons in personal change.* New York, NY: Simon & Schuster.

Davidoff, F., Batalden, P., Stevens, D., Ogrinc, G., & Mooney, S. (2008). Publication guidelines for quality improvement in health care: Evolution of the SQUIRE project. *Quality and Safety in Health Care, 17*(Suppl 1):i3–i9. Retrieved from http://squire-statement.org/resources/

Donabedian A. (1988). The quality of care: How can it be assessed? *Journal of the American Medical Association, 260,* 1743–1748.

Frick, T. W., Boling, E., Barrett, A., Dagli, C., Myers, R., Albayrak-Karahan, M., . . . Matsumura, N. (2014). *How to recognize plagiarism: Tutorial and tests.* Bloomington, IN: Department of Instructional Systems Technology, School of Education, Indiana University. Retrieved from: https://www.indiana.edu/~istd/

Giddens, J. F., & Lobo, M. (2008). Analyzing graduate student trends in written paper evaluation. *Journal of Nursing Education, 47*(10), 480–483.

Happe, B. (2005). Disseminating nursing knowledge: A guide to writing for publication. *International Journal of Psychiatric Nursing Research, 10*(3), 1147–1155.

Heyman, B., & Cronin, P. (2005). Writing for publication: Adapting academic work into articles. *British Journal of Nursing, 14*(7), 400–403.

Institute for Healthcare Improvement. (2015). How-to-guide: Sustainability and spread. Retrieved from http://www.ihi.org/resources/Pages/Tools/HowtoGuideSustainability Spread.aspx

Leddy, C. (2011). Advice from the master of the writing craft. *The Writer, 124*(6), 36–38.

Lee, N. J. (2010). Preparing for thesis and viva: Some practicalities. *Nurse Researcher, 17*(3), 52–59.

Moos, D. D., & Hawkins, P. (2009). Barriers and strategies to the revision process from an editor's perspective. *Nursing Forum, 44*(2), 79–92.

Morse, G. G. (2009). Faculty application of the American Psychological Association style. *Journal of Nursing Education, 48*(10), 542–551.

Nolinske, T. (1996). Writing a research proposal. *Journal of Prosthetics and Orthotics, 8*(4), 132–137.

Plagiarize. (2015). *Merriam-Webster.* Retrieved from http://www.merriam-webster.com/dictionary/plagiarize

Saunderlin, G. (1994). Writing a research proposal: The critical first step for successful clinical research. *Gastroenterology Nursing, 17*(2), 48–56.

Schmelzer, M. (2006). Research in practice. *Gastroenterology Nursing, 29*(2), 186–188.

Venolia, J. (2001). Write right! Berkeley, CA: Ten Speed Press

Watson, J. (2012). *Caring science ten caritas processes.* Retrieved from http://www.watson caringscience.org/index.cfm/category/60/definitions.cfm

Helpful Resources

APA style available at http://www.apastyle.org/

BioMedical Editor available at http://www.biomedicaleditor.com/ama-style.html

CONSORT statement available at http://www.consort-statement.org/consort-2010

Indiana University plagiarism module available at https://www.indiana.edu/-istd/plagiarism_test.html

International Committee of Medical Journal Editors (Uniform Requirements for Manuscripts) available at http://www.icmje.org/

Purdue Online Writing Lab (OWL) available at http://owl.english.purdue.edu/owl/section/2/10/

SQUIRE guideline available at http://www.squire-statement.org/

STROBE statement available at http://www.strobe-statement.org/Checklist.html

Appendix

Running head: SHORTENED TITLE ALL UPPERCASE   1

[Project Title – Upper and lowercase no more than 12 words]

[Student First Name Middle Initial(s) Last Name]

[Name of University]

[Date]

Abstract

The abstract is a brief summary of the proposal. Review the university requirements for specific instructions related to the abstract format, for example, word count, margins, and font size. The abstract generally does not exceed one page. Although the requirements for the abstract content may vary from institution to institution, most require a project purpose, the problem statement, description of the sample and overall project design, the proposed methods, analysis procedures, and significance.

Table of Contents

(Check with university to determine if a table of contents is required)

Abstract 2

List of Tables 4

List of Figures 5

    1. Introduction 6

        Problem Statement 6

        Purpose of the Project 6

        Clinical Question 6

        Review of the Literature 6

    2. Conceptual and Theoretical Framework 7

    3. Methodology 8

        Participants 8

        Setting 8

        Tools 8

        The Intervention and Data Collection 8

    4. Analysis 9

    5. Significance and/or Implications 10

References 11

Appendix A 12

List of Tables

Table 1. The table title belongs here

List of Figures

Figure 1. The figure title belongs here

1. INTRODUCTION

The introduction tells the reader why this topic is important; it sets the stage for what is to come. Even though a heading is provided in this example to illustrate placement, because a manuscript always begins with an introduction, the title *introduction* is not used in the actual proposal.

Problem Statement

The statement of the problem should be concise but clearly articulate the breadth and depth of the problem, why it is a concern, and why it should be evaluated.

Purpose of the Project

The project aim or purpose should be limited to one or two key areas that are clearly articulated. It should describe what the project will involve and what it will accomplish.

Clinical Question

The clinical question helps the student describe the phenomenon of interest, informs the reader about an issue, and clarifies previous research, or it can add to the body of knowledge already available (Nolinske, 1996).

Review of the Literature

The literature review is used to present the data that support the need for the DNP project, such as a gap in knowledge or flaws within the current literature. A comprehensive literature review provides the evidence to defend a *logical argument* supporting the need for and the value of the proposed scholarly project.

2. CONCEPTUAL AND THEORETICAL FRAMEWORK

A conceptual framework is similar to a map; it can be used to connect all the important aspects of the project. A theoretical framework helps inform the project.

3. METHODOLOGY

This section is used to describe how the project will be done; connecting it to the project purpose and describing how the clinical question will be answered. The project design will be determined based on the type of project being implemented. Any proposed project should have a project design *plan*.

Participants

When describing the project participants, it is important to discuss how they will be chosen, give a description of the participants, as well as indicate the total number of anticipated participant.

Setting

Describe the environment where the project will take place. This provides a clear picture of the setting for those who may want to replicate the project in the future.

Tools

In this section, describe the tools that will be used to evaluate the phenomenon of interest (if applicable).

The Intervention and Data Collection

When the DNP project includes an intervention, this section is used to describe the process step by step, from start to finish. It includes the rationale for the intervention, a broad overview of the description of the intervention, and an operational plan.

The purpose of this section is to describe what will be done (including the collection of data and the purpose), how it will be done (the approach or process that is appropriate for the project design), who will be responsible for implementing the process (including background and credentials), how many people are involved in the process, and the expected timeline. Think of this section as a plan that can be used to train the members of the project team.

4. ANALYSIS

This section of the proposal focuses on how the student plans to evaluate the results of the project and/or analyze the data. The evaluation plan identifies the criteria that will be used to evaluate what worked and what may not have worked in the project and may help the student determine the next steps or recommendations (i.e., what needs to occur after completion of the project). The project evaluation plan or approach may include key individuals who will be involved in the process, the overall goals of the project and/or the outcomes-based performance measures that will be used to assess change, the description of how the goal will be evaluated, and the reason for using the chosen evaluation method. An effective data analysis section presents a *summary* of how the results will be interpreted in logical succession.

5. SIGNIFICANCE AND/OR IMPLICATIONS

The significance and/or implications section should describe how the results of the project may impact practice, patient outcomes, and so forth. The student should describe how the project will provide new insight into the existing knowledge where there is currently a gap regarding the phenomenon of interest or regarding the clinical and cost-effectiveness implications of the project. It is also appropriate to discuss the potential for project sustainability and spread [replication], as well as subsequent clinical inquiry, how the project could influence current programs, or perhaps even healthcare policy.

REFERENCES

The following are a few examples of reference types available using APA sixth edition; refer to APA section 7.01–7.11. The student can also refer to http://www.apastyle.org/

References in APA format should start on a new page, the word *References* is centered at the top of the page using uppercase and lowercase letters. The references section is double-spaced and should begin with a hanging indent (as illustrated in this section).

Journal example:
Author, A., Author, B., & Author, C. (2012). Title of article. *Title of Periodical in Italics, xx*(x), xxx–xxx. doi:xx.xxxxxxxx (Please note: the volume number *is* italicized, but the issue [in parentheses] is not; the page numbers are not prefaced with pp. or p. The student should list only the page numbers; the student should include the digital object identifier [doi] if there is one assigned.)

Journal from online source (without doi) example:
Author, A., Author, B., & Author, C. (2012). Title of article. *Title of Periodical in Italics, xx*(x), xxx–xxx. Retrieved from http://www.xxx.xxxx

Special issue or section of a journal example:
Author, A. A., & Author, B. B. (Eds.). (2012). Title of article [Special issue or Special section]. *Title of Periodical in Italics, xx*(x), xxx–xxx.

Magazine article example:
Author, A. A., Author, B. B., & Author, C. C. (2012, Month). Title of article. *Title of Periodical in Italics, xx*(x), xxx–xxx.

Book example:
Author, A. A. (2012). *Title of the book.* City of publication, STATE abbreviation: Publisher.
Editor, A. A. (Ed.). (2012). *Title of the book.* doi:xx.xxxxxxx (Please note: Include the doi when it is available)

Online book example:
Author, A. A. (2012). *Title of book.* Retrieved from http://www.xxxxx.xxxx

Chapter in a book example:
Author, A. A., & Author, B. B. (2012). Title of chapter. In A. Editor, B. Editor, & C. Editor (Eds.), *Title of book* (pp. xxx–xxx). City of publication, STATE abbreviation: Publisher. (Please note: In this example, pp. does precede the page numbers for the chapter.)

APPENDIX A: THE TITLE OF APPENDIX GOES HERE

When additional information is needed to support the presented work but is too cumbersome to include in the body of the work (e.g., a tool used to evaluate outcomes), the information can be presented in the appendix section. The type of documents included in the appendices section will vary based on the project.

When only one appendix is included in the manuscript, it should be labeled *Appendix*. If more than one appendix is included, they are labeled with letters rather than numbers (i.e., Appendix A, Appendix B, Appendix C) in the order they appear in the manuscript. Each appendix should also have a title, and each should begin on a separate page (**Table 11-3**).

Table 11-3 A Clear and Concise Table Title Goes Here*

Heading 1	Heading 2	Heading 3
The data that will be illustrated below each heading belong here.	Use headings and labels that the reader will understand.	A table key may help provide clarity.
The information within a table must be able to stand alone.	Check with the university to verify format requirements.	Be sure to arrange the data in the table logically.

*Tables describe data using columns and rows.

Figure Example

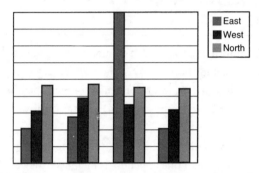

FIGURE 11-1   A clear and concise figure title goes here

Figures are used for visual presentation of data and may include charts, graphs, pictures, maps, and so on. A caption should follow the figure title that explains what the figure illustrates. A legend should be included to explain the information in the figure.

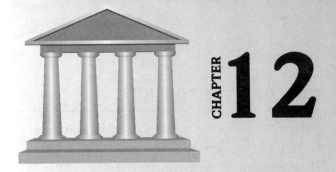

CHAPTER 12

The Scholarly Project Toolbox

Katherine Moran, Rosanne Burson, and Dianne Conrad

CHAPTER OVERVIEW

Multiple tools are available to help the doctor of nursing practice (DNP) student develop a plan for the project, ensure seamless implementation, and drive efficient project management. The goal of this chapter is to introduce the student to a sample of available tools to use throughout the DNP project development and implementation cycle.

CHAPTER OBJECTIVES

After completing this chapter, the learner will be able to:
1. Identify one assessment tool that may be useful for the DNP project
2. Select a tool to use for project management
3. Describe a tool used for budget management
4. Identify two tools appropriate for process improvement
5. Explain how scheduling tools may be used within the DNP project
6. List three examples of tools used for project evaluation
7. Identify information technology tools that can assist with management of the DNP project

UTILIZING THE TOOLBOX

The toolbox is designed to help the student identify the tools that will be most beneficial during the project development and implementation phases and that will ultimately help ensure a successful outcome. A description of each tool and/or intended purpose is provided, followed by an example and/or tool template.

1. Assessment Tools

Assessment tools include those items that help the student organize thoughts and work through conceptual ideas, as well as in the decision-making process. The following tools can be used early in the project planning phase.

Organizational Assessment Tools—Evaluating the organization in which the project will take place is a helpful exercise in project planning. Identifying the organization's strengths, weaknesses, resources, and other attributes can help in planning and implementing a project smoothly and successfully. **Table 12-1** lists

Table 12-1 Organizational Assessment Tools

Tool	Description	Resource
Free Management Library	Website with tools for evaluating and improving organizations	http://managementhelp.org/aboutfml/diagnostics.htm
Reflect and Learn	Over 60 tools for various types of organizational assessment	http://reflectlearn.org/discover/self-assessment-tools
Canadian International Developmental Agency	Organizational Assessment Guide presents a framework for conducting assessments and guidelines for shaping execution	http://www.acdi-cida.gc.ca/INET/IMAGES.NSF/vLUImages/Performancereview6/$file/OA%20Guide-E.pdf
Center for Nonprofit Management	CNM's Organizational Assessment is based on accepted best practices in the nonprofit sector that experts deemed critical as success factors for high-performing nonprofit organizations	http://cnmconnect.org/consulting/oa/
American Medical Association C-CAT	Communication Climate Assessment Toolkit	http://www.ucdenver.edu/academics/colleges/medicalschool/centers/BioethicsHumanities/academicactivities/Pages/C-CAT.aspx

resources for choosing an appropriate organizational assessment aid discussed in Chapter 7, Interprofessional and Intraprofessional Collaboration in the Scholarly Project.

Self-Assessment Tool–Competency Assessment for Practicum Design— This tool is used to assess the student's current skill set prior to the onset of the practicum. Completing this self-assessment based on the DNP *Essentials* helps the student develop a practicum plan that strengthens core competencies. It can also be used as a tracking tool throughout the DNP curriculum to show progression in the attainment of competencies related to the DNP *Essentials* (**Appendix A**).

2. Tools to Connect Relationships and Organize Thoughts

The following tools can help as the DNP student brings multiple ideas and data together to formulate a problem statement.

Concept Map—A concept map is used to show relationships or connections among words, ideas, or a general notion (concept) (see **Figure 12-1**). Using the concept of health as an example, one can quickly see that health encompasses more than the absence of disease; it involves physical, social, spiritual, and mental health. The concept map provides a means for the student to graph and organize knowledge in a way that promotes logical thinking and thus helps the student better understand ideas from a larger whole. Concept mapping is also a helpful tool in nursing to promote critical thinking (Schmehl, n.d.). A concept map template is provided in **Appendix B**.

Mind Mapping—Mind mapping is a technique used to organize data in an attempt to develop or visualize ideas, solve problems, or even make a decision.

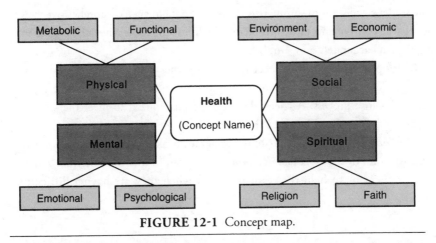

FIGURE 12-1 Concept map.

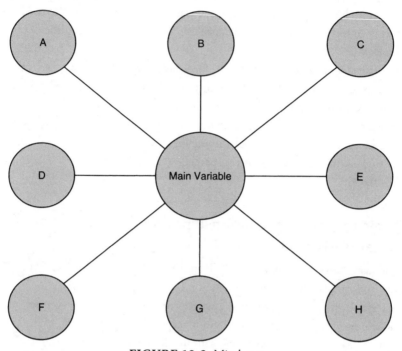

FIGURE 12-2 Mind map.
Reproduced with permission from QI Macros. http://www.qimacros.com

This tool is often used as a brainstorming approach to show connections between ideas. In **Figure 12-2**, multiple like variables are linked to the central or main variable to show possible associations.

3. Tools to Help Define the Problem

The student will want to summarize assessment data to get a comprehensive view of the true components of the problem. The following tools will assist in gathering the data accurately and simply.

Check Sheet—The check sheet is used to gather data about a process. The user typically places a check mark on the sheet to indicate observation of a specific point in a process. A check sheet can be customized to meet the specific needs of a project (see **Figure 12-3**).

Fishbone Diagram—The fishbone diagram is also known as the *cause and effect* diagram or the *Ishikawa diagram,* and is used to identify potential causes of a problem or to help the team members when they are having difficulty

Checkpoint One	Checkpoint Two	Checkpoint Three
Step/Item 1	Step/Item 1	Step/Item 1
Step/Item 2	Step/Item 2	Step/Item 2
Step/Item 3	Step/Item 3	Step/Item 3
Step/Item 4	Step/Item 4	Step/Item 4
Step/Item 5	Step/Item 5	Step/Item 5
Step/Item 6	Step/Item 6	Step/Item 6

FIGURE 12-3 Check sheet.

Reproduced with permission from QI Macros. http://www.qimacros.com

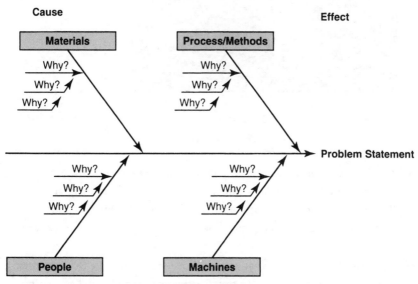

FIGURE 12-4 Fishbone diagram.

Reproduced with permission from QI Macros. http://www.qimacros.com

coming to a conclusion (see **Figure 12-4**). To use a fishbone diagram, the team must first agree on a problem statement, which is captured on the horizontal center line running through the diagram. The team then begins to brainstorm ideas about the cause of the problem. These ideas are captured on vertical lines running into the center (problem) line. As more and more ideas are added to the figure, it begins to take on the appearance of an arrow, or fishbone (hence the name). If it is difficult for the team to generate ideas, headings can be used to facilitate the process (e.g., materials, process/methods). As the team continues to drill down, subcategories that further describe the problem are generated.

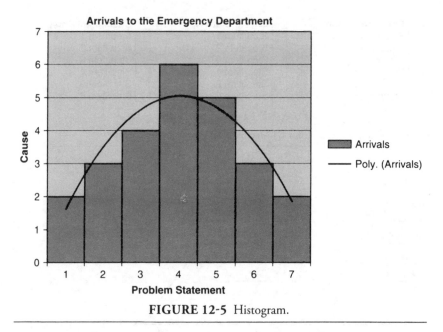

FIGURE 12-5 Histogram.

Another use for tools is to present data, including assessment or evaluation data, in a powerful and efficient manner. Basic graphs such as bar graphs will highlight differences between groups or categories. Other examples include radar or spider charts, frequency histograms, line graphs, pie charts, and run charts. A few specific examples follow.

Histogram—A histogram is a bar graph that is used to illustrate the frequency distribution of a phenomenon. It is a rough estimate of the probability distribution of the given variable. For example, **Figure 12-5** illustrates the frequency distribution of patient arrivals in the emergency department over a period of time. "A histogram can evaluate the capability of a process to meet specifications using variable data like time, money, weight" (Arthur, 2011, p. 11). In the example in Figure 12-5, time is used as the variable.

Scatter Plot—The scatter plot is a tool used to display the distribution of two variables to show relationship. In **Figure 12-6**, one can see that as speed increases, fuel consumption increases as well. Use a scatter plot when there is a believed relationship between two variables.

4. Project Management Tools

As mentioned in Chapter 9, Creating and Developing the Project Plan, project management involves planning, organizing, acquiring, managing, leading, and

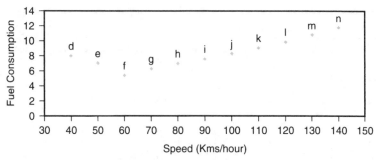

FIGURE 12-6 Scatter plot.
Reproduced with permission from QI Macros. http://www.qimacros.com

controlling resources to achieve the overall project goal(s). Clearly, multiple tools may be needed to manage a project effectively. The following tools will assist in determining alternate solutions to problems and will help identify the appropriate plan for implementing change. Finally, a project plan template is provided in **Appendix C**.

Action Plan—The project action (implementation) plan, in essence, articulates how to achieve the project goals. It controls the execution of the project plan and delineates the details of project implementation by addressing *who, what, where, when, why,* and *how* (see **Table 12-2**).

Balanced Scorecard—The balanced scorecard is a value-added management process that aligns the organizational mission and/or vision to project/business activities and other nonfinancial performance measures to help improve communication, monitor performance, and give managers a balanced view of the organization's performance (Balanced Scorecard Institute, 2012; see **Figure 12-7**). The balanced scorecard incorporates a variety of perspectives, including financial, customer, and internal business process perspectives (McLaughlin & Hays, 2008).

To be successful, companies need to measure and monitor four main results:

1. Financial–profit
2. Customer satisfaction
3. Quality–speed, quality, cost
4. Growth (Arthur, 2011, p. 47)

These items are key performance indicators (KPIs) and can be used to define values for measuring and monitoring achievement toward goals.

Table 12-2 Action Plan

Type	What	How	Who	When	Where	Why
Strategy						
People Organization						
Process						
Technology						

Reproduced with permission from QI Macros. http://www.qimacros.com

Process Flowchart—The flowchart is used to map a process showing all the steps involved (see **Figure 12-8**). This can be a very high-level chart or it can be a visual graphic depicting a very simple process. These flowcharts can also be used to improve a process by identifying opportunities for improvement.

5. Process Improvement Tools

Lean Methodology—Lean is a process management methodology based on the Toyota Production System. The aim of lean is to improve efficiency through the use of tools by removing waste, such as (Pinnacle Enterprise Group, 2012, para. 1):

- Overproduction—making too much
- Transportation—moving resources, that is, people, material, information

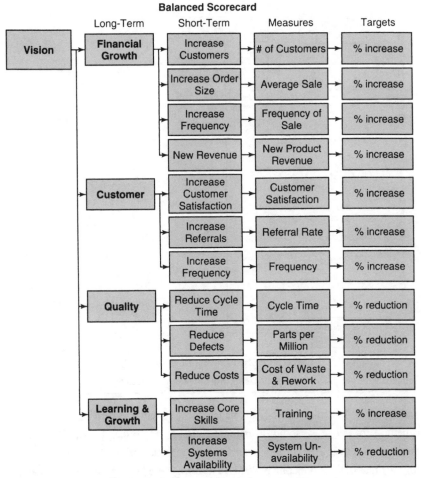

FIGURE 12-7 Balanced scorecard.

Reproduced with permission from QI Macros. http://www.qimacros.com

- Motion—unnecessary movement
- Correction—refers to a product/information that needs to be fixed
- Overprocessing—anything that is done to the product/information that does not add value
- Inventory—product/information that is waiting to be used
- Waiting—people waiting for product/information to arrive
- Unused Employee Ideas and Talent—people's ideas or talents not being used

Lean methodology involves various tools that help the project manager assess the project flow at a very detailed level with a goal of removing complex processes that are associated with higher costs.

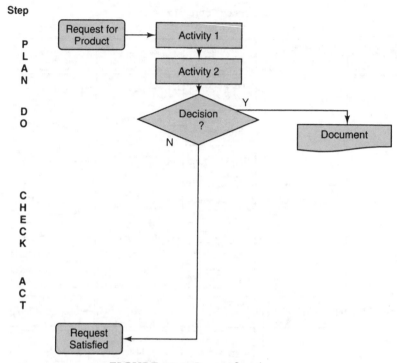

FIGURE 12-8 Process flowchart.
Reproduced with permission from QI Macros. http://www.qimacros.com

Six Sigma®—This methodology or management system was developed in 1986 as a method to reduce variability in manufacturing at Motorola. Today, Six Sigma methods are used in a variety of arenas ranging from manufacturing, to government, to healthcare organizations (Chapman, 2011). The term is used to evaluate quality based on a scale that aims to achieve no more than 3.4 defects per one million opportunities (DPMO). The focus of this methodology is improving quality and reducing errors and variation (McLaughlin & Hays, 2008). "A good Six Sigma implementation plan will identify what activities to implement, how to do them, who will do them, when they will be started and completed, and how they will be measured" (Arthur, 2011, p. 44).

DMAIC Process—The DMAIC process, which stands for define, measure, analyze, improve, and control, is a Six Sigma problem-solving method that uses the five stages of quality improvement:

> ***Define*** the opportunity for improvement, the project goals, and the key stakeholders
>> Tools that may be used: Project charter, project status report, issue log, process flowchart, work breakdown structure

Measure performance; the current state of the process. Determine what to measure and collect the data

Tools that may be used: Pareto chart, process flowchart

Analyze the data to identify opportunities, improve the process, or fix the problem

Tools that may be used: Pareto chart, fishbone diagram, histogram, scatter plot, statistical analysis, hypothesis testing

Improve the process by making the needed changes based on analysis

Tools that may be used: Brainstorming; failure modes and effects analysis (FMEA)

Control the outcome by making sure the changes are set in the process by developing and initiating a monitoring plan

Tools that may be used: Control plan

6. Budget Tools

Budget tools help estimate how much a project will cost based on the project activities as well as monitor the costs during project implementation. Generally, project budgetary tools include revenues (if applicable) and expenditures (costs) as outlined in the project plan.

Project Budget—The project budget includes both direct and indirect costs. Direct costs include items such as equipment and supplies. Indirect costs are those associated with the day-to-day operation of an organization, for example, electricity and heat. A budget template is provided in **Appendix D**.

Cost–Benefit Analysis—As the name implies, a cost–benefit analysis is used to determine the costs and/or benefits associated with implementing a change (see **Table 12-3**). To conduct a cost–benefit analysis, all the

Table 12-3 Cost–Benefit Analysis

Countermeasure	Cost	Benefit

costs (e.g., resources used) associated with the change (countermeasure) are listed, followed by all the potential benefits (e.g., time savings). Both columns are totaled, and then the costs are subtracted from the benefits. This decision-making tool helps the student identify which potential change is most cost-effective.

7. Risk Assessment Tools

As mentioned in Chapter 9, a risk assessment is suggested to identify and evaluate the potential impact of project risks. Conducting a risk assessment helps the student prioritize these risks and determine which may require a mitigation plan (see **Table 12-4**).

Force Field Analysis—The force field analysis is a decision-making tool used to identify all the potential forces driving and restraining a proposed change. Using the template in **Table 12-5**, the student would identify all the potential forces that will help him or her implement a project in the *driving forces* section, then fill in all the potential forces that would work against or impede the implementation of the project in the *restraining forces* section.

Table 12-4 Risk Assessment Matrix

Risk Description	Business Impact	Probability of Occurrence	Priority
	(1, 3, 5)	(1, 3, 5)	
			0
			0
			0
			0
			0
			0
			0
			0

1-low, 5-high

Table 12-5 Force Field Analysis

| Countermeasures Proposed Solutions | Forces | | Action to Be Taken |
	For (Driving Forces)	Against (Restraining Forces)	

Reproduced with permission from QI Macros. http://www.qimacros.com

In the *action to be taken* section, the student should list those actions that could be taken to strengthen the driving forces, as well as those that can be taken to weaken the restraining forces, thereby improving the chance of success. This tool is useful because it helps the student identify the potential for successfully implementing a project.

8. Disseminating the Plan—Communication Tools

Project Charter—The purpose of this document is to formally recognize the existence of a project. It is a valuable tool to use when securing commitment for project implementation within an organization. Even if the charter is not required by the institution, it is a useful tool to ensure that all aspects of the project, including potential constraints, are addressed. The project charter typically includes:

- Project title and high-level description
- Project lead/manager
- The overview/rationale—explains the problem being solved by completing the project (business case)
- Project scope—the features and functions of the project

- Risks—if the project is not done
- Stakeholders
- Project goals, objectives, and deliverables (metrics)
- High-level timeline
- Project risks/constraints
- Anticipated resources—team members, equipment, and so on
- Preliminary budget
- Project approval—signature required

A sample of a project charter is provided in **Appendix E**.

Communication Plan—As mentioned in Chapter 9, Creating and Developing the Project Plan, the purpose of the communication plan is to describe how communication will occur during the project. This plan includes how and when information will be communicated, who communicates the message, and what is communicated. A sample of a communication plan is provided in **Appendix F**.

Project Meeting Agenda/Minutes—When conducting a project meeting, having an agenda will help ensure that key points are addressed, efficiency is improved, and that the meeting is kept on schedule. Following the meeting, the team will need a synopsis of the discussion points, the assigned action items, the members responsible for the action items, and the timeline for completion. The meeting agenda and minutes can be combined into one succinct form to meet the needs of both. An example of a meeting agenda/minutes form is provided in **Appendix G**.

Project Milestones—As mentioned in Chapter 9, project milestones are important events or key deliverables that are completed during the life cycle of the project (see **Table 12-6**). A table can easily be used to describe and track the estimated time of completion for each milestone.

Project Status Report—Communication is the key to successful project management. The project status report helps maintain communication during the project implementation phase. The project manager or lead uses the report to

Table 12-6 Project Milestones

Milestones	Description	Estimated Completion Date

Table 12-7 Issues Log

Issue Number	Description of Issue	Date Reported	Assigned To	Status	Date Resolved	Resolution

communicate the status of the project against the project plan on a regular basis to the key stakeholders. The content of the report varies from project to project based on the project size and so on. The typical report will include information on the project milestone overview and status, issue summary, risks summary, and metrics. An example of a project status report is provided in **Appendix H.**

Issues Log—An issues log is simply a record of all the issues or problems that arise during a project that require some type of resolution. This record helps the student keep track of and effectively manage these issues during project implementation (see **Table 12-7**).

9. Scheduling Tools

Scheduling tools can be used to assign duties to team members so they know what they are expected to accomplish and by when (deadline). However, scheduling tools can also be used to plot out all the activities and resources required to complete a project. The following tools can be used to help the DNP student manage project resources and activities so the project goals are accomplished on time!

Project Time Worksheet—The project time worksheet is used to track project team members' time on the project. The example in **Table 12-8** identifies each team member, the date and hours worked, and the total hours that each team member and the team as a whole worked over a given period of time.

Project Schedule—This document is used to estimate the time and effort required to complete the project. In some cases, it is used to hold people accountable (see **Table 12-9**). However, it is important to note that the focus should be only on those activities that are important for achieving the overall project goal.

Table 12-8 Project Time Worksheet

Period Start					
Team Member	Date and Hours Worked	Date and Hours Worked	Date and Hours Worked	Date and Hours Worked	Total Hours
Project Lead					
Team member A					
Team member B					
Team member C					
Team Total					

Project Timeline—The project timeline is a visual representation of tasks to be completed related to calendar dates (see **Figure 12-9**). It helps organize the project and establish deadline dates for each task. When setting up a project timeline, it is often helpful to begin with the deadline for completion of the project and work backward to the present to establish the framework for realistic completion of the tasks.

Work Breakdown Structure—The work breakdown structure is also included in the *project scope*. This document helps identify how the objectives and goals of the project will be met. The work breakdown structure lists the tasks (or milestones) that must be completed to meet an objective and the resources that will be needed to accomplish the task (McLaughlin & Hays, 2008). In the example in **Figure 12-10**, the work breakdown structure is provided for building a bicycle.

10. Evaluation Tools

A wide variety of evaluation tools are available for use, and they can be used for a variety of reasons. For example, evaluation tools can be used to help the student problem solve, brainstorm ideas, determine risk, answer basic questions about a program, or even determine effectiveness of an action, intervention, or project. Many of the previous assessment tools can and should be used as part of the evaluation to compare pre- and post-intervention data.

Table 12-9 Project Schedule

Project Schedule for...

Tasks	Who	Hours	Start	End	1/1	1/8	1/15	1/22	1/29	2/5	2/12	2/19	2/26	3/5
Planning Phase		84.0	1/2	1/11	▓	▓								
Task 1		45.0	1/2	1/5	▓									
Task 2		15.0	1/5	1/8	▓	▓								
		24.0	1/8	1/11										

Reproduced with permission from QI Macros. http://www.qimacros.com

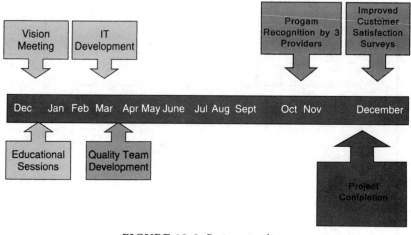

FIGURE 12-9 Project timeline.

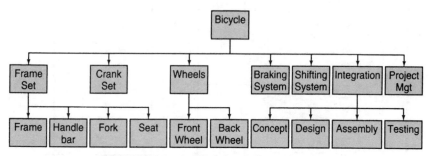

FIGURE 12-10 Work breakdown structure.

Reproduced with permission from QI Macros. http://www.qimacros.com

11. Information Technology Tools *(by Melissa Willmarth-Stec DNP, APRN, CNM, FACNM)*

There is evidence that technology-enhanced teaching and learning improves student outcomes (Beetham & Sharpe, 2013; New Media Consortium, 2012); however, a significant barrier to realizing technology's promise is the educational community's ability or willingness to capitalize on this opportunity. Adopting and integrating emerging technologies throughout teaching and learning culture relies on the successful diffusion of the innovations, and diffusion depends on acceptance of change (Rogers, 2003). As nursing is an interactive, kinesthetic profession that requires the use of both technological and visual expertise, it is believed that parallels between these attributes and use of technology will directly contribute to the preparation, success, and excellence of its students and their abilities to transform health care.

The infusion of technology in education has broad implications for DNP students. Tablet devices are providing students with a creation tool that allows for small-scale, application-based learning rather than the more traditionally directed software-based project tools that are often cumbersome and difficult to negotiate (Walters & Baum, 2011). Several opportunities are available for students to use informatics tools throughout the DNP project process. The informatics toolbox has provided a robust resource for students to consider when engaging in project development, implementation, and evaluation. **Table 12-10** outlines tools that work to enhance the project process and ensure a streamlined, comprehensive output that accomplishes the student's goals.

Table 12-11 features applications for Windows, iOS, and Android operating systems along with approximate costs.

Table 12-10 Informatics Tools to Enhance the DNP Project Process

Function	Application	Description
Annotation	iAnnotate Skitch	Used to read, markup, and share files in various file types; improves productivity
Sharing	Flipboard Box	Share information with others with secure file space or with interactive magazines
Logic Models	iThoughts Mindmap PureFlow	Create multidirectional flow charts and logic maps that can be color coded, easily edited, and exported in multiple file formats
Portfolios	Evernote	Allow users to write, present, collect, and use information in one place
Posters and Presentations	PowerPoint Keynote Google Slides Nearpod Explain Everything Presentation Maker	Create interactive posters and presentations with graphics, data, and voice-over components; used to create both static and dynamic presentations on a variety of platforms
Project Planning and Budget	Microsoft Project Planning Pro Plus	Produce complex project plans that include GANTT charts, resource usage tracking, budgets, risk management tools, and multitasking gestures
Risk Management	Risk Registrar	Used for organization risk assessment and as a repository for all identified risks of a project or business plan
White Boards	Collaborate Jot LiveBoard	Use electronic white space to write, draw, and collaborate; can be captured and used later

Table 12-11 Informatics Tools: Functions and Operating Systems

Functions	Tablet Applications		
	Windows	iOS	Android
Annotation	Skitch (NC)	iAnnotate ($$)	iAnnotate ($$)
Information Sharing	Flipboard (NC), web based, all devices		
Logic Models	Ithoughts HD ($$)	PureFlow ($)	iMindMap HD (NC)
Portfolios	Evernote (NC, $$$) web based, all devices		
Posters	PowerPoint (NC)	Keynote (NC)	Google Slides (NC)
Presentations	Nearpod ($$)	Explain Everything ($$)	Presentation Maker (NC)
Project Planning and Budget	Microsoft Project (NC) Planning Pro Plus ($)	Planning Pro ($$$)	Planning Pro ($$$)
Risk Management	Risk Registrar (NC)	Risk Register +-($)	Not available
Sharing	Box (NC), web based, all devices		
White Boards	Collaborate (NC)	Jot (NC)	LiveBoard (NC)
Key: NC: no charge	$: 0-$5	$$: $5-$10	$$$: $10-$20

The following excerpt, from Maria Johnson, highlights the value of using technology to enhance the learning experience.

Using Technology Tools to Assist in the Scholarly Project Process
Maria Johnson MSN, RN, CPNP

To assist in the DNP project process, I used many applications available on an iPad. Thanks to the portability of the iPad, I could work on my project anytime, anywhere! All of my coursework, including readings, assignments and discussion boards, are conveniently available on the iTunesU app. Additionally, I used the Evernote application to compile and organize all my completed coursework, including papers, videos, and presentations. The Evernote application allows the creation of many folders that can be used for different courses, and professors and peers can be invited to see your folder, ensuring easy transmission of coursework. Planning Pro allowed me to create an interactive project timeline and incorporate needed resources and budget on a per step basis. One of my favorite applications for the DNP program is Keynote. I have made all my presentations, study guides, and even labels for printing in this application. Lastly, Explain Everything is an application that allows you to add voiceover to presentations made in Keynote. Even if your program does not require an iPad as mine did, I would recommend iPad use for DNP students as it allows your coursework to be available at your fingertips for even the busiest of students.

SUMMARY

A vast amount of resources are available to assist the DNP student in the planning and implementation phase of the DNP project. This chapter provided only a sample of the potential tools available for use; a wealth of additional information is available via the Web and project management textbooks. The student should check with an advisor or his or her DNP project team to identify those resources that may be available through the university at no or reduced cost.

REFERENCES

Arthur, J. (2011). *QI macros example book*. Denver, CO: KnowWare International.

Balanced Scorecard Institute. (2012). *Balanced scorecard basics*. Retrieved from http://www.balancedscorecard.org/BSCResources/AbouttheBalancedScorecard/tabid/55/Default.aspx

Beetham, H., & Sharpe, R. (2013). *Rethinking pedagogy for a digital age*. New York, NY: Routledge.

Chapman, A. (2011). *Six sigma*. Retrieved from http://www.businessballs.com/sixsigma.htm

McLaughlin, D. B., & Hays, J. M. (2008). *Healthcare operations management*. Chicago, IL: Health Administration Press.

New Media Consortium. (2012). Horizon Report – 2012 Higher Education Edition. Retrieved from http://www.nmc.org/pdf/2012-horizon-report-HE.pdf

Pinnacle Enterprise Group. (2012). *Lean and six sigma*. Retrieved from http://www.pinnacleeg.com/shp-lean-and-six-sigma.php/page/services/service/lean-and-six-sigma

QI Macros. (2012). *The short-cut to lean six sigma results!* Retrieved from http://www.qimacros.com

Rogers, E. (2003). *Diffusion of innovations*. New York, NY: Free Press.

Schmehl, P. (n.d.). Concept mapping. Retrieved from: http://www.nursingconceptmapping.com/

Walters, E., & Baum, M. (2011). Point/Counterpoint. "Will the iPad Revolutionize Education?" *Learning and Leading with Technology, 38*(7), 6–7.

Appendix A: Competency Assessment for Practicum Design

Essential I: Scientific Underpinnings for Practice Competencies	DNP student competency rating (low-mod- high)	Needed for project	Needed for practicum
1. Integrate nursing science with knowledge from ethics and from the biophysical, psychosocial, analytical, and organizational sciences as the basis for the highest level of nursing practice.			

2. Use science-based theories and concepts to:
    a. determine the nature and significance of health and healthcare delivery phenomena;
    b. describe the actions and advanced strategies to enhance, alleviate, and ameliorate health and healthcare delivery phenomena as appropriate;
    c. evaluate outcomes;
    d. develop and evaluate new practice approaches based on nursing theories and theories from other disciplines.			

Essential II: Organizational and Systems Leadership for Quality Improvement and Systems Thinking Competencies	DNP student competency rating	Needed for project	Needed for practicum
1. Develop and evaluate care delivery approaches that meet current and future needs of patient populations based on scientific findings in nursing and other clinical sciences, as well as organizational, political, and economic sciences.			
2. Ensure accountability for quality of healthcare and patient safety for populations with whom they work. a. Use advanced communication skills/processes to lead quality improvement and patient safety initiatives in healthcare systems.			

b. Employ principles of business, finance, economics, and health policy to develop and implement effective plans for practice-level and/or system-wide practice initiatives that will improve the quality of care delivery. c. Develop and/or monitor budgets for practice initiatives. d. Analyze the cost-effectiveness of practice initiatives accounting for risk and improvement of health-care outcome. e. Have demonstrated sensitivity to diverse organizational cultures and populations, including patients and providers.			
3. Develop and/or evaluate effective strategies for managing the ethical dilemmas inherent in patient care, the healthcare organization, and research.			
Essential III: Clinical Scholarship and Analytical Methods for Evidence-Based Practice **Competencies**	DNP student competency rating	Needed for project	Needed for practicum
1. Use analytical methods to critically appraise existing literature and other evidence to determine and implement the best evidence for practice.			
2. Design and implement processes to evaluate outcomes of practice, practice patterns, and systems of care within a practice setting, healthcare organization, or community against national benchmarks to determine variances in practice outcomes and population trends.			
3. Design, direct, and evaluate quality improvement methodologies to promote safe, timely, effective, efficient, equitable, and patient-centered care.			

	DNP student competency rating	Needed for project	Needed for practicum
4. Apply relevant findings to develop practice guidelines and improve practice and the practice environment.			
5. Use information technology and research methods appropriately to: a. collect appropriate and accurate data to generate evidence for nursing practice, inform/guide database designs that generate meaningful evidence for nursing practice, analyze data for practice, design evidence-based interventions; and b. predict and analyze outcomes, examine patterns of behavior and outcomes, and identify gaps in evidence for practice.			
6. Function as a practice specialist/consultant in collaborative knowledge-generating research.			
7. Disseminate findings from evidence-based practice and research to improve healthcare outcomes.			
Essential IV: Information Systems/Technology and Patient Care Technology for the Improvement and Transformation of Healthcare **Competencies**	**DNP student competency rating**	**Needed for project**	**Needed for practicum**
1. Design, select, use, and evaluate programs that evaluate and monitor outcomes of care, care systems, and quality improvement, including consumer use of healthcare information systems.			
2. Analyze and communicate critical elements necessary to the selection, use, and evaluation of healthcare information systems and patient care technology.			
3. Demonstrate the conceptual ability and technical skills to develop and execute an evaluation plan involving data extraction from practice information systems and databases.			

	DNP student competency rating	Needed for project	Needed for practicum
4. Provide leadership in evaluation and resolution of ethical and legal issues within healthcare systems relating to the use of information, information technology, communication networks, and patient care technology.			
5. Evaluate consumer health information sources for accuracy, timeliness, and appropriateness.			
Essential V: Healthcare Policy for Advocacy in Healthcare **Competencies**	DNP student competency rating	Needed for project	Needed for practicum
1. Critically analyze health policy proposals, health policies, and related issues from the perspective of consumers, nursing, other health professions, and other stakeholders in policy and public information.			
2. Demonstrate leadership in development and implementation of institutional, local, state, federal, and/or international health policy.			
3. Influence policy makers through active participation on committees, boards, or task forces at the institutional, local, state, regional, national, and/or international levels to improve healthcare delivery and outcomes.			
4. Educate others, including policy makers at all levels, regarding nursing, health policy, and patient care outcomes.			
5. Advocate for the nursing profession within the policy and healthcare communities.			
6. Develop, evaluate, and provide leadership for healthcare policy that shapes healthcare financing, regulation, and delivery.			
7. Advocate for social justice, equity, and ethical policies within all healthcare arenas.			

Essential VI: Interprofessional Collaboration for Improving Patient and Population Health Outcomes Competencies	DNP student competency rating	Needed for project	Needed for practicum
1. Employ effective communication and collaborative skills in the development and implementation of practice models, peer review, practice guidelines, health policy, standards of care, and/or other scholarly products.			
2. Lead interprofessional teams in the analysis of complex practice and organizational issues.			
3. Employ consultative and leadership skills with intraprofessional and interprofessional teams to create change in healthcare and complex healthcare delivery systems.			
Essential VII: Clinical Prevention and Population Health for Improving the Nation's Health Competencies	DNP student competency rating	Needed for project	Needed for practicum
1. Analyze epidemiological, biostatistical, environmental, and other appropriate scientific data related to individual, aggregate, and population health.			
2. Synthesize concepts, including psychosocial dimensions and cultural diversity, related to clinical prevention and population health in developing, implementing, and evaluating interventions to address health promotion/disease prevention efforts, improve health status/access patterns, and/or address gaps in care of individuals, aggregates, or populations.			
3. Evaluate care delivery models and/or strategies using concepts related to community, environmental, and occupational health, and cultural and socioeconomic dimensions of health.			

Essential VIII: Advanced Nursing Practice Competencies	DNP student competency rating	Needed for project	Needed for practicum
1. Conduct a comprehensive and systematic assessment of health and illness parameters in complex situations, incorporating diverse and culturally sensitive approaches.			
2. Design, implement, and evaluate therapeutic interventions based on nursing science and other sciences.			
3. Develop and sustain therapeutic relationships and partnerships with patients (individual, family, or group) and other professionals to facilitate optimal care and patient outcomes.			
4. Demonstrate advanced levels of clinical judgment, systems thinking, and accountability in designing, delivering, and evaluating evidence-based care to improve patient outcomes.			
5. Guide, mentor, and support other nurses to achieve excellence in nursing practice.			
6. Educate and guide individuals and groups through complex health and situational transitions.			
7. Use conceptual and analytical skills in evaluating the links among practice, organizational, populations, fiscal, and policy issues.			

Key:

Assessment	Explanation
Low-moderate-high	Student self-rated competency
*	Competencies needed for the scholarly project
**	Identified professional growth need for the project
^	Additional identified professional growth need

Modified from American Association of Colleges of Nursing. (2006). The essentials of doctoral education for advanced nursing practice. Retrieved from http://www.aacn.nche.edu/publications/position/DNPEssentials.pdf

Appendix B: Concept Map Template

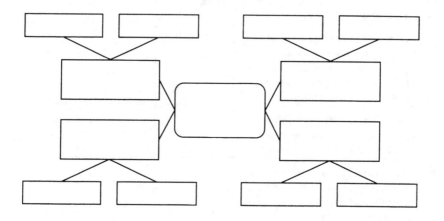

Appendix C: Template for Project Plan

(Project Name)

Project Plan

(Student Name)

(University)

(Date)

Table of Contents

1. Introduction
    1.1 Purpose of the Project Plan
2. Executive Summary
3. Project Goals and Objectives
4. Scope
5. Project Administration
    5.1 Structure
    5.2 Boundaries
    5.3 Roles and Responsibilities
6. Project Management
    6.1 Assumptions and Risks/Constraints
    6.2 Risk Management Plan
    6.3 Monitoring Plan
    6.4 Staffing Plan
    6.5 Communication Management Plan
7. Software and Hardware Requirements
    7.1 Security
8. Work Breakdown Structure
    8.1 Work Structure
    8.2 Relationships
    8.3 Resources
    8.4 Cost Management
    8.5 Schedule/Time Management
9. Quality Management
    9.1 Milestones
    9.2 Quality Indicators
10. Project Initiation Plan
11. Training Plan
12. Procurement Plan
13. Appendices

1. Introduction
   1.1 Purpose of Project Plan
2. Executive Summary
3. Project Goals and Objectives
4. Scope
5. Project Administration
   5.1 Structure

   5.2 Boundaries

   5.3 Roles & Responsibilities
6. Project Management
   6.1 Assumptions and Risks/Constraints

   Assumptions

   Risks/Constraints

   6.2 Risk Management Plan

   6.3 Monitoring Plan

   6.4 Staffing Plan

   6.5 Communication Management Plan
7. Software and Hardware Requirements
   7.1 Security
8. Work Breakdown Structure
   8.1 Work Structure

   8.2 Relationships

   8.3 Resources

   8.4 Cost Management

   8.5 Schedule/Time Management

9. Quality Management
   9.1 Milestones

Milestone	Description	Estimated Completion Date

   9.2 Quality Indicators
10. Project Initiation Plan
11. Training Plan
12. Procurement Plan
13. Appendices

This plan was adapted from the Centers for Disease Control (n.d.), North Carolina Enterprise (2004), and Project Management Docs (n.d.).

Appendix D: Sample Budget

Program Expenses

Salaries/Wages[a]

Itemize human resource costs in this section (i.e., administrative support, practitioner, etc.).

	Monthly	Total
•	$	$
•	$	$
•	$	$
•	$	$
Total Salary Costs		$

Startup Costs

Itemize startup costs in this section (i.e., copies, charts, display board, etc.).

•	$
•	$
•	$
Total Startup Costs	$

Capital Costs

Hardware	$
Equipment	$
Other	$
Total Capital Costs	$

Operational Costs

Itemize operational costs in this section (i.e., electricity, heat, etc.).

•	$
•	$
•	$
Total Project Expenses	$

Program Revenue[b]

Revenue Generation

Itemize potential revenue in this section.

•	$
•	$
•	$
	$
Total Project Revenue	$

Program Benefit/Loss

Total Revenue	$
Less Expenses	$
Total Program Benefit/Loss	$

[a] Include either actual wages paid (if available) or median full-time salary for the same position in the United States. An additional 30% may be added to wages to cover benefits.

[b] For example, revenue attained through billable evaluation and management codes, teaching codes, and so on.

Adapted from Moran, K., Burson, R., Critchett, J., & Olla, P. (2011). Exploring the cost and clinical outcomes of integrating the registered nurse certified diabetes educator in the patient centered medical home. *The Diabetes Educator, 37*(6), 780–793.

Appendix E: DNP Project Charter

Project Name:

Project Lead:

Date:

Project Overview (Including background)

Project Scope

Risks (If the project is not done)
1.
2.
3.
4.

Stakeholders
1.
2.
3.
4.

Project Team (List team members and roles each will play)
1.
2.
3.
4.

Desired Outcomes (Overall goals)
1.
2.
3.
4.

Objectives (Must be achieved to complete the project)
1.
2.
3.
4.

Project Deliverables (Those tasks that must be achieved to meet the objectives/complete the project)

<u>Metric</u>   <u>Target</u>
1.
2.
3.
4.

Project Timeline

Project Phase	Milestone	Estimated Month of Completion[a]					
		Jan	Feb	Mar	Apr	May	June
Initiation	Project charter approved						
Planning	Project planning meeting						
	Project plan completed →						
	Communication plan completed						
	IRB approved						
	Hardware and software approved						
Implementation	Training completed						
	Equipment approved						
Monitoring	Midproject evaluation complete						
Closing	Project completion meeting						

[a]An arrow (——→) is used to indicate the month the activity is estimated to be completed.

Project Risks/Constraints and Mitigation Plan (Any event that could have a negative impact on the project objectives and what will be done to address it proactively)

Risks	Mitigation
1.	
2.	
3.	
4.	
5.	

Assumptions (Factors that are assumed, for example, access to the setting, access to participants where applicable, and use of equipment)
1.
2.
3.
4.
5.

Project Resources (Staffing, equipment, etc.)
1.
2.
3.
4.
5.

Preliminary Budget

One-Time Costs		Project	Ongoing
Staff		$	$
Professional services		$	$
Other		$	$
	Total One-Time Costs	**$**	**$**
Capital Costs			
Hardware		$	$
Equipment		$	$
Other		$	$
	Total Capital Costs	**$**	**$**
Ongoing Costs			
Software license fees		$	$
Maintenance fees		$	$
Other		$	$
	Total Ongoing Costs	**$**	**$**

Signatures:

_____

Advisor/Chair [date]

_____

DNP Student [date]

Adapted from Stanford University Information Technology Services. (2008). *IT services project charter*. Retrieved from http://www.stanford.edu/dept/its/projects/PMO/files/pm_checklist.html

Appendix F: DNP Communication Plan

1. Introduction
In this section, briefly describe the project and communication goals.

2. Contact List

Team Member Name	Role	Work Number	Cell Number	Email Address

3. Reports

Document (Description)	Name of Recipients	Method for Distribution (email, etc.)	Who Is Responsible for the Distribution?	Frequency of Distribution

4. Project Meetings

Meeting	Purpose	Participants	Meeting Leader	Meeting Frequency

Adapted from North Carolina Enterprise. (2004). Project management plan template; IEEE. (1988). 1058.1-1987 IEEE Standard for Software Project Management Plans.

Appendix G: DNP Project Meeting

Date:

Location:

Facilitator:

Attendees:

Please review before the meeting:

AGENDA ITEMS

Discussion Topic
✓
✓
✓
✓
✓
✓
✓
✓
✓
✓

ACTION ITEMS

Description: **Assigned to:**   **Due date:**
✓
✓
✓

Appendix H: Project Status Report

Name:

Date:

Completed Activities
Complete/Date of Completion •   •

Activities in Progress
Activity/Estimated Date of Completion •   •   •   Issues •

Planned Activities
Planned Activity/Estimated Date of Completion •   •   •   •   Risks •   •

Modified from Centers for Disease Control and Prevention–Document Library. (n.d.). *Status reporting.* Retrieved from http://www2.cdc.gov/cdcup/library/matrix/default.htm

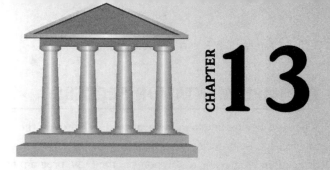

CHAPTER 13

Project Implementation

Katherine Moran and Rosanne Burson

CHAPTER OVERVIEW

The implementation phase occurs only after extensive development, planning, and communication. This chapter highlights aspects of the implementation phase that the doctor of nursing practice (DNP) student must consider to reach his or her intended goals.

CHAPTER OBJECTIVES

After completing this chapter, the learner will be able to:

1. Identify components of implementation success
2. Discuss the importance of project implementation planning
3. List the key factors associated with operationalizing the project plan
4. Define the most valuable characteristics of an effective leader
5. Describe the project implementation close-out phase

THE IMPLEMENTATION PROCESS

When it is finally time to implement the DNP project, the student will undoubtedly feel a sense of relief, excitement for what is yet to come, and possibly a little trepidation. Progressing to this point in the DNP program takes a lot of commitment and perseverance. It is likely that many months of planning have already been invested in conceptualizing the project. The phenomenon of interest has been identified, various project types have been explored, appropriate identification of measurable outcomes has occurred (see Chapter 14, Aligning Design, Method, and Evaluation with the Clinical Question), and finally a decision has been made and the project plan is developed.

> Operationalizing the plan is the action phase of the project plan.

Now it is time for the next step— operationalizing the plan. This is the action phase of the project plan.

How Leadership Influences Project Implementation

Most people would agree that the project leader/manager influences or at least has an impact on the overall project success, especially where project implementation is concerned. Right or wrong, good results or outcomes tend to be associated with good leaders. However, there is more to the story than meets the eye. Successful project management involves the coordination of project activities, team member needs, team needs, stakeholder needs, and organizational needs. The goal is to reach a balance with these competing priorities (see **Figure 13-1**).

There is a plethora of information in the literature on the topic of what it takes to be an effective leader. **Table 13-1** outlines a few of the characteristics

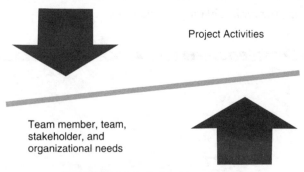

Project Activities

Team member, team, stakeholder, and organizational needs

FIGURE 13-1 Balancing priorities.

Table 13-1 Characteristics of an Effective Leader

Personal	Skills	Qualities
Charismatic	Leads by example	Enthusiastic
Confident	Persuasive	Assertive
Humble	Communicates effectively	Knowledgeable
Selfless	Manages multiple priorities	Flexible
Visionary	Motivational	Respectful
Caring	Active listener	Emotional intelligence
Positive attitude	Fiscally responsible	Imaginative
People oriented	Decisive	Driven to succeed

associated with effective leadership. A good leader is able to draw on his or her skill set and use the appropriate skills, at the appropriate time, to keep the project in balance. The skills used are based on the needs of the moment. For example, when there is an urgent matter that needs resolution, the leader will be assertive, confident, and decisive.

The skills or competencies the DNP student will need to demonstrate to be a successful project leader are incorporated in *Essential* II—Organizational and Systems Leadership for Quality Improvement and Systems Thinking (American Association of Colleges of Nursing [AACN], 2006). See Chapter 7, Interprofessional and Intraprofessional Collaboration in the Scholarly Project, for the National Center for Healthcare Leadership (2010)—defined leadership competencies for medicine, nursing, and administration. The project leader must have an understanding of his or her skill set as a leader and the behaviors that correspond to project implementation factors. A few critical leadership abilities include setting goals and objectives, project planning, team building, decision making, consulting with stakeholders, project ownership, problem solving, communicating, being enthusiastic, and motivating others.

A high degree of emotional competence is required to become a successful project leader (see Chapter 10, Driving the Practicum to Impact the Scholarly Project). Emotional competence behavior includes self-awareness, compassion, passionate optimism, mindfulness, personal humility, appreciation of ambiguity and paradox, appreciation of knowledge, willpower, resilience, and impulse control (Porter-O'Grady & Malloch, 2015). Self-awareness includes understanding self and others' unique perceptions and preferred styles of interaction. It also incorporates the ability to be comfortable with ambiguity and unclear paths, to be open to other viewpoints and new information. Compassionate leaders combine an understanding of the context of situations with the policies of an organization. In other words, a leader looks at the personal side of the equation, as well as what is best for the organization, to deliver a solution. Passionate optimism involves maintaining a positive mindset and resilience, even with the promise of disappointments. Mindfulness refers to being aware of recurring situations, how other members of the team responded, then being able to interpret these situations, and use what is learned to guide future behavior. Finally, impulse control is the ability to temper negative feelings while sharing feelings (Porter-O'Grady & Malloch, 2015). Chism (2016) discusses the aspects of emotional competence specifically in the DNP as an important leadership competency.

Project implementation is also the time during which the DNP student will demonstrate the characteristics and behaviors of all the DNP *Essentials*. Those involved with the project will have an opportunity to view the competencies of the DNP-prepared nurse. This is the time to begin marketing yourself and your degree. Chism (2016) states that the DNP-prepared nurse ". . . may develop a brand to share what unique talents, skills and knowledge they bring to their career environment" (p. 364). The DNP student should focus on articulating what a DNP degree *is* as well as the *strengths* the DNP-prepared nurse brings to the organization. This can be accomplished using an "elevator speech" (Chism, 2016). Be prepared to present a 1-minute, 3-minute, and 5-minute version of your elevator speech. There will be opportunities, often when least expected, to market the DNP degree and the skills that DNP-prepared nurses bring to the table.

WHAT CONSTITUTES PROJECT SUCCESS?

Whether a project is considered a success is largely dependent on the perception of the key stakeholders, including the student, university, organization where the project is implemented, and patients (when applicable). In Chapter 9, Creating and Developing the Project Plan, it was noted that if the project goals are met on schedule and within the budget, and there is a high level of satisfaction regarding the outcome, then the project will likely be considered a success. This makes sense, but what are the factors that are associated with successful projects? How can these factors be leveraged to improve outcomes?

FACTORS TO CONSIDER DURING PROJECT IMPLEMENTATION

Pinto and Slevin (1987) are well versed in project implementation and have been recognized for their interpretation of factors associated with successful project implementation. According to Pinto and Slevin (1987), the following factors are involved in project implementation:

- Top management support, mission, and schedule
- The client, personnel, and technical skills
- Monitoring, feedback, and communication
- Troubleshooting
- Client acceptance.

Project Planning
Management Support, Mission, and Schedule

As mentioned in Chapter 9, an important aspect of successful project implementation is a carefully considered plan. From this perspective, the most important piece of advice the doctoral student should consider when developing the DNP project is to *plan ahead*. The student really needs to take the time to carefully consider what he or she wants to achieve in the project and build a solid business case that will garner top management support. First, be clear regarding what the overall goal is; what is it that you want to achieve (i.e., the expected benefits), and then develop objectives that will lead to the desired outcome. These objectives need to be measureable (so that you know if you achieved the goal). When developing the project objectives, think about the 'critical success factors' and/or project deliverables that will be needed to assure project success (Haughey, 2014). The project deliverables should be relevant to the project, of course, but they should also be of interest to the stakeholders. From the organization's perspective, deliverables that relate to improving healthcare quality, the patient experience, efficiency, reducing costs, and so on are always important to keep in mind. Next, consider the time that will be needed to complete the project, and then *add time* to the schedule to account for unexpected delays. In other words, expect the unexpected.

There is an old carpenter saying, "measure twice, cut once"—which essentially means that a person has only one shot at cutting the piece of wood, so he or she

> The most important piece of advice the doctoral student should consider when developing the DNP project is to *plan ahead*.

should take the time to get it right the first time. In other words, it pays to do the legwork up front. As mentioned in Chapter 6, Developing the Scholarly Project, Pareto's principle is applicable to planning the DNP project; approximately 80% of the project is planning and 20% is implementation.

The first three factors of project implementation relate to the planning phase (Pinto & Slevin, 1987). These factors were addressed in Chapter 9 in more detail. However, the key messages here are to first make sure there is top management support for the project before even considering implementation. Without management support, the resources needed for the project are in jeopardy.

As mentioned, presenting a solid business case for the project is critical. The DNP student can strengthen the business case by taking the time to complete an organization needs assessment (see Chapter 5, The Phenomenon of Interest). Equally important is the need to communicate the project purpose and goals clearly to all of the stakeholders. Key stakeholders are more likely to support the project when they have a clear understanding of the project goals, including how the goals are aligned with the mission and vision of the organization; stakeholder support is critical (see Chapter 6, Developing the Scholarly Project).

> Key stakeholders are more likely to support the project when they have a clear understanding of the project goals, and stakeholder support is critical.

A White Paper, a 5–7 page document that is targeted at the organization, may be helpful in communicating the recommended project to the stakeholders. The purpose of a White Paper is to provide useful, practical, and educational content that helps stakeholders understand an issue, solve a problem, and/or make a decision regarding a project (Graham, 2013). The organizational needs assessment informs the following elements of the White Paper (Graham, 2013):

- Purpose
- Significance
- Current practice
- New evidence
- Intervention
- Considerations
- Recommendations.

Finally, the doctoral student should develop a project schedule that sufficiently and realistically outlines the various stages of the implementation process, including all activities, milestones, and team member roles and responsibilities in relation to the time needed for completion. The project schedule will be a useful document to help the student manage and meet the project deadlines. See Chapter 12, The Scholarly Project Toolbox, for an example of a project schedule. The next seven factors in the outline really involve operationalization of the project plan. This is the action phase of the project implementation process (Pinto & Slevin, 1987).

Operationalizing the Project Plan
The Client, Personnel, and Technical Skills

The next two factors to consider in the operationalization phase of project implementation relate to human resources. These include the client (defined as anyone who has an interest in the result of the project) and personnel recruitment, selection, and training (Pinto & Slevin, 1987). First, consider the client's needs. The student needs to make sure that the end users (i.e., key stakeholders or those who will be affected by the outcome of the project) are consulted during this process to help inform the project. See Chapter 6 for more information on identifying key stakeholders. Next, the student needs to gather the team. What is most important to note about the team is the need to select the *right person* with the *right skill set* for the *right job*. Certainly, the team includes the student's advisor and/or the project faculty mentor, and practice mentor, but the team may also include additional members whose primary responsibilities are implementing various aspects of the project. For example, certainly it is important to have the technology available to support the project, but it is also important that team members possess the ability to use technology to successfully meet the project goals and objectives.

In addition to having the right skill mix, team members also need to be committed to the project. When commitment is lacking on the part of any team member, the project outcome can be negatively impacted. Once the team is gathered, it is time to prepare for training. As mentioned earlier in this book, most projects will require some form of team member training or coaching prior to implementation. During this process, the training plan is considered and discussion regarding the need to work as a team to meet project goals is stressed. See Chapter 9 for more information on training the team.

Monitoring, Feedback, and Communication

Project monitoring and feedback are facilitated via a monitoring plan, which often involves further project refinement and/or adjustments to the plan. This

> The goal is to identify any potential problems early in the implementation phase and to address them before they become major issues.

includes tracking adherence to the project timeline, budget, and milestones. The goal is to identify any potential problems early in the implementation phase and to address them before they become major issues. For example, one problem that is sometimes encountered during project implementation is 'scope creep,' that is, the project grows in size. This can lead to a project running over budget or even not completing on time (Haughey, 2014). Having a well-defined project scope that all key stakeholders agree to is important; then you need to stick to it.

The monitoring process involves problem solving, decision making, and managing any project changes and/or risks; but, part of the monitoring process also involves making sure that team members are meeting project goals and expectations, while encouraging them to continue to meet objectives. This is important because an essential piece of monitoring and communication is motivation. Prabhakar (2008) states, "One of the biggest ways to motivate people and to convince them of the potential for successful outcomes is to communicate effectively" (p. 6). Therefore, when monitoring team members' productivity, it is important to give timely feedback, communicate effectively, and to be sensitive to individual team members' needs. In addition, as stressed by Pinto and Slevin (1987), it is critical to communicate effectively with key stakeholders, such as the organization where the project is being implemented.

Finally, the identification of issues and barriers is also part of the monitoring process. As mentioned in Chapter 10, Driving the Practicum to Impact the Scholarly Project, barriers may be identified prior to or during implementation. To keep the project on track, the DNP student should consider the following common barriers to project implementation (Flick, 2009):

1. Lack of clarity—when the project team or stakeholders do not understand the project goals and objectives and/or their respective roles and responsibilities.
2. Project requirements have not been defined—also a contributing factor to lack of clarity; make sure all of the stakeholders agree on the project requirements.
3. Resources are not adequate to meet project goals—a comprehensive project plan must include all of the resources needed to implement the project, including resources that may be needed to sustain the change once the project is completed.

4. Lack of stakeholder support—ongoing effective communication can help mitigate this barrier.

5. Biases (the stakeholder's and yours)—make sure you can deliver what you promise. Stakeholders may have had past experiences where outcomes were "over-promised and under-delivered." This can set a negative tone before the project begins; again, effective communication is the key.

6. Technology gap—as mentioned, it is important to have technology available to support the project, but it is also important that team members possess the ability to use technology to successfully meet the project goals and objectives. The DNP student will also want to consider whether a technology gap exists from the perspective of the stakeholders; especially if the project is technology based.

7. Resistance to change—as most projects involve interaction with other people, it is wise for the DNP student to assess the potential for resistance to change and consider ways to overcoming resistance when developing the project plan. One way to overcome resistance is to make sure all stakeholders understand the benefits of the project. A White Paper may be a useful tool in communicating succinctly to stakeholders.

8. Lack of time—this is a critical factor that can be mitigated with a realistic timeline.

9. Not invented here—this barrier relates to DNP students who attempt to implement a project in an organization where they do not have an established relationship. If this is the case, it is helpful for the student to choose a practice mentor who can open organizational doors and be a champion for the project early on.

10. Political barriers—organizational culture, strategic priorities, and so on, are examples of political barriers that are important to consider. Again, a thoughtful project plan prevents most problems.

As you can see, for the most part, successful project implementation begins and ends with effective communication as well as having a well-developed plan to address and hopefully overcome barriers. Prabhakar (2008) notes that it may be necessary to adjust the plan to improve opportunities for success and cites the following 10 key factors that can be used to improve project performance during implementation:

1. Bypass an obstacle
2. Cause people to stretch
3. Focus on the goal

4. Follow a standardized process
5. Learn from the past
6. Maintain ongoing communications
7. Document the work being done
8. Reuse previous work
9. Seek buy-in from all involved
10. Seek simplicity, not complexity, in goal and path (p. 6).

Following these recommendations will ensure a path to project success that will be identified in the close-out phase. Further, the identification and eventual overcoming of the barriers may actually strengthen the commitment of the key stakeholders and improve the final product.

Troubleshooting

It is virtually impossible to predict every potential problem that could come up during project implementation. The key is to monitor the implementation process carefully, troubleshoot any identified issues early, and develop a mitigation plan. Here is where the value of the student's problem-solving skills will be recognized, as he or she works with the team to develop a strategy to overcome barriers. Monitoring and troubleshooting could be necessary in the areas of the planning process, the budget, personnel issues, or identification of participants, to name a few. See Chapter 12, The Scholarly Project Toolbox, for information regarding the tools available for the student to use in the troubleshooting/problem-solving process.

> The key to successful project implementation is to monitor the process carefully, troubleshoot any identified issues early, and develop a mitigation plan.

Client Acceptance

At this stage in the process, the student will find out if the project end result was valuable to the key stakeholders. In most cases, the student will already have a good idea of how the project has been received. However, in some cases, even though the project was completed on time, stayed within its budget, and the student had communicated effectively and managed the project as expected, the end user of the project *may or may not* find the end result valuable. The best way to prevent an unexpected outcome is to include key stakeholders early in the process (Pinto & Slevin, 1987). The student should ensure that stakeholders are engaged in the project and that they feel they have some ownership in the outcome. As mentioned previously, stakeholder support is critical, even at the end of the project.

> Stakeholder support is critical, even at the end of the project.

Close-out Phase

Once the implementation phase is complete, the close-out phase begins. The close-out phase includes an evaluation of the process and the outcomes. Clearly delineating the evaluation tool that will be used in the project and identifying the measurable outcomes early in the project planning phase are essential. Certainly by now one can recognize how important it is to plan appropriately for each phase of the project. Choosing an evaluation method that is appropriate for the project and its purpose is necessary to effectively evaluate the final outcome of the project. Hickey and Brosnan (2012) state that "the form of an evaluation is based on its intended purpose and use" (p. xi). Areas of evaluation include:

1. Economic
2. Organization and system
3. Healthcare informatics and patient care technology
4. Patient care standard guidelines and protocols
· 5. Populations
6. Conceptual models (Hickey & Brosnan, 2012).

Other components of the evaluation plan should include communication of the findings, as well as participant satisfaction results, to all key stakeholders. "Lessons learned, barriers that were overcome during the implementation phase, and strategies used to overcome the barriers could further inform the project" (Beene, 2012, p. 83) and should be included in the final report.

At this point in the project implementation phase, it is important to acknowledge the team and other supporters for a job well done and to show appreciation for all efforts. Also acknowledge your own accomplishment and take time to reflect on the experience and satisfaction of completing the project.

In the following excerpt, Dr. Christina Worgess shares her DNP project implementation experience in a primary care practice.

Improving Diabetes Care Through Provider Adherence to Diabetes Practice Guidelines: A Primary Care Based Quality Improvement Project
Christina Worgess, DNP, FNP-C, RN

My final project was to evaluate and improve current provider adherence to the American Diabetes Association's Standards of Medical Care in Diabetes in a primary care practice using the Institute for Healthcare Improvement Model for Improvement. It was implemented in a practice that served greater than 4,500 recurrent patients with approximately 35% of the population having a primary or secondary diagnosis of diabetes. An initial randomized chart review provided data to the practice improvement team who determined the project goals, which included improving the percentage of patients obtaining urine microalbumin, ophthalmology referral, and comprehensive foot exam. Utilizing the Plan, Do, Study, Act (PDSA) process, initial results showed an improvement in all areas within 6 weeks: 41.6%, 51.6%, and 51.6%, respectively. In addition to improvement in adherence to practice guidelines, there was an increase in staff awareness of their value in the practice and a sense of accomplishment of their role in the project. But most importantly, it provided the ground work to improve patient quality of care, increase patient knowledge in the disease process, and decreased the potential risk of diabetes complications.

Although the DNP project brought many challenges and accomplishments, lessons were learned throughout the implementation phase. I realized my role as a leader was more pronounced than I could have imagined. I had to lead team members through a new process as effectively and efficiently as possible, which required assertiveness, confidence, and accurate decision making. It was important for the physicians in the practice and office staff to have a clear understanding of pre-implementation data in order to contribute to the planning and support the project. Team meetings were held to disseminate data, explain the project in detail, provide key players with a description of their role, and to coordinate all project activities. It was essential to conduct the meetings frequently in the beginning to assure a successful project completion. Once the team planning phase was completed and the project was underway, continued monitoring and communication were key elements. Nothing could be left to assumption. I continued to make daily contact with the team members, which allowed me to provide additional support and address concerns quickly. After the first week, the trepidation of tackling such a project began to subside and a team bond began to form. I became more confident and comfortable in my leadership role. I was able to share my knowledge with others and became empowered to reach higher and farther in order to benefit the population I serve.

If I were to offer advice or a recommendation to the DNP student who is ready to implement their project, communication with all stakeholders would be at the top of the list. High quality project planning is critical to the implementation of the DNP project and its success. This takes a considerable amount of time, evaluation, re-evaluation, project coordination, team building, perseverance, and above all open, effective and continuous communication with all stake holders involved. During the implementation of my DNP project, communication proved to be my most valuable tool. Each key player needs to have a clear understanding of their role in the project and it cannot be assumed that "no news is good news." The DNP student leader must be persistent in follow-up, available to answer questions, troubleshoot any conflict or barriers, and be prepared to redirect and reinstruct team members as needed. Assuring practice support is also essential to the success of this DNP project. Clear and precise goals must be defined in order to evaluate outcomes and project effectiveness. Finally, during the implementation stage it is critical to maintain ongoing assessment of the project progress and continue to communicate effectively with all stakeholders, so that adjustments can be made to ensure project goals are met.

Key Messages

- Include key stakeholders early in the planning and implementation process.
- Gather an effective team by selecting the *right person* with the *right skill set* for the *right job*.
- Identify any potential problems early in the implementation phase and address them before they become major issues.
- When monitoring team members' productivity, it is important to give timely feedback, communicate effectively, and be sensitive to individual team members' needs.
- Successful project management involves the coordination of project activities, team member needs, team needs, stakeholder needs, and organizational needs.
- A good leader is able to draw on his or her skill set and utilize the appropriate skills, at the appropriate time, to keep the project in balance.
- Emotional competence in the DNP is an important leadership competency.
- The close-out phase includes an evaluation of the process and the outcome.
- After the project is completed, it is important to acknowledge the team and other supporters for a job well done.

Action Plan—Next Steps

1. Plan ahead to implement your project.
2. Implement the project using leadership skills.
3. Monitor the progress of the project through implementation.
4. Close out the project by reporting the planned outcomes and lessons learned.
5. Plan an elevator speech.

REFERENCES

American Association of Colleges of Nursing. (2006). *The essentials of doctoral education for advanced nursing practice.* Retrieved from http://www.aacn.nche.edu/DNP/pdf/Essentials.pdf

Beene, M. S. (2012). Implementing a project. In J. L. Harris, L. Roussel, S. E. Walters, & C. Dearman (Eds.), *Project planning and management* (pp. 79–92). Burlington, MA: Jones & Bartlett Learning.

Chism, L. A. (2016). *The doctor of nursing practice: A guidebook for role development and professional issues.* Burlington, MA: Jones & Bartlett Learning.

Flick, S. (2009). How to reduce barriers to project implementation? Retrieved from http://www.bizmanualz.com/blog/top-ten-obstacles-to-project-implementation.html

Graham, G. (2013). *White papers for dummies.* Hoboken, NJ: John Wiley & Sons, Inc.

Haughey, D. (2014). Eight key factors to ensuring project success. Retrieved from http://www.projectsmart.co.uk/docs/eight-key-factors-to-ensuring-project-success.pdf

Hickey, J. V., & Brosnan, C. A. (2012). *Evaluation of health care quality in advanced practice nursing.* New York, NY: Springer.

National Center for Healthcare Leadership. (2010). *Health Leadership competency model summary.* Retrieved from http://www.nchl.org/Documents/NavLink/Competency_Model-summary_uid31020101024281.pdf

Pinto, J. K., & Slevin, D. P. (1987). Critical success factors in effective project implementation. Retrieved from http://gspa.grade.nida.ac.th/pdf/PA%20780%20(Pakorn)/8.Critical%20Success%20Factors%20in%20Effective%20Project%20Implementati.pdf

Porter-O'Grady, T., & Malloch, K. (2015). *Quantum leadership: Building better partnerships for sustainable health* (4th ed.). Sudbury, MA: Jones & Bartlett Learning.

Prabhakar, G. P. (2008). What is project success: A literature review. *International Journal of Business and Management, 3*(9), 3–10.

DOCTOR OF NURSING PRACTICE OUTCOMES

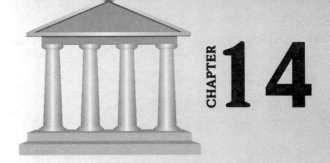

CHAPTER 14

Aligning Design, Method, and Evaluation with the Clinical Question

Patricia Rouen

CHAPTER OVERVIEW

The doctor of nursing practice (DNP) project process is an exciting and rich experience that sets the stage for future scholarship and contributions to nursing practice. Just as DNP projects vary in their designs and methods, implementation processes and evaluation are also diverse. The importance of a tight project that aligns the scientific approach with the appropriate design, methodology, and evaluation cannot be understated. The goal of this chapter is to introduce the DNP student to the general processes and most common components of project design, data collection, and evaluation. Resources that support DNP project work are identified, with an emphasis on interprofessional collaboration.

CHAPTER OBJECTIVES

After completing this chapter, the learner will be able to:

1. Select a design for the DNP project that is congruent with the project aim
2. Propose methods and outcome measures for the DNP project
3. Identify and describe the analytical approach for data evaluation in the DNP project
4. Describe the elements of interprofessional collaboration that contribute to DNP project implementation

IT STARTS WITH DESIGN

Design is a plan for arranging elements in such a way as best to accomplish a purpose.
—*Charles Eames*

The holistic nature of nursing practice invites DNP students to explore a wide variety of phenomena that eventually guide the DNP project. As such, DNP projects are diverse and may take on many forms, requiring different methodological approaches. In these situations, the DNP project team and student work together to determine the best design to guide the project and to ensure rigor and measure success. Just as DNP projects are diverse in scope and design, data collection methods and processes are also quite varied. A critical component of the DNP project is the congruence between the project aim(s) and study design, with the data collection and analysis plan. This congruence is a key factor in ensuring the veracity and accuracy of the DNP project outcome(s). The congruence between the design, methods, and analysis plan is discussed and evaluated by the doctoral project team as part of the project approval process. See Chapter 8, The DNP Project Team, for more information about DNP team functions.

> The designs and methods of the DNP project should be congruent with the purpose and goals.

DNP projects use a variety of approaches including quality improvement, program and policy evaluation, evidence-based practice (EBP) initiatives, and components of quantitative and qualitative research methodologies to evaluate, innovate, or improve practice (**Table 14-1**). The design choice for the project is always driven

Table 14-1 DNP Project Approaches

	Research	Quality Improvement (QI)	Evidence-Based Practice (EBP)	Program Evaluation (PE)
Definition	Systematic investigation including development, testing, and evaluation designed to develop or contribute to generalizable knowledge (U.S. Department of Health and Human Services [DHHS], 2009)	Systematic data-guided activities to monitor, evaluate, and improve quality and safety outcomes of health services and care processes (Adapted from Cronenwett et al., 2007; U.S. DHHS, 2011)	A systematic approach that integrates the review and appraisal of the best available scientific evidence combined with clinical expertise and patient/population circumstances to guide care delivery (Adapted from Melynk & Fineout-Overhold, 2011, Sackett, Rosenberg, Gray, Haynes & Richardson, 2000)	A systematic assessment of the processes and/or outcomes of a program, guided by standards, to make judgments regarding the program's effectiveness, improve its effectiveness, and guide further development (Centers for Disease Control and Prevention [CDC], 2011)
Purpose	Investigate or answer a research question relevant to nursing practice	Improvement or innovation in healthcare outcomes or workflow processes	Integration of evidence into practice (Shirey et al., 2011)	Evaluation of a program's achievements and effectiveness
Methods	Scientific method, clinical question, or hypothesis Quantitative, qualitative, or mixed methods approaches	Plan-Do-Study-Act Six Sigma LEAN Failure Mode Effects Analysis Root cause analysis Structure Process Outcome (Donabedian, 2005)	IOWA model (Titler et al., 2001) ARCC (Melynk & Fineout-Overholt, 2011) ACE (Stevens, 2004) PARIHS (Rycroft-Malone, 2004) Stetler Model (Stetler, 2001) Johns Hopkins Hospital Nursing EBP Model (Newhouse, Dearholt, Poe, Pugh & White, 2007) Rosswurm & Larrabee Model (1999)	CDC Framework (1999) Logic model (Millar, Simeone, & Carnevale, 2001) Balanced scorecard (Kaplan & Norton, 1992) CIPP (Stufflebeam, 1983)

(Continued)

Table 14-1 DNP Project Approaches (*Continued*)

	Research	Quality Improvement (QI)	Evidence-Based Practice (EBP)	Program Evaluation (PE)
Data Collection	Multiple options Surveys, standardized instruments, physiologic measures, registries or database extraction, interviews, observations, focus groups	Multiple options Surveys, check sheets, process flow diagrams, cause-and-effect diagrams, clinical record reviews or data extraction, interviews, observations, focus groups, key informants, system/stakeholder assessment	Literature search Literature review System/stakeholder assessment Baseline and/or post-implementation measures of outcomes relevant to the practice guideline integration	Multiple options to measure the program's execution, outcomes, and impact System/stakeholder assessment, resource review, surveys, interviews, focus groups, program costs and measures for the specific program goals
Data Analytics	Specific to the clinical question or hypothesis Emphasis on quantitative and qualitative techniques; fiscal analyses. Process and outcome evaluation for intervention and implementation projects	Specific to the quality issue Quantitative and qualitative techniques Run charts Pareto charts Statistical process control Fiscal analyses	**Practice Guideline Development** Evaluation of evidence strength: *Quantitative Data* Levels of Evidence: I–VII (Melynk & Fineout-Overholt, 2011) Levels of Evidence (Johanna Briggs Institute [JBI], 2014a) Grades of Recommendations (JBI, 2014b)	Diverse approaches to measure processes and outcomes that can include quantitative and qualitative techniques and financial analyses

Intersections*	Research informs QI, EBP, and program evaluation New research can be initiated from gaps in EBP reviews	QI informs EBP QI can identify needs for research and program development	*Qualitative Data* CERQual: Confidence in Evidence from Reviews of Qualitative research (www.cerqual.org). *Guideline Assessment* AGREE-II (www.agree.trust.org) **Practice Integration Evaluation** Analysis of achievement of designated outcomes with quantitative, qualitative, and fiscal techniques EBP informs QI EBP evaluation identifies need for additional research EBP can guide program development and evaluation	PE informs and identifies opportunities for research, EBP and QI
	Interprofessional collaboration	Interprofessional collaboration	Interprofessional collaboration	Interprofessional collaboration

Data from CDC, 2011; Newhouse, 2007; Shirey et al., 2011; Schaffer, Sandau & Diedrick, 2012.

351

by the clinical question or issue. For example, clinical inquiry to evaluate a population health outcome, risk factor prevalence in a community, needs of a client group, or to determine the priority health issue of a community or organization may use a research approach. Common designs for these clinical questions are exploratory, descriptive, or correlational. These designs are considered observational and nonexperimental (because the outcome variable is only measured or compared) (Plichta & Kelvin, 2013), but they are valuable in determining the characteristics or needs of a unique population. Descriptive and correlational projects can also be used to assess behaviors of healthcare professionals, patients, communities, and systems or to provide baseline data that can be used to drive practice improvements.

Examples of exploratory DNP projects include:

- Perceived barriers to pain management among nursing staff in a long-term care facility
- Perceptions of body image, body satisfaction, and knowledge of obesity-related health risks among African-American college students
- Environmental and situational factors related to job stress and turnover in staff nurses in critical care.

When the DNP project aim is to initiate change via an intervention, practice improvement, or implementation of an innovative new model of care delivery, the design choice includes a research or a quality improvement (QI) approach. Experimental designs range from the randomized controlled trial to a quasi-experimental study. In practice settings, the quasi-experimental approach is helpful because it does not require randomization or a control group (Plichta & Kelvin, 2013). This design is capable of measuring change in health-related outcomes after treatment or intervention when it is not feasible to use a true experiment (Polit & Beck, 2012). The quasi-experimental approach is practical and useful in the clinical arena. Examples of DNP projects using this approach include:

> Quality improvement uses data-based methods to improve clinical or healthcare systems outcomes (Batalden & Davidoff, 2007)

- A spirituality-based physical activity intervention to promote weight loss in African-American women
- Implementation of group medical visits to improve glucose control in persons with diabetes
- A social media intervention to promote healthy eating and physical activity in low-income urban women.

Practice improvements guided by QI models are an important source of DNP project opportunities. QI uses data-based methods to improve clinical or healthcare systems processes and outcomes (Batalden & Davidoff, 2007). There are several QI approaches that may guide the DNP project: the well-known Plan-Do-Check-Act (PDCA) cycle, Lean methodology, and the Six Sigma process (see Chapter 12, The Scholarly Project Toolbox). These methods focus on process refinements to control variation and ultimately improve the designated outcome. QI involves the systematic collection and analysis of data to measure change, with growing emphasis on rapid cycle change. Other QI methodologies such as root cause analysis (RCA) and failure mode effects analysis (FMEA) are feasible tools for the DNP project that focus on retrospective analysis of untoward events (RCA) or the prospective assessment of risk (FMEA) to promote safety and quality in clinical outcomes. Competence in QI is an expectation in today's healthcare environment, and DNP projects using this approach make important data-driven contributions to practice. Examples of DNP projects using a QI approach include:

> Competence in QI is an expectation in today's healthcare environment, and DNP projects using this approach make important data-driven contributions to practice.

- A process improvement in a primary care office to reduce wait times and improve patient and provider satisfaction
- Implementation of an RN patient navigator to support hypertension medication adherence among high-risk clients in primary care
- Improving provider compliance with the use of a symptom-based individualized written asthma action plan.

Qualitative inquiry is another perspective that contributes to a DNP project. These types of designs provide evidence for practice when little is known about the phenomenon of interest (Miller, 2010). At other times, the phenomenon of interest may have been described in a population or social setting, but there is a gap in practice knowledge with a new group of clients or a new setting. Qualitative data provide a holistic understanding of phenomena, capture the real-world context, and are congruent with the nursing paradigm (Leeman & Sandelowski, 2012). The qualitative approach is flexible and feasible for use in practice. A qualitative component can be included in program evaluation, quality improvement, or in a research project to enrich the understanding of the clinical issue, especially from the system or key stakeholder's perspectives. There are several different types of qualitative inquiry, such as ethnography or grounded theory (Polit & Beck, 2012).

If qualitative data collection is being considered for a DNP project, consultation with a researcher skilled in these methods is highly recommended. Examples of qualitative projects that provide evidence for practice include:

- Perceptions of family support of African-American women with type 2 diabetes
- Perspectives of caring nurse practice in highly technical and complex care environments.

> Program evaluation is a systematic process to gather evidence that a project, program, or policy is effective and efficient.

Program evaluation (PE) is another option for the DNP project. PE is a systematic process to gather evidence that a project, program, or policy is effective and efficient. Guided by standards, program evaluation examines the processes, outcomes, and impact of the project and includes the key stakeholders or systems who participate in or are affected by the project. There are several models for program evaluation, and the selected approach should be congruent with the type of program that will be evaluated. Common models used in healthcare include, but are not limited to, the Logic model (Millar, Simeone, & Carnevale, 2001), the Centers for Disease Control and Prevention (CDC, 1999) framework for public health programs, the Balanced Scorecard (Kaplan & Norton, 1992) and the Context-Input-Process-Product model (CIPP; Stufflebeam, 1983). Parameters of program evaluation differ slightly among the models, but most address stakeholder engagement, available resources, planned activities, outputs, and outcomes with an assessment of the impact of the program. Outcomes can be varied and should align with selected framework and the purpose of the project. Some processes of program evaluation are similar to intervention research or QI, including the types of data collected (quantitative, qualitative, fiscal) and the options for data analysis. An important distinction of program evaluation is the pivotal role of collaboration with key stakeholders in the development and evaluation process and the use of formative and summative evaluation during program implementation (CDC, 2012). Examples of DNP projects that address program evaluation include:

- Evaluation of a nurse-practitioner-led smoking cessation program for rural adolescents
- Evaluation of a patient navigation program for colorectal cancer
- Outcome evaluation of a college-based sexual assault prevention program.

DNP projects also enhance evidence-based practice (EBP). EBP is a decision-making approach that incorporates clinical expertise and patient preferences with the best scientific evidence to guide healthcare interventions (Sackett, Rosenberg, Gray, Haynes & Richardson, 2000; Melynk & Fineout-Overholt, 2011). EBP emphasizes the integration of existing knowledge (evidence) into contemporary healthcare practice (Titler, 2011).

> EBP emphasizes the integration of existing knowledge (evidence) into contemporary healthcare practice (Titler, 2011).

Evidence-based DNP projects are developed using a systematic process that includes a critical appraisal of the literature to determine the best available evidence along with knowledge of the organizational culture and resources needs of the practice environment, to implement a planned change. EBP projects often produce practice guidelines or best practices statements that direct healthcare service delivery for specific clinical concerns or populations (Brouwers et al., 2010). As with other DNP projects, EBP initiatives are evaluated post implementation to measure outcome attainment and opportunities for guideline revision.

There are several models for EBP (Table 14-1) that can guide the DNP project. The six major models have several common elements and some differences. In their overview of the major models, Schaffer and colleagues (2012) noted that most models are applicable to organizational settings, while others address building capacity for EBP among clinicians. In planning the DNP project, it would be important to consider the model features to select a "best fit" approach that addresses the practice issue. Examples of DNP projects that use an EBP approach include:

- Development of a practice guideline for childhood obesity in a pediatric primary care practice
- Best practices in HIV screening for Native Americans
- Development of a depression screening and management protocol for elders in an assisted living setting.

Policy analysis or evaluation is another domain for the DNP project. Health policy analysis projects address outcomes related to healthcare quality, cost, and access in the context of a specific topic or population group. Policy may be examined at the macro- or microsystem level and from different theoretical perspectives (epidemiology, sociology, etc.). Data is used to guide policy analysis via metrics that document the specific concerns with the policy's achievement of its intended actions. The methods for health policy analysis are varied but consistently require a systematic assessment (Weimer & Vining, 2005) that weighs the benefits and liabilities associated with the policy, and provides evidence related to cost and quality of the expected outcomes. One of the more well-known approaches to policy analysis is Bardach's (2011) model, which recommends a summary of the policy issues, evaluation of supporting and opposing arguments, analysis of stakeholders, and anticipated impact on sentinel outcomes including population health benefits, costs, equity, and administrative feasibility. A student considering a health policy analysis for a DNP project should work with the project team to determine the most appropriate method. Examples of DNP projects that employ policy analysis include:

- Policy analysis: Community-based services programs and implications for rural elder care
- Contraception and unintended pregnancy in adolescents: Policy analysis of regional school-based teen programs.

DIVERSITY IN DNP PROJECTS

DNP projects are diverse and use different methodologies that address the broad perspective of nursing practice. Yet, while differences among the approaches exist, all employ interprofessional collaboration (see Chapter 7, Interprofessional and Intraprofessional Collaboration in the Scholarly Project), and use a systematic process that is data driven, evaluates outcomes, and provides evidence for nursing practice. The rich diversity of DNP project work also generates opportunities for future work among the different approaches. For example, EBP projects have the potential to identify other QI opportunities (Newhouse, 2007; Shirey et al., 2011) and provide data that can guide program development and evaluation. Further, gaps in the evidence can prompt new research studies. QI provides contextual data that can inform EBP initiatives as well as uncover needs for research (Shirey et al., 2011) and program development. Program evaluation can identify other opportunities for QI, EBP, and research projects. Data from clinical research can suggest the need for QI (Newhouse, 2007; Shirey et al., 2011) or new program development, as well as contribute to the pool of evidence-based data for practice. Policy analysis can suggest the need for

> All DNP projects use a systematic process that is data driven, evaluates outcomes, and provides evidence for nursing practice.

QI actions to improve policy outcomes, provide data to support EBP, identify gaps in the literature that requires more research, or suggest the need for new program development and evaluation.

DRIVEN BY DESIGN: DATA COLLECTION METHODS

Once the design and the specific aim(s) for the DNP project is determined, the next step is to select the data collection method. DNP projects can involve the collection of new data via surveys and interviews or evaluation of stored data from repositories such as electronic health records (EHRs) and national registries. It is critical that the data collection method is congruent with the study design and the project purpose (**Table 14-2**). Data collection methods should be broad enough to encompass measurement of the outcome or dependent variable, as well as the relevant independent and confounding factors thought to be related to the outcome variable.

> It is critical that the data collection method is congruent with the study design and the project purpose.

The major data collection methods used in research and QI projects include self-report via survey or structured interviews, direct observation, and physiological measures (Polit & Beck, 2012). QI projects may also use prospective logs or tracking sheets to collect real-time data. In addition, QI initiatives include process flow diagrams and cause-and-effect diagrams to guide the data collection process. Extraction of data from EHRs or registries can be used to evaluate clinical outcomes such as disease prevalence rates or immunization compliance, costs, or patterns in service usage to identify opportunities for QI, EBP and research projects, or the need for new programs. The most common qualitative data collection methods are focus groups or individual interviews, in which participants respond to open-ended questions, and investigators observe responses. This data is important for QI, EBP, and program evaluation projects as it provides insight into the organizational stakeholder's perspectives regarding the practice issue. Storytelling and written narratives are other choices for collecting qualitative data.

It is important to select the data collection method that is best suited for the DNP project goals. The data collection method should be feasible, practical, and amenable for use in the clinical setting or with the population of interest. For example, an online survey would be a method of choice if working with young adults or collecting input from stakeholders regarding a QI opportunity, while

Table 14-2 Practice Projects: Sample Outcome Evaluation Plans

Approach	Design	Purpose	Intervention/Action/Process	Outcome Measures	Analysis
Research	Intervention	Improve (1) nutrition knowledge and (2) physical activity in low-income women at risk for CVD	6-week cooking class 6-week yoga and self-directed walking program Weekly motivational text messages Interprofessional team	Pre-/post-clinical measures: Nutrition knowledge tool Weekly steps log End of program: Participant satisfaction (open and closed questions)	Descriptive statistics Paired *t* tests Repeated measures ANOVA Percentages Content analysis of comments
Quality Improvement	LEAN	Reduce wait times to 10 minutes or less on phones for patients in a primary care clinic	Collected and reviewed baseline data: number of calls every hour, minutes of wait time to answer, number of complaints related to phone issues	Outcome Measures: Extracted data from phone system: A. Number of calls answered within 10 minutes between 8 a.m. and 9 a.m; and 1 p.m. and 2 p.m.	Frequencies
		Improve patient satisfaction related to ability to access office staff	Focus group with providers, staff, and managers to review data and discuss options. Identified excess wait times at 8 a.m. and 1 p.m. Process map of clinic activities at those times. Brainstorming, cause-and-effect diagram, solution selection matrix, and multivoting to select feasible improvements	B. Average number of calls measured every hour	Run chart
				C. Average number of minutes waiting	Run chart

			Implementation plan: Pull three of the six medical assistants to answer phones between 8 a.m. and 9 a.m. and 1 p.m, and 2 p.m. Collect daily data and reevaluate measures weekly for 6 weeks. Use a Kanban visual signal via a scrolling display loop in main office with the number of phone calls in the queue waiting.	Number of complaints offered during the phone conversation at 8 a.m. and 1 p.m. (Track sheet)	Run chart
				Patient satisfaction survey scores	Percentages
			Focus group with staff to evaluate continued feasibility	Staff perception of feasibility of change	Content analysis
Evidence-Based Practice	Evidence-based protocol Implementation	Decrease pain and distress for children aged 4–6 years and caregiver with immunization administration in primary care office (Burgess, Nativio, & Penrose, 2015)	Staff education program on pain and distress reduction and immunization compliance. Practice with the protocol materials for active distraction for patients. Team member training on use of the anesthetic spray protocol	Pre- and post-immunization survey that measured pain and distress level of caregiver and child completed by the caregiver and the healthcare provider	Paired t tests
				Staff perception of the feasibility of the protocol: Likert scale completed by RN and Medical Assistants	Mean scores

(Continued)

359

Table 14-2 Practice Projects: Sample Outcome Evaluation Plans (*Continued*)

Approach	Design	Purpose	Intervention/Action/Process	Outcome Measures	Analysis
Program Evaluation	Patient navigation program	Examine the value and effectiveness of a patient navigation program for newly diagnosed breast cancer patients (Koh, Nelson, & Cook, 2010).	Nurse navigator to coordinate care from time of diagnosis to time care is rendered in cancer treatment center with breast cancer specialist	1. Timely access to care: number of days from diagnosis to treatment in cancer center	Independent *t* tests Sample compared to historical controls
				2. Identify barriers to care and amount of time spent on resolution. National Cancer Institute patient navigation log	Frequencies and percentages by barrier category Minutes of navigator time per barrier
				3. Patient satisfaction with care: Hospital care questionnaire	Mean satisfaction scores

ANOVA, Analysis of Variance; CVD, cardiovascular disease; RN, registered nurse.

an elderly population might require survey questions to be asked aloud as part of a structured interview.

All methods have strengths and limitations, and these are carefully considered during DNP project planning (see Chapter 9, Creating and Developing the Project Plan). For example, while surveys are direct measures that are versatile, they are prone to bias when respondents provide the socially acceptable answer rather than their true opinion. Direct observation is a more objective approach than self-reported survey data, but this method is vulnerable to bias from the observer's personal interests in conducting the study. Extraction of data from EHRs is economical and efficient but may be limited by the missing data points in the records. In focus groups, the dialogue permits clarification of participant responses, but the presence of others and the risk for a breach in confidentiality may limit disclosure.

When selecting measures to gather quantitative data, it is important to choose tools that have documented reliability, validity, sensitivity, and precision so that they best approximate the true meaning of the concept or parameter being measured (Polit & Beck, 2012). It is also helpful if the instruments have previously been used with the population of interest in the DNP project. Measurement of theoretical concepts, such as self-efficacy, evidence of reliability, and validity should be documented in the project proposal (see Chapter 11, The Proposal). When biophysiological parameters are used, such as glucose, the precision (coefficient of variation) and sensitivity (lowest limit of detection) of the measure are usually reported.

In research, QI projects, EBP initiatives, and program evaluation, multiple measurement methods may be required to capture the relevant data that measures the expected outcomes of a QI or an EBP initiative, each objective of a program evaluation plan, or data that appropriately answers each clinical question of a research-oriented project. For QI, EBP, and program evaluation projects, economic measures of costs savings or burden may be included. DNP projects may also include a process and impact evaluation component that examines the actual development and implementation of a new program, quality improvement, or an EBP initiative. While outcome evaluation measures the changes that occurred with the project, process evaluation assesses whether the program met its target goals for enrollment, or that the interventions were implemented as planned; impact evaluation assesses the longer term benefits of the project's intended goals (Perrin, 2015). For example, outcome measures in an improvement project to reduce infection rates in postoperative hip replacement patients, measures may include direct observation of the surgeon's handwashing technique, direct measure of the temperature in the operating room, checklists recording the surgical process (time under anesthesia, dose of antibiotic medication, etc.), or extraction of relevant patient-related variables, such as body mass index, and glucose levels from the electronic health record that categorize the patient's risk status. Process measures in this project would include disruptions in the system or organization that compromised the project implementation, such as switching vendors for the handwashing product. Impact evaluation may show that after 3 years, the infection rates remain lower than the expected goal or were the lowest rates in the local community.

With EBP initiatives, a major data-driven component of the project is the evidence-based guideline development that requires a systematic process to search for relevant literature and evaluate the evidence. Criteria for rigor in the development of practice guidelines are described in the AGREE II (Brouwers et al., 2010) instrument and may be used to guide this type of DNP project. The AGREE II (Brouwers et al., 2010) criteria include the use of a systematic search strategy with inclusion and exclusion criteria, an assessment of the strengths and limitations of the evidence, and the process used to determine the recommendation decisions. The process of appraising evidence includes determination of the level and grade of evidence to determine the essential guideline components for the selected practice outcome, population group, and system setting (Melynk & Fineout-Overholt, 2011; Johanna Briggs Institute Levels of Evidence and Grades of Recommendations Working Party, 2014a). In addition, an assessment of the benefits and risks of the recommendations, a process for expert review, and the feasibility, appropriateness, and meaningfulness of the guideline (Johanna Briggs Institute Levels of Evidence and Grades of Recommendations Working Party, 2014b) is also required.

RESOURCES FOR DATA COLLECTION: REGISTRIES AND SURVEYS

When developing the DNP project, it can be helpful to search for reliable and valid surveys and tools that may be adapted for use. There are several online public resources that house well-written, previously tested survey questions from large multicenter observational studies. In addition, several national registries that can be mined for data to support a DNP project are available. A list of these resources for registries and surveys is included at the end of the chapter (see *Helpful Resources*).

IT TAKES A TEAM: DATA COLLECTION

The data collection phase of the DNP project is action oriented and involves collaborators to assist with participant recruitment, instrument development, and data collection. Depending on the project design, data collection may occur in different settings and require permission from organizational leadership and the engagement of staff at each location. Consultation with PhD-prepared researchers or statisticians may be needed for instrument construction, complicated analyses such as statistical process control, or strategies to mine data from data repositories. Information technology experts are another group of professionals that contribute to data retrieval and DNP project work.

There are several administrative dimensions to the data collection process (Polit & Beck, 2012). Procedures and forms for data collection need to be developed and may include surveys, chart abstraction tools, checklists, tracking sheets, or scripted interview guides. See Chapter 12, The Scholarly Project Toolbox, for information on tools to support the scholarly project. If direct assessments are used, forms to record the observations will be needed. Newly developed instruments should be attractive, legible, and formatted in a logical structure to facilitate use. An assessment of the literacy level of the tool may be needed. It is helpful to pilot test instruments before implementation to evaluate the ease of use, the clarity of the items, and the amount of time needed for completion.

Procedures to recruit, screen, and obtain consent from participants, if indicated, need to be established along with the protocol for data collection. It is helpful to produce project protocol books and Gantt charts for all personnel assisting with the study. As mentioned in Chapter 9, Creating and Developing the Project Plan, a project meeting is also highly recommended to review all procedures prior to the study start. If an intervention, QI improvement, or EBP guideline implementation is planned, training sessions for the project team members (investigators, project assistants, and system staff) are needed. In more complex or lengthy projects, periodic evaluation of the project team members is indicated to ensure fidelity of the intervention or the innovation.

QI projects may involve large groups of staff, rather than individual subjects, who participate in the data collection process. A series of meetings to review the project processes and engage staff may be needed. Periodic visits to the project site encourage collaboration and provide personnel the opportunity to ask questions or alert the DNP student to issues as they arise. These actions contribute to a successful project outcome. See Chapter 9 for a discussion on forming and training the project team.

Qualitative data collection uses smaller groups of subjects, and often only a single investigator and one assistant are needed for data collection. Subject recruitment is purposive to engage the specific types of participants required (Miller, 2010). Informed consent is needed; and if the study uses focus groups, a group commitment to confidentiality is required. Open-ended questions or interviews are commonly used as the primary data collection method, with responses recorded by audiotapes. The role of the investigator is to facilitate the discussion. The study assistant observes nonverbal behaviors, taking field notes as needed.

Not everything that can be counted counts, and not everything that counts can be counted.

—*William Bruce Cameron*

DATA MANAGEMENT

> Data security is an important issue to consider in any clinical inquiry project and requires a protocol to protect participants.

Data security is an important issue to consider in any clinical inquiry project and requires a protocol to protect participants. In projects that collect personal health information and require human subject review, participants are assigned an identification (ID) number, and a master list of participants with their study IDs is created. This master list is stored in a secure location, with access granted only to the primary investigator and trained study staff. When possible, data collection tools should be devoid of identifying information and stored in a different secure location away from the master list. QI, EBP, and program evaluation projects often collect data in aggregate form that may or may not include protected health information.

There are several strategies used during the data collection period to facilitate efficiency and accuracy. A process for tracking responses from participants should be developed and monitored. Maintaining a project log is recommended to document issues that arise and decisions that are made as the project progresses. A data codebook is created and includes the name or label for each data item, its level of measurement, and its numeric coding scheme. For example, if gender is the variable, the codebook would indicate this is a nominal-level variable, where a value of 1 indicates female and a value of 2 indicates male. A code for missing data is also commonly created for each item.

As they are received, data collection forms should be examined for completeness and legibility. Steps to retrieve pieces of missing data may need to be implemented. If this is not possible, decisions regarding the amount of missing data that warrants exclusion of the record from the study need to be considered. Sometimes participants creatively complete data collection forms. For example, they may write in an answer rather than selecting from the ones provided. At other times, they may change their answer several times, making it difficult to determine which answer they intended to select. The DNP student will need to make decisions about the interpretation of these items. One solution is to create a new code for these variant items that is labeled "other" to distinguish these data. These concerns would invite collaboration with a PhD-prepared researcher or statistician. Decisions made should be entered into the project log to ensure consistency in the evaluation of all data forms.

When dealing with numerical data, approximately right is better than precisely wrong.
                                                                    —*Carl G. Tor*

DATA ENTRY

When all data collection forms have been reviewed, verified, and cleaned, they are coded using the schema established in the codebook. Coded data are then entered into the selected statistical program. There are several statistical software programs available, including the Statistical Package for the Social Sciences, (SPSS), the Statistical Analysis System (SAS), and Stata. Microsoft Excel is also capable of descriptive data analysis and graphics. With additional software, Excel can perform inferential statistics and produce QI metrics. The choice of statistical software should be driven by the analyses needed to accurately measure the DNP project outcome.

Data entry is a tedious, time-intensive process, and errors are common. Consequently, it is necessary to verify or check the entries to correct mistakes prior to data analysis. One option for data verification is to print all data set values and compare the numbers visually to each original data record (e.g., survey). Another option is double data entry. In this case, the data are entered twice and the two data sets compared for errors. The comparison can be done visually or, if available, the statistical computer program can compare both data sets.

> Data entry is a tedious, time-intensive process, and errors are common. Therefore, it is important that the student verify the entries to correct mistakes prior to data analysis.

Qualitative data include audiotapes from interviews and focus groups, field notes with observations of nonverbal behaviors, or written narratives. Verification of data often occurs during the data collection process, in which the researcher checks with the participant to affirm the interpretations. Management of qualitative data includes the transcription of audiotaped interviews into text for analysis. Computerized software products (e.g., NVivo) are also available to manage verbal and written narrative data.

The processes of both data management and analysis are complex and challenging. This is another dimension of the DNP project where interprofessional collaboration is paramount. Consultation with expert researchers and statisticians experienced in quantitative and qualitative inquiry is highly recommended when selecting analytical software or making decisions that affect data veracity.

However exhausted I might be, the sight of long columns of numbers was perfectly reviving to me.

—Florence Nightingale

DATA ANALYSIS

> Statistical analyses organize and transform the numbers that represent the project outcome data into meaningful information that can be interpreted.

Data analysis is an exciting phase of the DNP project! Statistical analyses organize and transform the numbers that represent the project outcome data into meaningful information that can be interpreted. As with the other components of the DNP project, there is a systematic process to evaluate and interpret data. The

> The data analysis plan will differ based on the DNP project approach and can be diverse including a broad array of outcome measures.

data analysis plan will differ based on the DNP project approach and can be diverse including a broad array of outcome measures.

The first step in data analysis is to evaluate the distributions of the dependent/outcome and independent variables for normality using histograms and frequency distributions (See Chapter 12, The Scholarly Project Toolbox). If the distributions are normal, parametric analyses can be used. If distributions are not normal, variables can be transformed to try to achieve normality. If this is not successful, nonparametric analyses are used. The next wave of data analysis includes descriptive analysis with measures of central tendency (mean, median, and mode) and variation (range and standard deviation). These data provide an overall picture of the participants' characteristics and measures of the independent, confounding, and outcome variables.

The second set of analyses examines the relationships between the variables. These analyses usually include scatter plots, chi-square tests (crosstabs), and bivariate Pearson or Spearman rank-order correlations depending on the measurement level of the variables. Additional analyses may include regression or the assessment of differences between groups using parametric (independent or pair *t*-tests, ANOVA) or nonparametric (Mann Whitney *U*, Kruskal Wallis) tests if congruent with the project aim and type of data that were collected. Additional statistical tests may be conducted to answer questions related to the DNP project outcome.

QI data can be analyzed using histograms, scatter plots, pie charts, line graphs, frequencies, and descriptive statistics using the same analytical programs. Change in the dependent variable from an innovation can also be measured with traditional statistical analyses. Additional QI analyses such as control and run charts, Pareto charts, or value stream maps can be created using Excel with QI macros if congruent with the DNP project plan. For well-developed QI processes, statistical process control is the sentinel analytic technique. See Chapter 12, The Scholarly Project Toolbox for examples created using QI Macros.

Qualitative data analysis involves thoughtful reviews of transcribed audio-taped data or written narratives to identify themes or patterns in the data. Statistical programs such as NVivo can be used to corroborate and support the investigator's suppositions. Data are analyzed inductively via specific, rigorous techniques to organize answers around the clinical inquiry question (Miller, 2010). Qualitative analysis seeks understanding about a phenomenon rather than a specific answer.

When analyses are complete, the challenge is to interpret the findings and apply them in the context of the clinical question as outcomes. What is the meaning in the data? How does it inform the clinical phenomenon? What are some of the possible explanations for the findings? What are the implications of the findings? Are there opportunities for systems improvements? How might these data be used to change practice? How does this work contribute to nursing practice?

At the same time, the limitations of the data are evaluated. Where is the bias or error in the study? How does this impact the conclusions? If the study were repeated, what improvements could be made? This phase of data analysis requires dedicated thinking time to reach thoughtful conclusions. It is also another time in the scholarly process where consultation with the DNP team and collaboration with other researchers and statistical or QI specialists can be helpful.

In God we trust, all others bring data.

—*W. Edwards Deming*

TELLING THE STORY

The last part of the project is the dissemination of findings. Dissemination can include an article for publication, or presentations at professional or community meetings (see Chapter 15, Disseminating the Results). If the project was conducted in a specific setting or with a special population, the findings should be shared with those groups. If the data inform policy, they should be shared with the relevant stakeholders. The diffusion of the project outcome is just as important, if not more important, than the actual work itself.

When preparing papers or presentations to share the project data, a structured format is helpful (Oermann, Turner, & Carman, 2014). There are specific guidelines for the reports of experimental and observational research, program evaluation (CDC, 2013), as well as for QI reports and EBP initiatives. The recommended formats are included in the *Helpful Resources* section at the end of this chapter.

> There are specific guidelines for the reports of research, program evaluation, QI reports, and EBP initiatives.

As is mentioned in Chapter 15, Disseminating the Results, in general, most papers and presentations begin with an introduction and background to establish the need for the project and its significance to nursing practice or healthcare delivery. This is followed by the methods section, which describes the project design, the sample or population studied, Institutional Review Board or Quality Council approval, and the protocols for data collection and measurements.

The project findings are also reported in a systematic fashion, starting with the participant response, if indicated, and a description of the sample characteristics or the clinical setting for a QI or an EBP project report. This is followed by the data outcomes organized around the clinical issue, program goals, or the improvement process. It is important to focus on the major points in this section. It is not necessary to provide every piece of data; the main outcomes are sufficient. If there were unanticipated findings that are relevant, they should be noted.

The last part of the paper or presentation is the discussion. This is the opportunity to give meaning to the findings for the audience or reader. The discussion should include the implication of the data for practice and opportunities for future change or improvement. The major findings and their implications should be discussed first, followed by other results considered important. The data are often compared to other studies in the literature or other improvement processes. The limitations of the data are summarized and the next steps for future innovation are presented.

The doctoral project is the summative scholarly product in DNP programs, and it demonstrates the synthesis of the student's academic work and achievement of the essential DNP competencies. The project, when viewed as a program outcome, should make a substantive contribution to nursing practice. DNP projects are diverse and address relevant patient, systems, or population issues with an emphasis on improving health- and healthcare-related outcomes. The project deliverables are disseminated professionally and provide a foundation for continued practice scholarship.

Key Messages

- The DNP project design drives the selection of methods, measures, and the data evaluation plan.
- DNP projects are diverse and encompass multiple different perspectives.
- Interprofessional collaboration is essential for a successful DNP project.
- The DNP project is the work of many, not the work of one—it takes a team!

Action Plan—Next Steps

1. Ensure that all appropriate team members have been brought to the table.
2. Verify that there is congruence between the clinical issue, selected design, and methods.
3. Choose a statistical software program to use for data analysis.
4. Consult with a PhD colleague or statistician when analyzing the data and interpreting the results.

REFERENCES

Bardach, E. (2011). *A practical guide for policy analysis: The eightfold path to more effective problem solving* (4th ed.). Washington, DC: CQ Press.

Batalden, P. B., & Davidoff, F. (2007). What is quality improvement and how can it transform health care? *Quality and Safety in Health Care, 16,* 2–3. doi:10.1136/qshc.2006.022046

Brouwers, M., Kho, M. E., Browman, G. P., Burgers, J. S., Cluzeau, F., Feder, G., Zitzelsberger, L. for the AGREE Next Steps Consortium. (2010). AGREE II: Advancing guideline development, reporting and evaluation in healthcare. *Canadian Medical Association Journal, 82,* E839–E842. doi:10.1503/090449. Retrieved from http://www.agreetrust.org

Burgess, S., Nativio, D., & Penrose, J. E. (2015). Quality improvement project to reduce pain and distress associated with immunization visits in pediatric primary care. *Journal of Pediatric Nursing, 30,* 294–300. http://dx.doi.org/10.1016/j.pedn.2014.09.002

Centers for Disease Control and Prevention. (1999). Framework for program evaluation in public health. MMWR 1999; 48 (No. RR-ID). Retrieved from http://www.cdc.gov/eval/framework/index.htm

Centers for Disease Control and Prevention. (2011). Introduction to program evaluation for public health programs: Self study guide. Accessed August 2, 2015 from http://www.cdc.gov/eval/guide/introduction/

Centers for Disease Control and Prevention. National Center for Chronic Disease Prevention and Health Promotion, Office on Smoking and Health, Division of Nutrition, Physical Activity and Obesity. (2013). Developing an effective evaluation report: Setting the course for effective program evaluation. Atlanta, Georgia: Author. Accessed August 11, 2015 from http://www.cdc.gov/eval/materials/developing-an-effective-evaluation-report_tag508.pdf

Cronenwett, L., Sherwood, G., Barnsteiner, J., Disch, J., Johnson, J., Mitchell, P. . . . Warren, J. (2007). Quality and safety education for nurses. *Nursing Outlook, 55*(3), 122–131.

Donabedian, A. (2005). Evaluating the quality of medical care. *Milbank Quarterly, 83,* 691–729. doi:10.1111/j.1468-0009.2005.00397.x

Johanna Briggs Institute. Levels of Evidence and grades of Recommendations Working Party. (2014a). New JBI levels of evidence. Accessed January 15, 2015 from http://www.joannabriggs.org/assets/docs/approach/JBI-Levels-of-evidence_2014.pdf

Johanna Briggs Institute. Levels of Evidence and Grades of Recommendations Working Party. (2014b). New JBI grades of recommendations. Accessed January 15, 2015 from http://www.joannabriggs.org/assets/docs/approach/JBI-grades-of-recommendation_2014.pdf

Kaplan, R. S., & Norton, D. P. (1992). The balanced scorecard – measures that drive performance. *Harvard Business Review, 70*(1), 71–79.

Koh, C., Nelson, J. M., & Cook, P. (2010). Evaluation of a patient navigation program. *Clinical Journal of Oncology Nursing 15,* 41–48. doi: 10.1188/11.CJON.41-48

Leeman, J., & Sandelowski, M. (2012). Practice-based evidence and qualitative inquiry. *Journal of Nursing Scholarship, 44*(2), 171–179.

Melynk, B. M., & Fineout-Overholt, E. (2011). Evidence-based practice in nursing and healthcare: A guide to best practice. Philadelphia, PA: Wolters Kluwer.

Millar, A., Simeone, R. S., & Carnevale, J. T. (2001). Logic models: A systems tool for performance management. *Evaluation and Program Planning, 24,* 73–81.

Miller, W. R. (2010). Qualitative research as evidence: Utility in nursing practice. *Clinical Nurse Specialist, 24*(4), 191–193.

Newhouse, R. (2007). Diffusing confusion among evidence-based practice, quality improvement and research. *Journal of Nursing Administration 37*(10), 432–435.

Newhouse, R. P., Dearholt, S. L., Poe, S. S., Pugh, L. C., & White, K. M. (2007). Johns Hopkins hospital nursing evidence-based practice model and guidelines. Accessed

August 5, 2015 from http://nursing.jhu.edu/news-events/news/archives/2009/evidence_based_model.html

Oermann, M. H., Turner, K., & Carman, M. (2014). Preparing quality improvement, research and evidence-based manuscripts. *Nursing Economics, 32*(2), 57–69. Accessed January 15, 2015 from https://www.nursingeconomics.net/ce/2016/article32025769.pdf

Perrin, K. M. (2015). *Principles of evaluation and research for health care programs.* Burlington, MA: Jones & Bartlett Learning.

Plichta, S. B., & Kelvin, E. (2013). *Munro's statistical methods for health care research* (6th ed.). Philadelphia, PA: Lippincott Williams & Wilkins.

Polit, D., & Beck, C. (2012). *Nursing research: Generating and assessing evidence for nursing practice* (9th ed.). Philadelphia, PA: Lippincott Williams & Wilkins.

Rosswurm, M. A., & Larrabee, J. (1999). A model for change to evidence-based practice. *Journal of Nursing Scholarship, 31*(4), 317–322.

Rycroft-Malone, J. (2004). The PARIHS framework: A framework for guiding the implementation of evidence-based practice. *Journal of Nursing Care Quality, 19*(4), 297–304.

Sackett D. L., Rosenberg, W. M., Gray, J. A., Haynes, R. B., & Richardson, W. S. (2000). Evidence-based medicine: How to practice and teach EBM (2nd Ed). London: Churchill Livingstone, p1.

Schaffer, M. A., Sandau, K. E., & Diedrick, L. (2012). Evidence-based practice model for organizational change: Overview and practical applications. *Journal of Advanced Nursing, 69*(5), 1197–1209. doi: 10.1111/j.1365-2648.2012.06122x

Shirey, M. R., Hauck, S. L., Embree, J. L., Kinner, T. J., Schaar, G. L., Phillips, L. A. . . . McCool, I. A. (2011). Showcasing differences between quality improvement, evidence-based practice and research. *Journal of Continuing Education in Nursing, 42*(2), 57–68.

Stetler, C. B. (2001). Updating the Stetler model of research utilization to facilitate evidence-based practice. *Nursing Outlook, 49*, 272–278.

Stevens, K. R. (2004). ACE star model of EBP: knowledge transformation. Academic Center for Evidence Based Practice. The University of Texas Health Science Center at San Antonio. Accessed July 30, 2015 from http://www.acestar.uthscsa.edu

Stufflebeam, D. L. (1983). The CIPP model for program evaluation. In G. F. Maddaus, M. Scriven, & D. L. Stufflebeam (Eds.), *Evaluation in health and human services* (Vol 6, pp. 117–141). Boston: Kluwer-Nijhoff.

Titler, M. G., Kleiber C., Steelman, V., Goode C., Rakel, B. Budreau G. . . . Goode, C. J. (2001). The IOWA model of evidence based practice to promote quality care. *Critical Care Nursing Clinics of North America 13*(4), 497–509.

Titler, M. (2011). Nursing science and evidence-based practice. *Western Journal of Nursing Research, 33*(3), 291–295.

United States Department of Health and Human Services. Office of Human Research Protection. (2009). Protection of human subjects. Title 45 Code of Federal Regulations. Part 46. Washington, DC. Department of Health and Human Services. Accessed July 29, 2015 from http://www.hhs.gov/ohrp/humansubjects/regbook2013.pdf.pdf

United States Department of Health and Human Services. Health Resources and Services Administration. (2011). Quality improvement. *Journal of Nursing Care Quality 19*(4), 297–304. Accessed August 1, 2015 from.http://www.hrsa.gov/quality/toolbox/508pdfs/qualityimprovement.pdf

Weimer, D. L., & Vining, A. R. (2005). *Policy analysis: Concepts and practice* (4th ed.). Upper Saddle River, NJ: Prentice Hall.

Helpful Resources

Evidence Based Practice Resources

Appraisal of Guidelines Research & Evaluation. AGREE-II. International tool to assess the quality of practice guidelines Available at http://www.agreetrust.org/agree-ii/

Johanna Briggs Institute. Provides resources on evidence-based practice including systematic review methods, levels of evidence, and grades of recommendations. Available at http://www.johannabriggs.org

Johns Hopkins Nursing Evidence-based Practice Tool kit. Provides resources including guides for appraising research and nonresearch evidence for nursing practice. Available at http://www.nursingworld.org/DocumentVault/NursingPractice/Research-Toolkit/Johns-Hopkins-Nursing-Evidence-Based-Practice.html

National Data Registries

Agency for Healthcare Research and Quality (AHRQ): Medical Expenditure Panel Survey. Online query system for the Medical Expenditure Panel Survey data maintained AHRQ. Available at http://www.meps.ahrq.gov/mepsweb/data_stats/meps_query.jsp

AHRQ: Healthcare Cost and Utilization Project data. Online query system for the Healthcare Cost and Utilization Project data. Available at http://hcupnet.ahrq.gov/

American Fact Finder—U.S. Census Bureau. A source for population, housing, economic, and geographic information. Available at http://factfinder2.census.gov/faces/nav/jsf/pages/index.xhtml

CDC Wonder. Online query system for data maintained by the Centers for Disease Control and Prevention. Available at http://wonder.cdc.gov/

National Center for Health Statistics. This site has links to survey instruments, methods, public use data sets, online data summaries, and reports. Available at http://www.cdc.gov/nchs/

United Kingdom (UK) Data Archive. Collection of digital research data in the social sciences and humanities. Available at http://www.data-archive.ac.uk/

Program Evaluation Resources

Centers for Disease Control and Prevention. Several resources on models for program development and evaluation on a variety of health initiatives. Available at http://www.cdc.gov/eval/resources/

RAND corporation. Provides exemplars of evaluation of healthcare programs Available at http://www.rand.org/topics/health-care-program-evaluation.html

Quality Improvement Resources

Institute for Healthcare Improvement. Available at http://www.ihi.org/

US Department of Health and Human Services. Health Resources and Service Administration. Quality Improvement Tools and Resources. http://www.hrsa.gov/quality/toolsresources.html

Survey Resources

Agency for Healthcare Research and Quality Surveys. Available at http://www.ahrq.gov/data/Centers for Disease Control Division of Adolescent and School Health.* Available at http://www.cdc.gov/HealthyYouth/data/surveillance.htm

National Behavioral Risk Factor Study Survey. Available at http://www.cdc.gov/brfss/

National Center for Health Statistics, Surveys and Data Collection Systems. Available at http://www.cdc.gov/nchs/express.htm

RAND Corporation. Health surveys are available from RAND, a nonprofit institution that helps improve policy and decision making through research and analysis. Available at http://www.rand.org/health/surveys_tools.html

Survey Monkey. Free for 10 questions per survey with 100 responses per survey; $17/month for unlimited questions and unlimited responses. Available at http://www.surveymonkey.com

Recommended Manuscript Formats

Reports of Nonrandomized Educational, Behavioral, and Public Health Interventions. Transparent Reporting of Evaluations with Nonrandomized Designs (TREND) statement. Available at http://www.cdc.gov./trendstatement

Reports of Observational Studies. Strengthening the Reporting of Observational Studies in Epidemiology (STROBE) statement. doi:10.1371/journal.pmed0040296

Reports of Quality Improvement Interventions or Programs. Standards for Quality Improvement Reporting Excellence (SQUIRE). *Available at http://www.squire-statement.org*

Reports of Qualitative Research. Consolidated Criteria for Reporting Qualitative Research (COREQ) checklist. Tong, A., Sainsbury, P., & Craig, J. (2007). Consolidated criteria for reporting qualitative research: A 32 item checklist for interviews and focus groups. *International Journal of Quality in Health Care, 19*(6), 349–357. doi:10.1093/intqhc/mzm042

Reports of Randomized Controlled Trials. Consolidated Standards of Reporting Trials (CONSORT) statement. Available at http://www.consort-statement.org/index.aspx?o=1065

Reports of Systematic Reviews. Preferred Reporting Items for Systematic Reviews and Meta-Analysis (PRISMA). Available at http://www.prisma-statement.org/

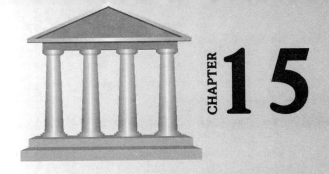

CHAPTER 15

Disseminating the Results

Rosanne Burson

CHAPTER OVERVIEW

Some of the first items the doctor of nursing practice (DNP) student should consider as he or she is preparing for the project are the required deliverables within the specific DNP program. Keep the end in mind. What are the requirements for graduation in relation to disseminating the results of the DNP project? Some type of dissemination will be required, although there is variability across programs. The requirements typically include a public presentation, a defense of the project, and a written manuscript for the university. A journal article may also be a requirement. Finally, there should be dissemination of the project outcomes as an executive summary or a written report within the organization that supported the project (AACN, 2015). Each of these formats will require very different approaches; they need to be considered early to avoid unnecessary rework. This chapter will review the various options that can be developed as part of disseminating the results of the DNP project.

CHAPTER OBJECTIVES

After completing this chapter, the learner will be able to:

1. Discuss the available options for disseminating the results of the DNP project
2. Understand the specifics for publicly presenting the results
3. Review pointers for manuscript submissions
4. Verbalize the importance of communicating and disseminating the results of the DNP project

WHAT ARE THE DELIVERABLES?

Dissemination of findings from evidence-based practice and research to improve health outcomes is described in DNP *Essential III*, Clinical Scholarship and Analytical Methods for Evidence-Based Practice (American Association of Colleges of Nursing [AACN], 2006). The use of evidence to improve practice or patient outcomes is highlighted by deliverables prior to graduation in a DNP program. A deliverable is a term used in project management to describe a tangible or intangible object produced as a result of the project that is intended to be delivered to a customer (Cutting, 2008). As mentioned in Chapter 3, Defining the Doctor of Nursing Practice: Current Trends, some recommended deliverables (AACN, 2015) include:

- Publishing in a peer reviewed print or online journal
- Poster and podium presentations
- Presentation of a written or verbal executive summary to stakeholders and/or the practice site/organization leadership
- Development of a webinar presentation or video
- Submission and publication to a nonrefereed lay publication
- Oral presentation to the public-at-large
- Development and presentation of a digital poster, grand rounds presentation, and/or a PowerPoint presentation.

It is critical that the DNP student has an understanding of the expected time frame from completion of the final deliverables to graduation. For example, when must the project be completed to be eligible for graduation? When must

> It is critical that the DNP student has an understanding of the expected time frame from completion of the final deliverables to graduation.

all deliverables be accepted by the project team and graduate or nursing school to be ready for graduation? Can deliverables, such as a final presentation, be completed after this date? The DNP program may require that the full project team or faculty mentor sign off on all written work, that the work be submitted to the university, and/or a journal 6 weeks prior to graduation, while allowing the presentation to occur in the month prior to graduation.

PUBLIC PRESENTATIONS

Public presentation of the DNP project may be a graduation requirement, so be sure to have a thorough understanding of the requirements for your specific DNP program. The public presentation may occur as a *proposal* prior to the implementation of the project or as a *presentation* after the completion of the project. The overall look of the presentation changes on the basis of its timing (before or after the project is implemented).

A presentation that occurs prior to the project is often considered a verbal defense of the project. A verbal defense includes:

- Introduction
- Background to the problem
- Literature review
- Hypothesis
- Project plan
- Methodology
- Projected sample requirements
- Tools for evaluation
- Expected implementation process
- Time for questions and comments from the audience.

See Chapter 11, The Proposal, for details in preparing the proposal. Sometimes the defense occurs in front of the project team only, and team members can add suggestions, ask questions, and finally approve the defense. The proposal may also be a public defense. In this format, there is often a public declaration of the presentation, with an invitation to the university to attend. The audience asks questions and may make additional comments. Audience members may consist of nursing faculty from the university or other universities, faculty from outside the school of nursing, graduate program faculty, deans from various colleges within the university, students from various programs, interested persons from healthcare organizations, or other interested parties.

A presentation that occurs after the project is completed has the purpose of disseminating results, and so it will also include the results of the project, an interpretation of the results, and sustainability, recommendations, and implications for practice. Forums used for disseminating results include conferences sponsored by the university, or podium and poster presentations outside the university in various local, regional, or national venues, including within the organization where the project was implemented.

Regardless of the timing or the place, there are a few items to consider in relation to the development of the presentation. The DNP student should understand:

- the purpose of the presentation (defense of the proposal vs. dissemination of results)
- the makeup of the audience attending the presentation
- when the presentation should occur during the education process
- how much time is allowed for the presentation
- the required format of the presentation.

The student will work with his or her DNP project team to negotiate a date for the defense. Several meetings with the DNP project faculty mentor, or project team, can be expected as the student fine-tunes his or her writing and develops all of the components of the project. The evaluation of the final DNP project is the responsibility of the faculty (AACN, 2015); hence, the faculty mentor will confirm with the project team that the student is indeed ready to defend.

In preparing the presentation, it is important to know the time allotted and the presentation format. A typical time allotment is 30 minutes, with an additional 30 minutes for questions. It can be challenging to focus on the high points of all the work that has been done in this brief time frame. A PowerPoint format can assist the presenter in staying focused on the points that must be considered and presented.

PowerPoint Pointers

In preparing a PowerPoint presentation, there are a few standard expectations to consider.

1. Express appreciation to the agencies, the project team members, and others who have been instrumental to the project.
2. Identify grant support or other funding sources, if any.
3. Cite references on your slides and list references at the end.

4. Use graphs and charts to make a point.

5. Use 32-point font or larger.

6. Do not crowd slides with too much information.

7. Follow the topic items to keep the presentation on track.

8. Practice, so that you stay in the time frame available.

Remember that although competency in developing a slide set is important, the PowerPoint presentation is just a tool to assist the presenter in providing information to the group. The way the presenter stands and his or her tone of voice, eye contact, and professional attire contribute to the entire package (Lim, 2012). The depth of knowledge regarding the topic,

> The depth of knowledge regarding the topic . . . will enhance the presentation far beyond the features of PowerPoint.

supported by the literature, as well as the creativity of the innovation and attention to the detail of the project plan, will enhance the presentation far beyond the features of PowerPoint.

Podium Presentations and Posters

Another mechanism for disseminating the results of the DNP project includes podium presentations and posters. For either format, the presenter must submit an abstract to the conference review committee and have it accepted. The process of preparing for either method is described by Boullata and Mancuso (2007) and is summarized as follows:

1. Identify what meeting would be most appropriate for the presentation.

2. Read/evaluate abstract submission guidelines regarding the format, word limits, space constraints, and deadline.

3. Most abstracts are submitted online, where one will cut and paste or upload the final version.

4. Be concise in your message, which should be carefully thought out.

5. The title should represent the content.

6. Project abstracts will contain five sections:
   - Background: Introduction to the topic and what is currently known
   - Objective: The aim or purpose of the project
   - Methods: How one addressed the purpose
   - Results: Pertinent results presented in text or table/figure
   - Conclusions: Focus on the response to the objective and how it fits in with future practice.

There are a few key recommendations to consider for the podium presentation. First, one must have a good understanding of the time allotted for the presentation. Always consider the audience and the purpose of the presentation in developing it. For a short presentation of 10–15 minutes, the following points by Weber and Cobaugh (2008) are recommended:

1. Present concisely and be specific to the audience.
2. Share the most important objectives and results.
3. Relegate background information to one or two points.
4. Use graphic presentation of results.
5. Avoid "busy" tables that take too long for the audience to absorb.
6. Always take the time to discuss the limitations of the study.
7. Request peer review prior to the presentation, both of the slide set and the actual presentation.

A poster is a presentation that provides a visual means of communicating information (Boullata & Mancuso, 2007). For poster presentations, the visual aspect is critical for success and is prepared with two areas in mind: content and display.

For poster content, use the same title as the abstract. Material should be organized, concise, and free of spelling or grammar errors. When considering the display, it is recommended to use the "10-10 rule." Keep in mind what a participant can look at in 10 seconds from 10 feet away (Boullata & Mancuso, 2007).

> Keep in mind what a participant reviewing a poster may look at in 10 seconds from 10 feet.

Color, layout, and well-placed graphs can be instrumental in attracting participants to the poster. Other conference specifications to consider include (Christenbery & Latham, 2013):

1. Poster format and size—freestanding or attached to a wall or corkboard
2. Location of the posters—conference room, hall, lobby
3. Number of posters/presenters, number of conference attendees
4. Bring copies of abstracts, contact information, push pins, business cards
5. Know dates that the poster must be delivered.

There are multiple poster templates available online, as well as companies that will produce a poster at a reasonable charge. Consider the type of material for the poster. If one is traveling a distance and may use the poster several times, consider a cloth poster that can be rolled up in the suitcase. Some conferences are moving to electronic posters to provide more space. Be sure that poster submissions meet all requirements of the specific conference that is being attended, especially in relation to formatting criteria which can include PowerPoints, website live demonstration and other web-focused media (Christenbery & Latham, 2013).

Podium and poster presentations are important, because they are great ways to disseminate information in areas of practice. These types of presentations can be a precursor to a journal article or a follow-up to the article. Another feature is that podium and poster presentations are a connection to other potential opportunities that can occur only through networking.

> Podium and poster presentations are a connection to other opportunities that can occur only through networking.

For example, one of the authors of this book was invited to be a guest lecturer to a DNP program in Utah to present the poster material to a leadership class because of a conversation with a professor who attended a poster session at a national conference. Finally, presentations are another aspect of scholarship that can be used for promotion and tenure evaluation for individuals working in academia.

PORTFOLIOS

A portfolio may be an expected deliverable within the DNP program, although it is not considered a DNP project (AACN, 2015). "Portfolio evaluation is an efficient and effective strategy to objectively demonstrate the accomplishment of program objectives using students' perceptions of their academic experience" (Kear & Bear, 2007, p. 109). The practice portfolio is described in the AACN (2006) DNP *Essentials* document. It is recommended that the portfolio documents, the final practice synthesis and scholarship, include the impact or effect on practice. Examples of representation in the portfolio include pilot studies, program evaluation, quality improvement (QI), evaluation of a new practice model, consulting projects, integrated research reviews, and manuscripts submitted for publication. Reflections may be a portion of the portfolio that exemplify synthesis of the DNP *Essentials*.

Once again, it behooves the DNP student to be aware of this requirement early in the program. Knowledge of the required documents for the portfolio helps the DNP student to begin preparation throughout the educational process and saves tremendous time in rediscovering the needed documents at a later time.

WRITTEN MANUSCRIPT

Understanding the written requirements of the university will be important for graduation as well. Written manuscripts will have requirements related to format and submission. Often there is a required date that the manuscript must be submitted by to be ready for graduation—this may be 4–6 weeks prior to actual graduation, so planning is essential. Be sure to get a list of the submission requirements. Manuscript submission requirements may include specific formatting such as that of the American Psychological Association (APA), as well as how the manuscript should be submitted, such as hard copy or bound.

For many programs, a requirement for graduation is submission of an article for publication, which integrates well with the purpose of the DNP to disseminate evidence-based practice.

Journal Submissions

Reasons to write for publication include:

1. Dissemination of evidence
2. Sharing initiatives and innovation with others
3. Keeping nurses updated
4. Communicating research findings
5. Developing the science base of nursing
6. Directing the future of the profession
7. Communicating the importance of clinical practice findings to build evidence (Oermann & Hays, 2016).

> Too often, the journal submission is the last item on the list separating the DNP student from graduation.

Too often, the journal submission is the last item on the list separating the DNP student from graduation, if this is a requirement of the university. If this submission is considered in the planning phase, it will be done well and there will be an improved opportunity for successful publication of an article on the DNP project.

TIPS FOR SUCCESSFUL JOURNAL SUBMISSION

Recognizing that students sometimes struggle when preparing a manuscript for submission to a peer-reviewed journal, several editors were interviewed for guidance. The editors share their perspectives on publishing specifics for the DNP student and practitioner.

Mary Fran Tracy, PhD, RN, CCNS, FAAN, is the editor for *AACN Advanced Critical Care.*

Denise O'Brien, DNP, ACNS-BC, FAAN, was past editor of the *Journal of Post-Anesthesia Nursing.* She recalls that the biggest change that occurred during her tenure in the publishing world related to electronic developments and overcoming the delays that occurred because of the need to copy and mail submissions. Now, with electronic submissions, "hot topics can rise to the top more quickly." Dr. O'Brien is a DNP graduate and an experienced author.

Marilyn H. Oermann, PhD, RN, ANEF, FAAN, is the editor of *The Journal of Nursing Care Quality. The Journal of Nursing Care Quality* is a quarterly journal. Most quarterly journals have a lower impact than monthly journals, although the impact factor for this journal is in the top 25.

The *impact factor,* often abbreviated *IF,* is a measure of the frequency that articles from the journal are cited, which reflects the journal's importance. This website gives a step-by-step direction on how to identify the IF in the journals of interest: http://www.hsl.virginia.edu/services/howdoi/hdi-jcr.cfm.

Dr. Oermann is the past author and editor for a newsletter titled *Nurse Author Editor* (www.nurseauthoreditor.com), which offers articles and tips on writing. She is also a past editor for *Outcomes Management for Nursing Practice* and *Annual Review of Nursing Education.* In addition, she coauthored *Writing for Publication in Nursing* (2016), which is an excellent reference for authors looking to develop writing skills for publication.

In the discussion that follows, the editors will share their knowledge of the editing process to assist the reader in understanding the important facets of journal submission.

What are the most important points for a writer to understand when choosing the appropriate peer-reviewed journal for publication?

Dr. O'Brien believes that the most important point relates to the focus of the DNP project. Does the project have a clinical or quality focus, or does it fit into a specialty journal? The author needs to consider if the topic is appropriate for the journal. For instance, if the article is more about the process than the disease state, consider a journal based on quality.

She also stresses the importance of considering the makeup of the target audience by reviewing recent issues of the journal to identify topics of interest and depth of content. Dr. O'Brien suggests perusing journals that were included in the literature review for the project. In addition, she recommends scanning journals that have published articles on topics that are related to the DNP project. It is plausible that the student's article could be considered a follow-up to some of those articles. Finally, one should also consider what he or she wants to present to the world. It is important to look at the IF for each journal that one is considering. IFs were discussed earlier in this chapter.

Dr. Oermann suggests preparing the manuscript for a specific journal. In other words, do not find a journal for the article, but write the article specifically for that journal. She recommends selecting five journals based on the type of journal, the articles in the journal, and its readership and audience, and then writing with those journals in mind. The submitted manuscript must be consistent with the journal's mission.

Dr. Tracy states that most journals say what they are looking for in a manuscript. The author should look at the mission and/or vision statement of the journal, the type of topics in the journal's call for papers, and who the readers are, all of which will identify the level of content that is required. Other recommendations include looking at the type of articles that are published in the journal and considering who the author feels would use the information that is in the manuscript. Questions to ask include: Does the journal publish articles like the manuscript in hand? For example, is this a research article or a case study? Does the journal target the population the author would like to reach?

As an editor, what are you looking for in an article?

Dr. O'Brien states that one of the editor's most important considerations in article submission relates to timing. In other words, what else has been published in this journal and other journals? What manuscripts does the editor already have for publication? How does this manuscript add to the body of nursing knowledge? The editor is not just trying to fill space but is creating an issue that is of interest to the audience and is important for building nursing's body of knowledge.

Dr. Oermann states that the editor is evaluating the author's writing skills from the first contact. There are specific clues that the editor keys into from the writer. How does the query letter read in relation to composing a sentence? If the article was submitted online without a query letter, the editor will look at the topic identified in the abstract as well as the writing skill. The title is critical—does it say what the article is about? In other words, the portrayal of content in the title is important.

Dr. Oermann states that when an editor reviews a manuscript, there are several important factors that are considered:

- Is the article consistent with the journal?
- Is the topic timely and innovative, or is it a twist on an older topic?
- Is the article unique?

Dr. Tracy also comments that the article must be timely, but adds that the topic should not be overdone (i.e., there are too many recent similar articles). The author may not know what is in the pipeline, but a review of recent articles in the journal may give perspective on what topics have already been published. A query letter may also give the author insight into what the journal is looking for in unsolicited articles. The editor reviews the manuscript to identify a match for the readership. The editor also looks at readability and whether the topic is developed. Occasionally, she will send an article back to the author for further development prior to being forwarded for peer review.

What recommendations do you have for future authors?

Dr. O'Brien recommends *jumping into* publishing. "You have to be bold enough to step in!" She encourages new authors, stating that skills improve the more one writes. She compares writing to golf—very few people walk out and are perfect from the start.

Another recommendation is to pay close attention to methodology and design, which will be reviewed very carefully by the reviewers. As planning for the project occurs, think about how unique it is relative to the literature. It may be helpful to review the table of contents of journals to help in this process.

Dr. Oermann recommends writing specifically for five selected journals. The number one recommendation is to follow directions—the author guidelines should be followed prior to submission. For example, it is important to write to match the journal, which includes the length of paragraphs, headings, and depth of content. The final product should look like a paper that would fit in that journal. It may be helpful to have the article reviewed by others before submission—the student should put forth his or her best effort.

Dr. Tracy states that if one has not yet authored, it may be helpful to check resources that are available. Read articles in other journals to see how others are developing and presenting case studies, for example. Present sections in the manuscript that are based on research guidelines if the manuscript is a research article or performance improvement guidelines for QI manuscripts.

Consider a literature search on how to write for publication. She also recommends www.nurseauthor.com for tips on writing. Finally, find a mentor for authorship. This should be someone who understands what mentorship entails.

The mentor does not have to be geographically located near the writer—mentoring can occur via the Internet. If the writer does not have a mentor in mind, consider academic connections or contacting professional nursing organizations that have journals. Often universities have writing centers or other mentoring support. Some of the organizations will have resources to match new authors with senior writers or may even have a formal mentoring program.

What recommendations do you have if an article is turned down?

Dr. O'Brien states that everyone has been rejected or had to undertake a major revision at some point in time. The writer should expect direction or clarification and give himself/herself permission to grieve—this is a normal process related to the sense of ownership of an article. One should expect good feedback and recommendations from the reviewers. Take all of the input and move forward. The writer should see that it is okay to need to revise an article. It is important to make the requested revisions and resubmit the manuscript. It is frustrating for editors when the author does not follow through. The editor feels that he or she has failed in encouraging the author. One thing the writer never knows is how many other submissions the journal has had or what is in "the hopper."

Dr. Oermann suggests taking the reviewer comments, incorporating the relevant ones, and sending the manuscript to the next journal on the list. She notes that less than one-half of authors resubmit. The key message here is to be persistent in making revisions and to keep submitting the article. She stresses that there are 500 nursing and healthcare journals and that there is no reason the work should not be published. She recommends that when three reviewers make the same comments, it is important to incorporate the recommendation in the next submission. However, after four rejections, the author may need to reframe the topic. Consider the recommendation and add a twist. Perhaps not enough preliminary work was done. It is also important to think about the project design. If there is no control group, perhaps the article is a report of a QI, a project, pilot, or initiative, rather than a research project.

Dr. Tracy recognizes that a rejection is difficult to experience but states it is important for the writer to understand why the manuscript was turned down. Take a deep breath and objectively consider the comments from the editor and the reviewers. If the comments state that the manuscript is well written but is not a match for the journal, the writer needs to resubmit to an appropriate journal. If there are content or writing recommendations, the author should take the feedback and make changes to strengthen the article before submitting it to another journal.

What is the process involved for selecting an article for publication?

Dr. O'Brien states that first the editor does a quick review to determine the worth in looking at the piece. The article will be assigned to a section editor for journals that have multiple editors. On the second pass, a call goes out for a panel of three reviewers. Timeliness is important: 2–3 weeks is allotted for reviews. The editor then examines the reviews and recommendations before putting a summary together.

According to **Dr. Oermann,** after the editor does the initial review, the manuscript is sent out for peer review. The editor matches the manuscript with the expertise of three reviewers. For instance, is a qualitative or quantitative expert needed? The editor will seek out reviewers who have specific expertise on the topic of the manuscript design. If the manuscript is using benchmarking data for QI, the editor will ask two reviewers who have expertise in quality. If there are no relevant reviewers on staff, he or she may search outside of the review staff. The reviewer has 21 days to complete the review.

Dr. Tracy shared that the process is the same for *AACN Advanced Critical Care.* After the initial editor review, two or three reviewers are identified depending on the content and the expertise needed. The reviewers will send back comments, as well as an opinion of acceptance/not acceptance or acceptance with revisions. The editor then compares the comments, reads the article in more depth, and makes a decision. Not as many articles are accepted as are written. The article may be accepted with minor revisions, the article may be sent back to the writer asking him or her to revise and resubmit the manuscript, or the article may be rejected.

Dr. Tracy writes a letter to the author, collating the comments from the reviewers. Her role as editor is to remove conflicting comments. She will encourage the author to revise. However, if the writer does not agree with the recommendations, he or she needs to document why there is a disagreement. She will request that the author respond to the reviewers and detail what has and has not been incorporated in the revision. The editor may send the article back out to one or two reviewers if the manuscript was a review/resubmit. The author may even need to revise again. The article may be rejected even later in the process if the author and reviewers cannot agree on revisions.

After submitting an article for consideration, what is the average amount of time one should expect to wait before receiving a response from the journal?

Dr. O'Brien states that this depends on how fast reviewer turnaround time is. The minimum time for turnaround is 6 to 8 weeks; however, it may take up to 3 months, depending on the journal.

Dr. Oermann states that it should be no more than 6 to 8 weeks. If it has been more than 8 weeks, she recommends calling the editor. She also states that this is a question the author can ask the editor prior to submission. An even more important question is how long after acceptance will it be before the article is published? It should be an immediate publication; however, some journals have been known to hold onto articles for 1 or 2 years after acceptance.

Dr. Tracy agrees that the initial response may take up to 8 weeks. Sometimes obtaining a reviewer may be a challenge. Reviewers are very busy; and even once assigned, it may take some additional time to complete the review.

If you haven't heard from the journal in that period of time, what do you recommend as next steps?

Dr. O'Brien states it is appropriate to send an email requesting an update if months have gone by with no response.

Dr. Oermann recommends an email after 8 weeks. She also recommends checking with the "writing grapevine" prior to submission by asking how long the journals of interest take to review. The "writing grapevine" includes those individuals who are well published and have experience with the journals in which one has interest. She recommends not sending the manuscript to those journals that take 6 to 8 months to review.

Dr. Tracy also agrees that it is appropriate to send an email to the editor after 8 weeks for a status update.

What is the percentage of submitted articles chosen for publication?

Dr. Oermann states that about 25% of all articles submitted are chosen for publication. Unfortunately, there is no one source for this information. She recommends emailing the editorial office to find out the percentage of articles chosen for publication, how long the review process is, and how long after acceptance articles are generally published—some take 2 years. This information can be obtained prior to a query letter and put in a file for future review prior to actual submission to the journal.

Dr. Tracy states that there is great variation between journals based on the competitiveness of the journal and the number of manuscripts that are submitted. The AACN acceptance rate is about 60%. Some journals may publish only solicited articles; many, including the AACN, are a combination of solicited and unsolicited manuscripts.

Are there strategies to improve one's chances of being selected for publication?

Dr. O'Brien states that there is no reason to be hesitant about submitting a manuscript, because there are a lot of journals and thus many opportunities. At the same time, the author must be thoughtful and research the best fit for the article, including the possibility of journals outside of nursing.

Dr. Oermann states that the topic must be an innovative project that has not been done, or done with a new twist. The manuscript should fit the journal. For example, if the article was originally developed for an academic setting, it must be rewritten to fit the journal. She also recommends not including a model in the article unless the paper is about a model. She reiterates the importance of following the author guidelines explicitly.

Dr. Tracy reinforces that matching the article to the appropriate journal is key. The author should also use resources for improving writing skills. At a very minimum, follow the guidelines. If the journal has a high influx of manuscripts, the editor will not even look at an article that does not follow journal guidelines.

Other recommendations include writing to the editor to propose a topic for a series of articles and suggesting your article as one of the published topics, or offering to write a column for the journal on your topic. Typically, an article in the AACN journal is 15 to 20 pages long, while a column is 6 pages long.

What are your views on the influx of DNP projects to a journal?

Dr. O'Brien states that even if it's not a requirement for graduation, DNP students and graduates need to have a commitment to publishing. Disseminating results provides others with information that is needed for evidence-based practice and success for other writers to build on. Also, time and resources from the journal have gone into the DNP's article review, so be sure to follow through and resubmit the manuscript if changes are required.

Dr. Oermann states that many more manuscripts are being submitted than in the past, and many are not publishable as submitted. For instance, an author may not follow the previously discussed recommendation of using a specific reference style like the American Medical Association (AMA) or APA format. Some topics are not innovative or the new practice initiative was only studied for a month. Some articles have errors in references, which raises a flag about the content. References may be incomplete, incorrect, or too old. She recommends that others, such as committee/chair/other faculty, read the paper. Another suggestion is to get an editor to assist with writing.

Dr. Tracy identifies that there has been a substantial increase in unsolicited manuscripts and she is grateful for the increase. However, she mentions that it is important for students, faculty, and advisors to recognize the need to rework the article for publication versus an academic manuscript. She also notes that the DNP skill and content level should match other manuscripts that are received by the journal. She encourages authors to consider offering to be a reviewer because they will often learn a great deal about clear writing and publishing.

Author Guidelines

Understanding the process and important pointers for manuscript submission will assist the author in producing a polished paper and provide a smoother journey to publication. In summary, the following points were expressed by the editors:

1. Choose the journal carefully based on its mission, readership, and types of articles.
2. Match the manuscript to the journal.
3. Follow all author guidelines for:
   - Manuscript style and format
   - Abstract guidelines
   - Development of tables, figures, and graphs.
4. Expect recommendations from reviewers and be willing to resubmit.
5. If needed, develop writing skills by using written resources.

A helpful tool to use when considering potential journals for an article is http://biosemantics.org/jane/index.php. This tool allows the author to submit an abstract, and then, based on the information received, provides the author with a list of journals that have accepted similar topics. The author can then access the recommended journals to review the types of articles that have been published.

When choosing a journal for submission, be sure to follow the author guidelines explicitly in relation to format, font, citations, and length of article. Most journals will have guidelines for various types of submission. The author will identify the specific type of article that is being submitted and will follow those specific guidelines. Here is an example of the requirements within a specific journal: **Authors.jblearning.com.**

When a manuscript presents timely and important content that is of interest to the specific journal's readership in the appropriate style, the opportunity for publication becomes a reality!

Online Manuscript Submission

In addition to the important concepts discussed by the editors, most journals will have an online submission process. Be sure to follow the directions explicitly. Typically, the article will be submitted in separate pieces that include the title page, abstract, body of the manuscript with references, and tables and figures. The directions will include whether the manuscript should be sent in PDF or other format. Each of these components may have word limits. Using a tool like Microsoft Word's word count feature can ensure that the submitted piece is well within the specified limits. There may be a letter to the editor submission area as well, where the author highlights why this is an important article to consider. Finally, make sure to plan for enough time to upload the submission accurately.

Other Journal Considerations

Another area to consider prior to journal submission is using a plagiarism program like SafeAssign. There are many plagiarism programs available for use. For example, journals may use a program like iThenticate to initially review the article. Manuscripts may be rejected before the editor does an initial review based on the results of the program. Even when references are cited correctly, a percentage over a predetermined level will suggest that the article is not original material. Too many direct quotes will increase the percentage level. The writer should strive for a result less than 15% using SafeAssign.

Often manuscripts will be accepted for publication, but they will be offered online prior to being published in print. The Appendix to this chapter includes a sample of an article that was published online and in print by authors Dianne Conrad, Patricia A. Hanson, Susan M. Hasenau, and Julia Stocker-Schneider. Note that Dr. Conrad was a DNP student at the time this article was written and submitted. Coauthors include the committee chair and members. See Chapter 8, The Project Team, for a discussion regarding authorship of submitted manuscripts.

In summary, an important aspect of journal submission is communicating the writer's experience or findings to contribute to the body of knowledge within nursing and health care. Collectively, the value of DNP-prepared nurses work will be discussed in the final chapter (Chapter 16, The Rest of the Story—Evaluating the Doctor of Nursing Practice).

In addition, there is great personal value in submitting for publication. This includes development of the author's own knowledge, personal satisfaction, sharing with a wider audience, and the potential benefits of promotion and tenure in a university setting (Oermann & Hays, 2016).

Executive Summary

The executive summary is another written method of dissemination that may be used to present the project outcomes within the organization that the project was implemented. This document is typically 1–2 pages and is a great tool to have available with an oral presentation. The format of the document will include:

- Description of the current status and why change is needed
- Presentation of the project details and how it aligns with the organization's goals, and objectives, mission, vision, and values
- Market analysis findings
- Implementation process
- Evaluation metrics
- Project outcomes as related to metrics:
  - clinical
  - financial
  - satisfaction
  - other as identified in the evaluation plan
- Sustainability
- Implications.

The following excerpt by Diane Grimaldi DNP, PMHCNS, BC describes her dissemination experiences with her DNP project:

The title of my DNP project is Association of Psychiatric History, Attendance of Postoperative Support Groups, and Outcomes Following Gastric Bypass Surgery: A Pilot Study. I was interested in pursuing this field of inquiry because treating bariatric surgery patients is a clinical specialty for me. I had been providing full-spectrum psychiatric and psychopharmacologic services, both preoperatively and postoperatively for this population for years prior to enrolling in my DNP program. A longstanding concern of mine has been the lack of standardized, evidence-based, psychological treatment protocols for patients undergoing bariatric surgical procedures.

A knowledge deficit regarding how to best meet the postoperative psychological needs of this population exists. Therefore, the aim of the project was to identify descriptors of long-term weight loss correlated with attendance of postoperative support groups following gastric bypass (GBP) surgery. Findings of this study revealed that approximately two-thirds of participants who underwent GBP screened positive for one or more Axis I diagnoses on the Psychiatric Diagnostic Screening Question-naire. Furthermore, higher numbers of comorbid psychiatric conditions were associated with less robust weight loss outcomes. It became clear that a more comprehensive understanding of the impact of a patient's psychiatric history on surgical outcomes might inform the development of evidence-based treatment protocols. Also, early identification of such conditions could reduce weight recidivism and improve outcomes.

The dissemination of project findings is an essential part of the process of sharing knowledge, translating outcomes, and deciphering implications in a local context for clinical application in a meaningful way. Since abstract submissions for dissemination was a requirement for successful completion of the DNP program I attended, I took ad-vantage of several opportunities to present the outcomes of my project in various venues. For example, a university-sponsored symposium for nursing faculty and students, including DNPs, enabled me to present a poster at the university and Lowell community toward the end of my program. I was also able to present my poster at the New England Chapter of the American Psychiatric Nurse's Association conference. During this conference I also presented a concurrent session entitled, *Psychosocial Issues Following Bariatric Surgery*, where I incorporated an ex-ecutive summary of my project.

Results of my project were also disseminated to clinical and com-munity audiences. Shortly after graduation, I was asked to present the project to a multidisciplinary group of staff members at a local psychiatric hospital and again at an informational session for people who were contemplating bariatric surgery as a possible treatment in-tervention. These different venues provided me with the opportunity to diversify the presentation of data and project outcomes in a way that addressed the interests of these audiences most effectively.

I also disseminated my work in a professional journal. To increase the likelihood of acceptance by a professional journal, I first identified my target audience, and then I searched for journals that were likely to reach that audience. The intention was to publish the manuscript in a journal that was read by healthcare professionals from different disciplines who provide treatment for bariatric surgery patients. I chose the Bariatric Surgical Practice and Patient Care journal because the journal met the criteria of having a multidisciplinary editorial staff, contributors, and readership. Acceptance of publication with minor revisions was achieved within 2 months of submission. Publication of the project in this peer-reviewed journal was accomplished 4 months after graduation.

Key Messages

- The DNP student should understand all of the university requirements for disseminating the results of the DNP project.
- The results of the DNP project may be disseminated in verbal presentations, such as an oral defense, or podium or poster presentations.
- The results of the DNP project may be disseminated in written documents that are submitted to the university or as a manuscript submitted to an appropriate journal.
- Follow all specific guidelines for verbal or written dissemination.
- Plan for the time it takes to develop and submit the results of the DNP project.
- Consider manuscript submission to a journal, even when it is not a graduation requirement.
- Consider the executive summary format to disseminate project outcomes to the organization where the project was implemented.

Action Plan—Next Steps

1. Know the requirements for communicating the results of the DNP project.
2. Plan how the results of the DNP project will be disseminated.
3. Develop a timeline to incorporate the planned communication.
4. Consider journal submission of a manuscript, even if it is not a requirement.

5. Review potential journals for the manuscript.
6. Write the manuscript with the journal in mind.
7. Happy writing!

REFERENCES

American Association of Colleges of Nursing. (2006). The essentials of doctoral education for advanced nursing practice. Retrieved from http://www.aacn.nche.edu/publications/position/DNPEssentials.pdf

American Association of Colleges of Nursing. (2015). The doctor of nursing practice: Current issues and clarifying recommendations. Retrieved from http://www.aacn.nche.edu/aacn-publications/white-papers/DNP-Implementation-TF-Report-8-15.pdf

Boullata, J. I., & Mancuso, C. E. (2007). A "how-to" guide in preparing abstracts and poster presentations. *Nutrition in Clinical Practice, 22,* 641–646. doi: 10.1177/0115426507022006641

Christenberry, T. L., & Latham, T. G. (2013). Creating effective scholarly posters. *Journal of the American Association of Nurse Practitioners, 25,* 16–25.

Conrad, D., Hanson, P. A., Hasenau, S. M., & Stocker-Schneider, J. (2012). Identifying the barriers to use of standardized nursing language in the electronic health record by the ambulatory care nurse practitioner. *Journal of the American Academy of Nurse Practitioners, 24*(7), 443–451. doi: 10.1111/j.1745-7599.2012.00705x

Cutting, T. (2008). Deliverable-based project schedules: Part 1. Retrieved from http://www.pmhut.com/deliverable-based-project-schedules-part-1

Kear, M. E., & Bear, M. (2007). Using portfolio evaluation for program outcome assessment. *Journal of Nursing Education, 46*(3), 109–114.

Lim, F. A. (2012). Wake up to better PowerPoints. *Nursing 2012,* 47–48.

Oermann, M. H., & Hays, J. C. (2016). *Writing for publication in nursing.* 3rd edition. New York, NY: Springer.

Weber, R. J., & Cobaugh, D. J. (2008). Developing and executing an effective research plan. *American Journal of Health System Pharmacists, 65,* 2058–2065.

APPENDIX*

Identifying the Barriers to Use of Standardized Nursing Language in the Electronic Health Record by the Ambulatory Care Nurse Practitioner

Dianne Conrad, DNP, RN, FNP-BC
Cadillac Family Physicians, PC, Cadillac, MI

Patricia A. Hanson, PhD, RN, GNP
Professor, College of Nursing and Health,
Madonna University, Livonia, MI

Susan M. Hasenau, PhD, RN, NNP-BC, CTN-A
Professor, College of Nursing and Health,
Madonna University, Livonia, MI

Julia Stocker-Schneider, PhD, RN
Associate Professor, McAuley School of Nursing
University of Detroit Mercy, Detroit, MI

Key words: nurse practitioners, nurse practitioner communication, language, computers

Corresponding Author:
Dianne Conrad, DNP, RN, FNP-BC
4825 E. 32 RD
Cadillac, MI 49601
231-920-7686
231-775-2570 (fax)
Email: conraddi@gvsu.edu

---

*Journal of the American Academy of Nurse Practitioners, 24(7), 443–451. DOI: 10.1111/j.1745-7599.2012.00705x.

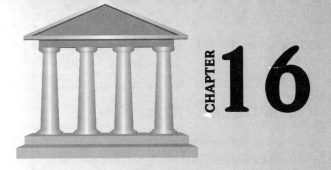

The Rest of the Story—
Evaluating the Doctor
of Nursing Practice

Dianne Conrad and David G. Campbell-O'Dell

CHAPTER OVERVIEW

Throughout this textbook, the doctor of nursing practice (DNP) project has been highlighted as an important product of DNP education that reflects the attainment of the skill set that launches the DNP graduate into scholarly practice. However, it is also important to recognize that the practice doctorate degree for nursing will need to be evaluated for effectiveness in accomplishing the goals of improving the nursing profession, health care, and society. In an attempt to begin this process, a model of evaluation of the practice doctorate is proposed using a framework that focuses on structure, process, and outcome measures. Current trends reflected in DNP practice are explored to support this evaluation model. Finally, an exemplar by Dr. Lisa Chism illustrates how the *Essentials* of DNP education are reflected in her DNP practice and scholarship.

CHAPTER OBJECTIVES

After completing this chapter, the learner will be able to:

1. Discuss the impact of the practice doctorate on the nursing profession, health care, and society
2. Explain the evaluation of the impact of the DNP in terms of the structure of DNP education, the process of advanced nursing practice, and the various types of outcomes expected
3. Review how contributions to the literature and practice are made by DNP-prepared nurses, beginning with the DNP project as a launching pad to practice scholarship

"DNP programs prepare leaders who will improve the quality of care, patient outcomes, and health policy that expands their impact on the health of society" (National Organization of Nurse Practitioner Faculties, 2005, para 3).

As discussed in Chapter 3, Defining the Doctor of Nursing Practice: Current Trends, the DNP educational program is the foundation for the practice doctorate and is built on the American Association of Colleges of Nursing (AACN, 2006) *Essentials* of DNP Education. The DNP project reflects the culmination of the attainment of the *Essentials* by the DNP student. However, the ultimate impact of the DNP graduate on nursing as a profession, health care, and society will be "the rest of the story . . ."

> The DNP project reflects the culmination of the attainment of the DNP *Essentials*.

Montgomery and Porter-O'Grady (2010) summarize the value of the scholarly project in DNP education by stating that it "provides students with an opportunity for rigorous and scholarly development of a clinical issue, demonstrating the ability to apply knowledge, translate learning and exhibit evidence-driven outcomes in their areas of practice expertise" (p. 45).

Marie Annette Brown (2011) challenges us to imagine the reality where the DNP project accomplishes multiple goals, such as

- building student expertise in practice inquiry
- contributing to advancing and improving care in institutions, local communities, and all types of healthcare settings by affecting care delivered and assisting agencies to innovate better models of care delivery, thus improving outcomes of care

- contributing to advancing the practice of registered nurses (RNs) and advanced practice registered nurses (APRNs)
- contributing to the nursing profession and nursing science
- contributing to practice inquiry, translational science, and comparative effectiveness research.

The completion of the DNP project prepares the graduate for the art and science of practice scholarship, as well as to contribute to the body of translational research knowledge and clinical practice knowledge development for the nursing profession. The ultimate value of practice scholarship in advanced nursing practice will be reflected in a variety of healthcare outcomes.

THE DNP: CONTINUOUS QUALITY IMPROVEMENT OF THE DEGREE, DNP GRADUATE PRACTICE, AND THE IMPACT ON OUTCOMES

Fontaine and Langston (2011) state that DNP programs are "forging new territory for translational science" and that "outcomes will need to be assessed in a robust manner" (p. 122). As the practice doctorate continues to mature, the present and future of the DNP degree and its impact on health care can be examined in the context of a quality improvement framework such as the Donabedian model. The Donabedian model focuses on three main categories: *structure, process,* and *outcomes* (Donabedian, 1988). *Structure* refers to the quality of the attributes of an organization or entity. *Process* refers to how care is delivered, and ultimately the test of quality is in the product produced. *Outcomes* refer to the improvement of the health status of patients and populations (see **Figure 16-1**).

This threefold approach to assessing quality acknowledges the linkage between all the components: good structure leads to good process, which in turn increases the likelihood of good outcomes. In assessing the impact of the DNP degree now and in the future, the *structure* of how DNP students are prepared and educated, the *process* of how care is delivered by the DNP-prepared nurse, as well as the *outcomes* of that care and how it impacts patients and society can be explored using the Donabedian framework (see **Figure 16-2**).

STRUCTURE—DNP EDUCATION

As the nursing profession grows, matures, and stretches to meet the evolving needs of patients in an evolving healthcare delivery system, the terminal practice degree in nursing is also evolving. Though the intentions of improving healthcare

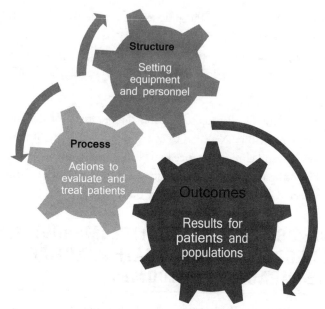

FIGURE 16-1 Donabedian model.

outcomes are understood, the question is how well are DNP graduates succeeding in this challenge? How has nursing education evolved to meet the growing demands of educating practice doctorates?

The foundation of the practice doctorate is the DNP *Essentials of Doctoral Education for Advanced Nursing Practice* (AACN, 2006) (see **Figure 16-3**). Regardless of the role in advanced nursing practice that the graduate undertakes, the core competencies attained are in the areas of leadership, advanced practice based on an evidence-based science, working in interprofessional teams, and influencing policy. All competencies are enhanced by the use of information technology. The roles of advanced nursing practice will continue to develop, and DNP education will evolve to meet the demands of these roles. The scholarly project is the first venture of the DNP student into practice scholarship and demonstrates that the student has met the DNP *Essentials outcome expectations*.

Evaluation of the DNP degree in terms of *structure* will involve assessment of the quality of DNP education. As more university DNP programs attain accreditation, quality and consistency across programs will continue to improve. One example of an accreditation body is the Commission

> Evaluation of the DNP degree in terms of *structure* will involve assessment of the quality of DNP education.

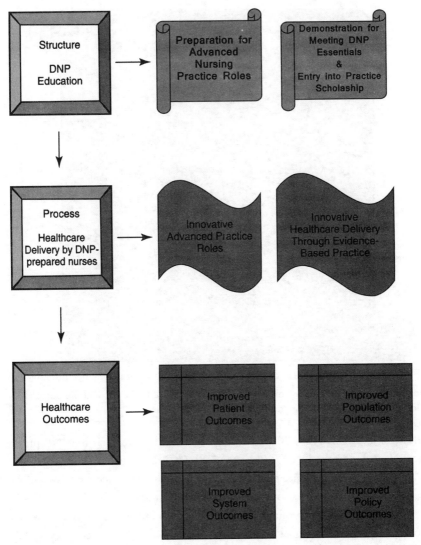

FIGURE 16-2 Evaluation of the impact of the Doctor of Nursing Practice degree.

on Collegiate Nursing Education (CCNE, 2012) that began accrediting DNP programs in 2008 and 2009.

Currently, the CCNE accredits only the practice doctorate; research doctorates such as the PhD and Doctor of Nursing Science (DNSc) are not eligible for CCNE accreditation.

DNP programs presented for accreditation are required to demonstrate incorporation of *The Essentials of Doctoral Education for Advanced Nursing Practice*

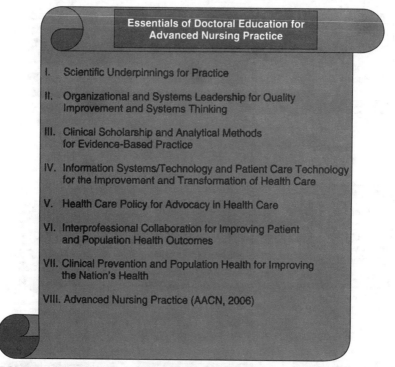

Essentials of Doctoral Education for Advanced Nursing Practice

I. Scientific Underpinnings for Practice

II. Organizational and Systems Leadership for Quality Improvement and Systems Thinking

III. Clinical Scholarship and Analytical Methods for Evidence-Based Practice

IV. Information Systems/Technology and Patient Care Technology for the Improvement and Transformation of Health Care

V. Health Care Policy for Advocacy in Health Care

VI. Interprofessional Collaboration for Improving Patient and Population Health Outcomes

VII. Clinical Prevention and Population Health for Improving the Nation's Health

VIII. Advanced Nursing Practice (AACN, 2006)

FIGURE 16-3 Essentials of doctoral education for advanced practice nursing.
Data from American Association of Colleges of Nursing. (2006). The essentials for doctoral education for advanced nursing practice. Washington, DC: Author.

(DNP Essentials) (AACN, 2006). In keeping with the two foci for DNP programs identified in the DNP *Essentials* (p. 18), CCNE accredits DNP programs with (1) an advanced practice nursing direct care focus, (2) an aggregate/systems/organizational focus, or (3) both foci (CCNE, 2012, para 2).

Accreditation has traditionally signified quality in curriculum and university resources to achieve the goal of preparing students for the degrees they seek. Students evaluating DNP programs can investigate the accreditation status of the program, as well as the standards of the certifying body to help choose a quality educational experience.

The University of Washington has undertaken a comprehensive approach to DNP program evaluation that includes both program effectiveness and the transition experience described by faculty and students (Kaplan & Brown, 2009). The evaluation process includes not only the traditional benchmarks of grade point average (GPA) retention and graduation rates but also data collected from students and faculty perspectives. Curriculum evaluation is based on successful achievement of the DNP *Essentials* as outlined by the

AACN. Evaluation of the nursing profession's transition to DNP education is explored using both qualitative and quantitative methodology in this comprehensive plan.

Evaluation of the quality of DNP education also involves assessment of the achievement of the *Essentials* of DNP education outcomes by DNP graduates. The Implementation of the DNP Task Force (AACN, 2015a) emphasizes that DNP programs must demonstrate that the graduate has attained all of the DNP *Essentials* outcomes. Evaluation tools such as the *Self-Assessment Tool–Competency Assessment for Practicum Design* found in Chapter 12, the Scholarly Project Toolbox, can be used for documentation of student progression toward attaining the DNP *Essentials* throughout the curriculum. Competency-based evaluation for the DNP-prepared nurse practitioner (NP) that aligns with the AACN DNP *Essentials* has also been addressed by the National Organization of Nurse Practitioner Faculties (NONPF). NONPF has developed a DNP Nurse Practitioner Toolkit for programs that have NP tracks to address specific knowledge, skills, and attitudes students should possess at the culmination of an educational program, including scientific foundation, leadership, quality, practice inquiry, information technology literacy, policy, health delivery system, and ethical and independent practice competencies (NONPF, 2013).

Another process for tracking the growth and development of DNP education and outcomes was created by an organization dedicated to enhancing the caliber of the DNP graduate. Doctors of Nursing Practice, Inc. was founded in 2006 by a group of DNP students at the University of Tennessee Health Science Center College of Nursing in Memphis, Tennessee. An online discussion about the growth and needs of the DNP-prepared professional began in 2005 during an assignment for one of the first courses in the program. Issues of sharing and growing as a group were discussed. There were less than 10 universities offering the DNP degree at the time, and the classmates recognized that, as a cohort, there were few colleagues nationally to connect to and share insights and challenges associated with this degree. In the fall of 2006, during an Advanced Leadership class, classmates agreed to develop a business plan with the mission of enhancing the DNP degree. This plan led to the development and implementation of DNP, Inc.

The mission of DNP, Inc. is to improve healthcare outcomes by promoting and enhancing the doctoral-prepared nursing professional.

The organization is dedicated to:

- providing accurate and timely information
- supporting, developing, and disseminating professional practice innovation

- collaborating in a professional manner that demonstrates universal respect for others, honesty, and integrity in communications
- responding with open discussions and dialogues that promote the evolution of advanced nursing practice and the growth of the DNP degree.

In 2010, DNP, Inc. began collecting data regarding DNP outcomes and education via the first national DNP outcomes survey. The goal of the initial surveys was to determine the *state of the practice* of DNP graduates and collect information about existing DNP programs in universities and colleges. In 2015, an updated DNP Practice Outcomes Survey was developed by DNP, Inc. to capture the perceptions of DNP graduates regarding their practice after earning the degree. Over 850 DNP graduates responded; over 90% were graduates of MSN to DNP programs. See **Table 16-1** for the characteristics of the survey respondents.

The questions in the 2015 DNP Practice Outcomes Survey addressed demographic data, and reports of practice activities, including dissemination of DNP-prepared nurses work since graduation. The 2015 DNP Practice Outcomes Survey graduate respondents clearly indicated a vital educational program outcome: the incorporation of the eight DNP *Essentials* into their practice (DNP, Inc., 2015) (see **Table 16-2**).

Table 16-1 Characteristics of 2015 DNP Practice Outcomes Survey Respondents

Gender (*n* = 683)	Female: 88% (*n* = 603) Male: 10% (*n* = 68) Preferred not to respond: 2% (*n* = 12)
Degree program entry (*n* = 683)	MSN-DNP: 94% (*n* = 639) BSN-DNP: 6% (*n* = 44)
DNP program track (*n* = 778)	APRN track: 61.4% (*n* = 478) Health Systems Leadership/Administration: 15.4% (*n* = 120) Education in academia: 9.5% (*n* = 74) Public Health: 2.4% (*n* = 19) Education in a healthcare system: 1.8% (*n* = 14) Informatics: 1.8% (*n* = 14) Health policy: 1.8% (*n* = 14) Others not identified: 5.8% (*n* = 45)

MSN, Master of Science in Nursing; DNP, Doctor of Nursng Practice; BSN, Bachelor of Science in Nursing; APRN, advanced practice registered nurses.

Data from 2015 DNP Practice Outcomes Survey, Doctors of Nursing Practice, Inc.

Table 16-2 DNP Practice Outcomes Survey: DNP Graduate Integration/Application of the DNP *Essentials* (*n* = 697)

Please indicate your level of agreement to the following statements using a 4 point likert scale, with 4 indicating strongly agree, 3 indicating agree, 2 indicating disagree and 1 indicating strongly disagree.

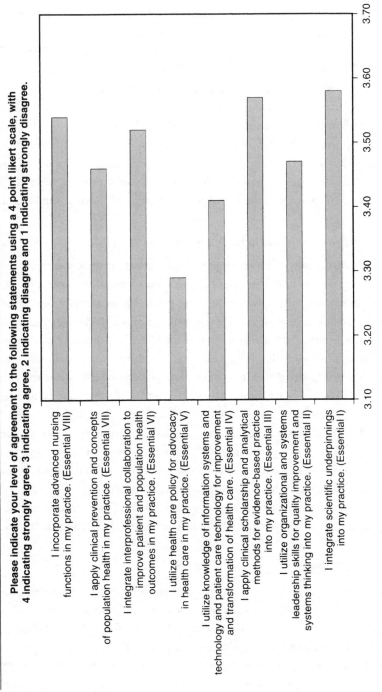

Data from 2015 DNP Practice Outcomes Survey, Doctors of Nursing Practice, Inc.

The results of the survey indicate that the DNP-prepared nurse can clearly articulate the main structural elements of DNP education as it relates to postgraduate practice. Incorporation of the skills and knowledge related to the *Essentials* are critical for the DNP graduate to develop and evaluate models of care delivery that can be sustained at multiple organizational levels in the healthcare system (AACN, 2015a).

Attainment of the *Essentials* of DNP education by DNP students is one of the first steps in evaluating the effectiveness of the degree to prepare nurses for advanced nursing practice roles. Further, by evaluating the *structure* of the DNP degree through various mechanisms, adherence of DNP educational programs to prepare the practice doctorate is assured by accreditation status, program self-evaluation, and commitment to continuous quality improvement of the educational process.

Preparation for Advanced Nursing Practice Roles

Though the majority of DNP programs have tracks to prepare students for established roles such as nurse practitioner, clinical nurse specialist, nurse midwife, and nurse anesthetist, other advanced nursing practice roles are now needed for the practice doctorate to assist in the transformation of health care. Alternative DNP educational tracks are evolving to prepare graduates with specialty knowledge beyond the traditional APRN roles. The AACN conducts a survey of DNP programs periodically to assess the various major areas of study offered across the country (see **Table 16-3**). The data from 2014–2015 AACN (2015b) survey illustrates the numbers of programs, students, and graduates from the APRN majors of study in both post-baccalaureate and post-MSN DNP programs. In addition to preparation for APRN roles, the surveyed DNP schools offer additional programs of study in administration/management, health management and policy, informatics, community/public health, leadership, advanced practice, and other majors. With in-depth preparation for innovative practice roles, the DNP graduate has the skill set to respond to the challenges of leading change in healthcare organizations.

The DNP Project

The DNP Project is also evolving to meet the changing needs of the nursing profession, practice, and society. The scholarly project is the entry into practice scholarship by the nurse with the DNP degree. With the rapid growth of DNP programs since 2004, a wide variation in requirements for the DNP projects was noted across the nation. As a result, the AACN Implementation of the DNP Task Force (2015a) was charged with clarifying the purpose of the DNP final project and the clinical learning expectations for DNP programs to require of their graduates. See Chapter 3 for a summary of the Implementation of the DNP Task Force recommendations

Table 16-3 Enrollment in BSN-MSN DNP Programs by Major Areas of Study

Enrollment (Fall 2014) and Graduations (August 1, 2013, to July 31, 2014) in Doctor of Nursing Practice (DNP) Programs by Major Area of Study (n = 264).

| MAJOR AREA OF STUDY[1] | NUMBER OF SCHOOLS OFFERING MAJOR | POST-BACCALAUREATE DNP | | | | | | GRADUATIONS | |
| | | FULL-TIME | | PART-TIME | | TOTAL | | | |
		NUMBER	Percentage (%)	NUMBER	Percentage (%)	NUMBER	Percentage (%)	NUMBER	Percentage (%)
Nurse-Midwifery	10	67	1.2	29	0.9	96	1.1	19	2.7
Nurse Anesthesia	23	847	15.1	65	2.0	912	10.2	72	10.1
Clinical Nurse Specialist (CNS)	27	42	0.7	56	1.7	98	1.1	7	1.0
Nurse Practitioner (NP)[2]	124	4,419	78.6	2,762	83.9	7,181	80.5	573	80.1
Administration/Management	22	33	0.6	31	0.9	64	0.7	0	
Informatics	4	11	0.2	4	0.1	15	0.2	4	0.6
Community Health/Public Health	14	25	0.4	35	1.1	60	0.7	10	1.4

(Continued)

Table 16-3 Enrollment in BSN-MSN DNP Programs by Major Areas of Study (*Continued*)

Enrollment (Fall 2014) and Graduations (August 1, 2013, to July 31, 2014) in Doctor of Nursing Practice (DNP) Programs by Major Area of Study (*n* = 264).

POST-BACCALAUREATE DNP

MAJOR AREA OF STUDY[1]	NUMBER OF SCHOOLS OFFERING MAJOR	FULL-TIME NUMBER	Percentage (%)	PART-TIME NUMBER	Percentage (%)	TOTAL NUMBER	Percentage (%)	GRADUATIONS NUMBER	Percentage (%)
Leadership	34	41	0.7	159	4.8	200	2.2	7	1.0
Advanced Practice	14	114	2.0	125	3.8	239	2.7	22	3.1
Other Majors	6	24	0.4	11	0.3	35	0.4	1	0.1
Major Area Not Specified	19	0		16	0.5	16	0.2	0	
TOTAL		*5,623*		*3,293*		*8,916*		*715*	

POST-MASTER'S DNP

		FULL-TIME NUMBER	Percentage (%)	PART-TIME NUMBER	Percentage (%)	TOTAL NUMBER	Percentage (%)	GRADUATIONS NUMBER	Percentage (%)
Nurse-Midwifery	12	4	0.1	7	0.1	11	0.1	8	0.3
Nurse Anesthesia	24	40	1.3	49	0.8	89	0.9	35	1.5

Functional or professional role		n	%	n	%	n	%	n	%
Clinical Nurse Specialist (CNS)	31	24	0.8	95	1.5	119	1.3	29	1.2
Nurse Practitioner (NP)[2]	125	675	21.3	1,683	26.8	2,358	25.0	708	30.1
Administration/Management	44	257	8.1	425	6.8	682	7.2	170	7.2
Health Management & Policy	2	9	0.3	1	0.0	10	0.1	2	0.1
Informatics	7	1	0.0	13	0.2	14	0.1	2	0.1
Community Health/Public Health	20	46	1.5	86	1.371	132	1.4	16	0.681
Leadership	82	571	18.0	1,584	25.3	2,155	22.8	550	23.4
Education	7	46	1.5	81	1.3	127	1.3	36	1.5
Advanced Practice	37	325	10.3	463	7.4	788	8.4	263	11.2
Other Majors	14	116	3.7	139	2.2	255	2.7	34	1.4
Major Area Not Specified	62	1,050	33.2	1,646	26.2	2,696	28.6	497	21.1
TOTAL	3,164		6,272		9,436		2,350		

[1] Functional or professional role.

[2] Information in this report pertaining to nurse practitioners is the result of a collaborative effort between the American Association of Colleges of Nursing and the National Organization of Nurse Practitioner Faculties.

Note: *n* = number of schools which reported a DNP enrollment and graduations. Percentages may not total 100 due to rounding.

Reproduced from American Association of Colleges of Nursing. (2015b). *2014–2015 Enrollment and graduations in Baccalaureate and graduate programs in nursing.* Washington, DC: Author.

regarding the DNP project. The task force outlined critical recommendations for standardizing the name of the final product as "The DNP Project" and clarified the expectations for the foci, content, and dissemination of DNP projects. The leadership of the AACN took action to standardize expectations for the DNP project with this report. This is a crucial outcome in the evolution of the DNP degree to insure quality and rigor for the final product of DNP education. Continued evaluation of the final deliverable by the DNP student, the DNP project, will be important in the evaluation of this structural element of DNP education.

PROCESS—HEALTHCARE DELIVERY BY THE DNP

> Evaluation of the DNP-prepared nurse in the *process* category will include assessment of healthcare delivery by the DNP graduate.

Innovative Advanced Practice Roles

Evaluation of the effectiveness of the DNP-prepared nurse in the *process* category will include assessment of health care delivery by the DNP graduate. Currently, the roles of the nurse in advanced practice are varied, ranging from the traditional APRN clinical roles to administrative roles. The DNP graduate is employed in a variety of settings including academic, hospital, and ambulatory clinical positions as well as nontraditional settings such as governmental/military, business, and private consulting firms (AACN, 2015b) (see **Table 16-4**).

Not only will the current advanced nursing practice roles assumed by the DNP graduate require evaluation but the emerging, innovative roles such as the advanced practice informatics nurse and advanced practice policy nurse will also require scrutiny for quality of care delivered and impact on outcomes. Delivery of care, via whatever role is assumed by the DNP graduate in new and traditional types of organizations, needs to be assessed for use and generation of evidence-based science as well as effectiveness in improving outcomes.

To explore the evolving roles of DNP-prepared nurses, Clark and Allison-Jones (2011) surveyed recent graduates regarding their practice environments and organizational factors that impact their roles. The graduates confirmed that their practices had changed with incorporating DNP competencies of evidence-based practice utilization, clinical leadership, advanced practice clinician, and change agency. Even if the DNP graduates were in faculty roles as educators, they were maintaining a clinical role as well. However, the acceptance of the DNP-prepared nurse in both academic and research environments was identified as a concern as the unique contributions of the DNP-prepared nurse continue to evolve.

Though the recommendations from the Implementation of the DNP Task Force (2015a) state that DNP programs are not to focus on preparing the nurse educator role, the nurse with a practice doctorate has a critical presence in nursing education. See Table 16-4 for numbers of DNP graduates accepting faculty positions in colleges of nursing (AACN, 2015b). Nursing is a *practice profession* that requires educators with nursing practice expertise to educate and mentor future nurses at all educational levels. All doctorally prepared nurses, including research doctorates, should have additional training in the pedagogy of teaching as the discipline of education encompasses an entirely separate body of knowledge and competence (AACN, 2015a).

Table 16-4 Employment Commitments of Doctor of Nursing Practice Graduates

Employment Commitment	DNP Graduates	
	Number	Percentage (%)
Faculty position: School/College of Nursing	400	13.1
Faculty position: Other type of school/college	9	0.3
Post-Doctoral Fellowship	2	0.1
Hospital clinical position	502	16.4
Hospital administrative or executive position	216	7.0
Ambulatory (nonhospital) clinical position	533	17.4
Ambulatory (nonhospital) administrative or executive position	33	1.1
Private consultation or consulting firm	18	0.6
Federal or state governmental agency	40	1.3
Military	37	1.2
Business or industry	13	0.4
No employment commitment	80	2.6
Other	77	2.5
Do not know	1,105	36.1
TOTAL	3,065	

Note: Percents may not total to 100.0 due to rounding.

Reprinted with permission from the American Association of Colleges of Nursing. (2015). The doctor of nursing practice: Current issues and clarifying recommendations. Retrieved from: http://www.aacn.nche.edu/aacn-publications/white-papers/DNP-Implementation-TF-Report-8-15.pdf

Innovative Healthcare Delivery Through Evidence-Based Practice

Changes in practice related to healthcare delivery were assessed in DNP, Inc.'s 2015 Practice Outcomes Survey of DNP graduates (see **Table 16-5**). DNP graduates responded that they are better able to incorporate the following activities in their roles as a practice doctorate more often since obtaining their degree:

- Translate evidence into new practice initiatives
- Incorporate evidence into their practice
- Incorporate health promotion and disease prevention
- Develop, implement and/or evaluate practice initiatives.

These practice initiatives by DNP graduate respondents occurred for most while participating in and/or leading interdisciplinary teams. These are important expectations of the practice doctorate in transforming health care. Recognition of the value of DNP graduates was reflected in the 2015 DNP Practice Outcomes survey, with over 43% of respondents indicating that they had experienced an increase in salary with the same or different employer. These important changes in areas of practice will need to be addressed in future surveys to assess both post-BSN and post-master's-prepared DNP graduate effectiveness as these practitioners develop healthcare delivery innovations.

However, the reported ability to apply evidence to practice by the respondents in the 2015 DNP Practice Outcomes Survey cannot be minimized. The number of respondents reporting increased skills in evidenced-based practice is important and reflective of the continuing potential for improving healthcare outcomes as a result of this skill learned as a DNP student. These changes in practice outcomes by the DNP graduate are also reflective of achievement of the goals of the Institute of Medicine's (2003) call for improved healthcare professional educational competencies to impact and transform care, signaling the nursing profession's ability to prepare qualified practitioners responsive to healthcare challenges now and in the future.

OUTCOMES—THE IMPACT OF THE DNP-PREPARED NURSE ON PATIENTS, SYSTEMS, POPULATIONS, AND POLICY

> The ultimate goal of the practice doctorate is to improve *outcomes*.

The ultimate goal of the practice doctorate is to improve *outcomes*. The type of outcomes to be evaluated include how DNP-prepared nurses affect patients and their care, how DNP-prepared nurses affect health policy, how DNP-prepared nurses improve care at

Table16-5 Changes in DNP Practice (*n* = 697)

Since earning your DNP degree, please indicate how often you engage in the following compared to prior to earning your DNP degree, using the 4 point likert scale, with 4 indicating considerably more often, 3 indicating more often, 2 indicating slightly more often, 1 indicating no change.

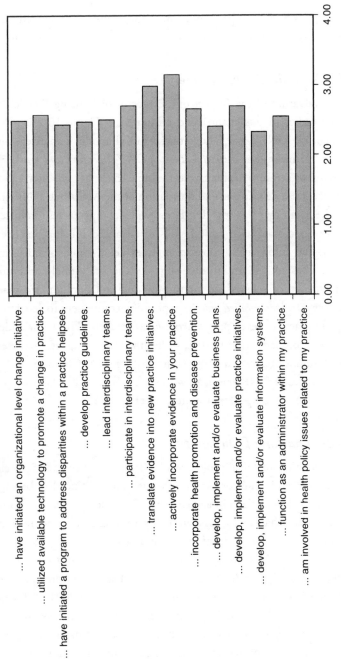

Data from 2015 DNP Practice Outcomes Survey, Doctors of Nursing Practice, Inc.

the systems level to improve outcomes, and how DNP-prepared nurses improve the quality of care delivered to populations to improve health outcomes.

The Actualized DNP Model

The Evaluation of the Impact of the Doctor of Nursing Practice model introduced earlier in this chapter and illustrated in Figure 16-2 is a framework to evaluate the DNP *degree*. The Actualized DNP model is an extension of this process in examining the *critical features of DNP education and practice that produce outcomes* to improve health care at multiple levels. See Chapter 4, Scholarship in Practice, for a description and illustration of the Actualized DNP model.

The attainment of the DNP *Essentials* competencies produces a nursing practice doctorate with critical skills in advanced nursing practice, leadership, policy, and informatics who can apply evidence-based practice in the clinical arena. Through the use of leadership skills in traditional and innovative roles, implementation science and interprofessional collaboration, the practice doctorate uses an *evidence-based practice* application component to generate new knowledge in practice, developing *practice-based evidence*. This is the added value that the DNP-prepared nurse brings to health care to impact outcomes in patient, population, systems, and policy (Burson, Moran, & Conrad, 2016).

Examples of DNP graduates with their roles, DNP project titles, and impact on practice outcomes are illustrated in **Table 16-6**.

Dissemination of Outcomes

Dissemination of DNP project results is critical to impacting health care outcomes. Dissemination of the project outcomes will need to become more systematic to close the gap in evidence-based practice implementation at the point of care. See Chapter 15, Disseminating the Results, for more information on communicating the results of the DNP project.

As more DNP graduates enter the workforce equipped with this skill set and knowledge of practice inquiry, the impact on improving outcomes with evidence-based practice has continued to grow. From 2001–2012, DNP authors published over 300 papers in 59 journals (Broome, Riner, & Allum, 2013). The publications included practice and patient-focused database papers, evaluation of clinical interventions and evidence-based practice guidelines, clinical teaching, and organizational/systems improvement studies. A more recent analysis of publication activity was conducted by Redman, Pressler, Furspan, & Potempa (2014) that found over 690 publications from 417 different authors with a DNP

Table 16-6 DNP Exemplars

Name/Preparation	Role	DNP Project	DNP Practice Impact
Sue Sirianni Nurse Practitioner	• Hospital Lead for Sepsis Quality Improvement Project and other QI efforts • Resident and Nursing Education	An Interprofessional Approach to Sepsis Care	• Improved application of evidence • Decreased mortality rate • Decreased costs • Increased collaboration • Saved $1 million – Choose Wisely Campaign
Denise O'Brien Clinical Nurse Specialist	• Perianesthesia nursing quality care	Intraoperative Risk Factors Associated with Pressure Ulcer Development in Critically Ill Patients	• Focused on perioperative outcomes; national and international dissemination • Collaborated with a PhD-prepared faculty member at the University of Michigan-School of Nursing, exploring the development of a clinically useful risk stratification tool to identify patients at risk for development of pressure ulcer intraoperatively and to determine best practices for positioning, padding, and protecting patients from skin injury in the perioperative and perianesthesia setting. • Developed and tested nurse-sensitive outcomes associated with care in the perianesthesia setting
Lisa Fetters Clinical Nurse Specialist	• Director Quality and Patient Safety • Emergency Physicians Medical Group: 35 Emergency Department and 8 Urgent Care sites	Fall Risk Factors in Emergency Department (ED) Patients	• Increased patient satisfaction • Increased collaboration, • Improved systems that increase safety • Decreased cost within the ED setting

(Continued)

415

Table 16-6 DNP Exemplars (*Continued*)

Name/Preparation	Role	DNP Project	DNP Practice Impact
Kristel Ray Nurse Practitioner	• Associate Professor	High Fidelity Simulation As A Strategy for Inter-professional Education: A Teaching Innovation Within the Community College	• Development of Interprofessional education using simulation in combination with other technology
Judy Paull Nurse Executive	• Chief Nurse Executive	An Examination of Nurse Caring and Hospital Acquired Pressure Ulcers	• Used program design best practice, capitalized on opportunities to meet population health needs • Drove organizational business objectives to achieve regulatory requirements • Centralized telemetry, which improved efficiency and increased patient safety
Ann Sheehan Nurse Practitioner	• Assistant Dean for Practice	Growing Grassroots Advocacy: Implementation of a Legislative Tracking Tool	• Multidimensional role: university faculty-, student-, and nurse-managed clinic responsibilities. • Strategic planning has resulted in a 60% increase in patient visits and revenue. • State NP organization, President elect
Stephanie Brady Mental Health Clinical Nurse Specialist	• Nurse Executive, Vice President of Care Transitions	The impact of mindfulness meditation on a culture of safety on an inpatient psychiatric unit	• Spearheaded 5 CMS demonstration projects • Was awarded $6 million dollars to evaluate 5 care coordination models (Community Care Transitions, High Intensity Care Model, Patient Care Liaison Role, Telephonic Case Management Program with 24/7 Nurse Rescue Line, Telephonic High Intensity Care Management to reduce readmissions).

Name	Positions	Publications	Achievements
Susan Burke-Bebee Informatics	• Senior Health Informatician • Office of the Assistant Secretary for Planning and Evaluation at the U.S. Department of Health and Human Services (HHS).	Building Health Information Technology Capacity: They May Come but Will They Use It?	• Restructured ambulatory rehabilitation services saving $500,000 • Wrote business plan for Senior Services—resulting in $250,000 additional revenue • Health informatics policy specialist • Part of the original team organizing and facilitating the HHS activities promoting the National Health Information Infrastructure (NHII) leading to the creation of Office of the National Coordinator for Health Information Technology (ONC)
Kim Kuebler Nurse Practitioner	• Associate Professor • Owner, Advanced Disease Concepts LLC • Director, Multiple Chronic Conditions, Resource Center	Comparing perceived knowledge of chronic disease management to quantitative knowledge measurement in a sample of baccalaureate nursing students: Implications for palliative care nursing education	• Principal Investigator: Systematic review to evaluate evidence to support chronic disease, symptom and self-management content in graduate nursing curriculum. • Principal Investigator: National graduate nursing survey queried 800 US nursing programs on self-knowledge and actual knowledge of chronic disease, symptoms and self-management. • Developed the Multiple Chronic Conditions Resource Center—virtual center with the most current evidence to support the care management of patients with symptomatic chronic conditions and policy specific topics

Source: Burson, R., Moran, K., & Conrad, D. (2016). Why hire a DNP? The value-added impact of the practice doctorate. *Journal of Doctoral Nursing Practice, 9*(1).

credential. The DNP-prepared nurse was a solo or first author on 79.5% of the publications. More than half of the articles dealt with clinical practice and included the areas of research, evidence-based guidelines, program evaluation, reviews, case studies, and opinions.

The Implementation of the DNP Task Force (AACN, 2015a) has also recommended that a digital repository for DNP projects be formed to advance nursing practice by archiving and sharing project outcomes. The goal of this repository is to showcase practice outcomes of the DNP-prepared nursing professional in an interactive format. The foundations of this database are in place, yet enhancements are still being developed. Since 2007, DNP, Inc. has continued to collect and catalog DNP project data via their website (http://www.doctorsofnursingpractice.org/resources/dnp-scholarly-projects/). To date, there is no other collection of national data reflecting a listing of DNP projects.

However, evaluating the impact of the DNP-prepared nurse on practice should not be determined solely by the amount of publications, as the literature may not reflect the added value of DNP project outcomes and the contributions by DNP graduates at the organizational, public, and societal level.

Through the 2015 DNP Practice Outcomes Survey, data was obtained related to the dissemination practices of DNP graduates (see **Table 16-7**). Clearly, the dissemination modalities are mostly related to publication, but also include poster and podium presentations, book contributions, and health-related information presentations to the public. These alternative modalities are important avenues that demonstrate the breadth and depth of the practice doctorate impact on health care.

THE IMPACT OF THE DNP GRADUATE IN PRACTICE

Graduates of DNP programs are impacting the nursing profession and the people they serve. Montgomery and Porter-O'Grady (2010) find that "in health care delivery systems, many DNP nurse leaders are disrupting traditional practices by evidencing their value; offering a broader, more integrated perspective on practice or system issues; and using innovation to positively impact patient and system outcomes" (p. 45).

The definitive impact of evaluating the effectiveness of the practice doctorate must come from the practice arena. The Rand Corporation Report (Auerbach, et al., 2014) recommended that the next steps in promoting and evaluating the DNP-prepared nurse are to conduct outcome studies to better understand the impact of DNP graduates on patient care; and secondly to provide outreach data to help employers and healthcare organizations understand the comprehensive competencies and capabilities of DNP-educated nurses.

Table 16-7 2015 DNP Practice Outcomes Survey: Dissemination Activities of DNP Graduates

Indicate what type of dissemination you have been involved in during and after earning the DNP degree (*n* = 688)

	While Earning or after Earning DNP Degree
Published a research article	49.0% (*n* = 337)
Published an evidence-based guidelines article	26.3%% (*n* = 181)
Published an integrative review	13.1% (*n* = 90)
Published a case study	17.6% (*n* = 121)
Presented a poster	88.7% (*n* = 610)
Provided a podium presentation	88.1% (*n* = 606)
Contributed to a book or professional journal	48.3% (*n* = 332)
Authored, edited or contributed to a book	26.0% (*n* = 179)
Provided a health-related information presentation outside of a professional organization	65.0% (*n* = 447)

Data from 2015 DNP Practice Outcomes Survey, Doctors of Nursing Practice, Inc.

The DNP graduate must be able to continually articulate, define, and promote their added value to practice leaders to demonstrate in practice the skill set attained with the DNP degree. To maximize their impact on health care, DNP graduates must reach out and partner with health care leaders, scientists, clinicians, patients, families, and community members. The practice doctorate also must demonstrate the ability to balance the demands of population data with individualized, patient-centered care, connecting research into care systems with an informed local context. Most importantly, the DNP graduate must courageously demonstrate the DNP *Essentials* to move organizations forward. The impact of the DNP-prepared nurse will need continuous and intentional evaluation by the profession. How the DNP graduate will affect patients, populations, systems, and policy will need systematic evaluation focusing on the impact and outcomes realized in practice. The ultimate impact will be the change in how health care is delivered and how the health of society is improved by innovative DNP-prepared nurses practice.

Dr. Lisa Chism was one of the first DNP graduates in the United States. She shares her story of how the DNP *Essentials* are reflected in her daily nursing practice.

A Personal Journey
Lisa Chism, DNP, GNP, BC, NCMP, FAANP

I began researching DNP degree programs in 2005. At the time, there were less than 10 DNP programs in the country. I was the first applicant at Oakland University in Rochester, Michigan, and I began my DNP program in the fall of 2006. It was a pilot program and the first in Michigan. My cohort and I were supported through a wonderful grant provided by the state of Michigan and experienced novel approaches in distance learning. We met for workshops across the state, stayed on campus for a week of concentrated coursework, and participated in Web-based "live" meetings and traditional online coursework. It was a wonderful experience. I met my first mentor in my DNP program, Dr. Morris Magnan, and with his guidance and support I graduated from my program 18 months later.

It was about two months after graduation when I realized that I wasn't sure how to develop my role as a DNP graduate. I figured that if I had questions about my new role, so did others. This notion sparked the idea for a resource I thought was needed for DNP students and graduates. This was my first opportunity to spread my leadership wings and incorporate *Essential II* (Organizational and Systems Leadership for Quality Improvement and Systems Thinking) of the *Essentials of Doctoral Education for Advanced Nursing Practice* (AACN, 2006) into my role as a DNP graduate.

Understanding the importance of interprofessional collaboration *(Essential VI*, Interprofessional Collaboration for Improving Patient and Population Health Outcomes) (AACN, 2006), I consulted with another of my mentors, Dr. Elizabeth Johnston Taylor, regarding the process of writing and publishing a book. Dr. Taylor had published a book on spiritual care and helped me formulate a query letter to send to publishers. This query letter led to a meeting with Jones & Bartlett Learning, and later, a contract. I incorporated *Essential VI* (Interprofessional Collaboration for Improving Patient and Population Health Outcomes) (AACN, 2006) and collaborated with colleagues to contribute chapters and interviews for the project. Through collaboration and leadership, I completed the project and the first edition of

The Doctor of Nursing Practice: A Guidebook for Role Development and Professional Issues was published in May 2009. The third edition of this text was recently published in February, 2015 (Chism, 2016). As the first DNP-related text written by DNP graduates for DNP graduates, this project truly exemplified leadership and collaboration.

I continued to develop my scholarship through regular presentations and guest lectures. I also partnered with my mentor, Dr. Morris Magnan, and published my DNP research project, which included the development and testing of a middle-range nursing theory. For myself and other DNP graduates, completing, publishing, and presenting the DNP project is an example of *Essential III* (Clinical Scholarship and Analytical Methods for Evidence-Based Practice) (AACN, 2006).

As a DNP graduate practicing as a nurse practitioner in a comprehensive breast center, I credit my DNP degree for expanding my perspective regarding my clinical knowledge. I had an interest in menopause and became certified as a menopause practitioner through the North American Menopause Society (NAMS). Developing scientific knowledge related to my practice is an example of *Essential I* (Scientific Underpinnings for Practice) (AACN, 2006). This experience led me to another mentor, Dr. Diane Pace, who is dean of Faculty Practice at the University of Tennessee Health Science Center and immediate past-president of NAMS. Dr. Pace mentored me and invited me to join the Patient Education and Scientific Programming Committees through NAMS. This experience was invaluable and led me to be able to develop *Essential V* (Health Care Policy for Advocacy in Health Care) (AACN, 2006). My work on these committees allowed me to impact policy regarding patient education materials program development and membership in the organization. In October 2015, I was elected to the NAMS Board of Trustees.

My work in menopause also led me to develop a practice dedicated to meeting the needs of women experiencing menopausal symptoms who have cancer or who are at risk for cancer. Through caring for these patients, I recognized the need to care for their sexual health concerns as well. I recently completed a certificate as a sexual health counselor and educator. Currently this dedicated clinic has transitioned to a Menopause and Sexual Health Clinic caring for patients with menopause- or sexual-health-related concerns. I credit my DNP degree for helping me recognize the need for a clinic dedicated to meeting the needs of these patients. This is an example of *Essential VII* (Clinical Prevention and Population Health for Improving the Nation's Health) (AACN, 2006).

Finally, I credit the skills I developed in leadership *(Essential II,* Organizational and Systems Leadership for Quality Improvement and Systems Thinking) (AACN, 2006) through the DNP degree to enable me to develop my current position. I practice within a comprehensive breast center in a clinic called the Women's Wellness Clinic (WWC) staffed by three nurse practitioners. We are the only independent nurse-managed clinic within the organization. I sensed a need for leadership within the clinic and developed a proposal for a Clinical Director position. I approached my nursing leadership with the proposal and received invaluable support. I was fortunate enough to write my own job description and have been in this role for approximately 2 years. I continue to grow within this role and develop additional skills related to the finances and productivity of the WWC clinic.

Seven years after graduating from a DNP program, I realize that my role as a DNP graduate continues to develop. With each year, I gain new perspectives about patient care and solutions to complex, challenging healthcare problems. I offer this advice to graduating DNP students: Take the time to allow yourself to grow and develop. You will need time to actualize your roles as DNP graduates. Be ready to change your perspective and widen your views. You will view health care through a different lens and be challenged in new ways to find new solutions. It is a journey, one most definitively worth taking.

SUMMARY

The practice doctorate in nursing is evolving to meet the needs of the society it serves. Evaluation of this new preparation for nurses at the practice doctorate level requires scrutiny and systematic evaluation to assess its value. One standard of quality assessment includes using the Donabedian approach to evaluate structure, process, and outcomes. Assessment of the DNP degree is needed to determine the quality of education delivered and to produce practitioners who are prepared to deliver high-quality, innovative, evidence-based care. Assessment of the impact of outcomes achieved with patients, populations, systems, and policy is also needed to evaluate the DNP-prepared nurse at multiple levels. This will be an ongoing process that will improve the quality of education and care delivered, as well as impact outcomes for society. It is an exciting time for nursing to take an active part in transforming healthcare. Donabedian (1988) acknowledges the journey with the statement, "I hope it is clear that there is a way, a path worn rather smooth by many who have gone before us. I trust it is equally clear that we have, as yet, much more to learn" (p. 1748).

Key Messages

- The DNP project reflects the culmination of the attainment of the DNP *Essentials*.
- Evaluation of the impact of the DNP-prepared nurse can be framed in terms of structure, process, and outcomes.
- DNP education provides the structure for developing an advanced nursing practice role as well as developing scholarly practice through the completion of the DNP project.
- Innovative healthcare delivery in advanced nursing practice roles is the process through which the DNP-prepared nurse will impact evidence-based practice.
- The impact of DNP practice will be realized in improved policy outcomes, improved patient outcomes, improved population outcomes, and improved system outcomes.

Action Plan—Next Steps

1. Successfully complete your DNP project.
2. Disseminate the results of the project.
3. Use the competencies gained in attaining the *Essentials* of DNP education in an advanced nursing practice role to impact healthcare outcomes.
4. Continually articulate, define, and promote the value-added impact of the DNP-prepared nurse to practice leaders, colleagues, and society.
5. Transform health care!

REFERENCES

American Association of Colleges of Nursing. (2006). *The essentials of doctoral education for advanced nursing practice.* Retrieved from www.aacn.nche.edu/publications/position/DNPEssentials.pdf

American Association of Colleges of Nursing. (2015). *The doctor of nursing practice: Current issues and clarifying recommendations.* Retrieved from: http://www.aacn.nche.edu/aacn-publications/white-papers/DNP-Implementation-TF-Report-8-15.pdf

American Association of Colleges of Nursing. (2015b). *2014–2015 Enrollment and graduations in Baccalaureate and graduate programs in nursing.* Washington, DC: Author.

Auerbach, D., Martsolf, G., Pearson, M., Taylor, E., Zaydman, M., Muchow, A., Spetz, J., & Dower, C. (2014). *The DNP by 2015: A study of the institutional, political, and professional issues that facilitate or impede establishing a Post-Baccalaureate Doctor of Nursing Practice Program.* Retrieved from http://www.aacn.nche.edu/DNP/DNP-Study.pdf

Broome, M. E., Riner, M. E., & Allam, E. S. (2013). Scholarly publication practices of doctor of nursing practice-prepared nurses. *Journal of Nursing Education, 52*(8):429–34.

Brown, M. A. (2011, January). Advancing practice through the DNP capstone. Paper presented at American Association of Colleges of Nursing Doctoral Conference, San Diego, CA.

Burson, R., Moran, K., & Conrad, D. (2016). Why hire a DNP? The value added impact of the practice doctorate. *Journal of Doctoral Nursing Practice, 9*(1).

Chism, L. A. (2016). *The doctor of nursing practice: A guidebook for role development and professional issues.* Sudbury, MA: Jones & Bartlett Learning.

Clark, R. C., & Allison-Jones, L. (2011). The doctor of nursing practice graduate in practice. *Clinical Scholars Review, 4*(2), 71–77.

Commission on Collegiate Nursing Education. (2012). Frequently asked questions on DNP programs and DNP accreditation. Retrieved from http://www.aacn.nche.edu/ccne-accreditation/DNP-FAQs.pdf

Doctors of Nursing Practice, Inc. (2015). 2015 DNP practice outcomes survey.

Donabedian, A. (1988). The quality of care: How can it be assessed? *Journal of the American Medical Association, 260,* 1743–1748.

Fontaine, D. K., & Langston, N. F. (2011). The master's is not broken: Commentary on "The doctor of nursing practice: A national workforce perspective." *Nursing Outlook, 59,* 121–122. doi: 10.1016/j.outlook.2011.03.003

Institute of Medicine. (2003). Health professions education: A bridge to quality. Retrieved from http://www.nap.edu/openbook.php?record_id=10681&page=45

Kaplan, L., & Brown, M. A. (2009). Doctor of nursing practice program evaluation and beyond: Capturing the profession's transition to the DNP. *Nursing Education Research, 30*(6), 362–366.

Montgomery, K. L., & Porter-O'Grady, T. (2010). Innovation and learning: Creating the DNP nurse leader. *Nurse Leader, 8,* 44–47. doi: 10.1016?j.mn/2010.05.001

National Organization of Nurse Practitioner Faculties. (2005). Sample curriculum templates for practice doctorate education. Retrieved from http://www.nonpf.com/associations/10789/files/DNP-NPCurricTemplates0907.pdf

National Organization of Nurse Practitioner Faculties. (2013). DNP NP toolkit: Process and approach to DNP competency based evaluation. Retrieved from: http://www.nonpf.org/?page=27

Redman, R. W., Pressler, S. J., Furspan, P., & Potempa, K. (2014). Nurses in the United States with a practice doctorate: Implications for leading in the current context of health care. *Nursing Outlook, 63*(2), 124–129.

Index

Page numbers followed by *f* and *t* indicate material in figures and tables, respectively.

A

abstract, 254–255
abstractness levels, in nursing theory, 97–98, 97*f*
accreditation, investigating status of program, 402
action (implementation) plan, 293, 294*t*, 330, 335
active voice, 269
Actualized DNP Model, 71, 72*f*, 414
advanced nursing knowledge, 71
advanced nursing practice
  defined, 17, 38, 50, 75
  Essential VIII, 75
  roles of, 39, 400, 410
    preparation for, 406, 407–409*t*
advanced practice registered nurses (APRNs), 18, 39
  Clinical Training Task Force report, 46–49
  model for APRN regulation, 28–29
Affordable Care Act (ACA), 28
AGREE II instrument, 362
Alfredson, Katie, 184–186
American Association of Colleges of Nursing (AACN), 6, 7, 15, 18–19, 44, 49, 64

AACN-AONE principles, 48, 54
  report on APRN education, 46–49
American Medical Association (AMA)
  C-CAT tool, 288*t*
  Manual of Style, 267
American Psychological Association (APA), 250, 382
  format, 270–271
analysis procedures, 265–266
annotated bibliography, 269
appendices, 267–268
application scholarship, 66, 69*t*
areas of interest, 94
article submissions, for publication, 382. *See also* journal submissions
assessment phase, 191, 192*t*
assessments, organizational, 123–124, 162
  tools, 288–289, 288*t*
Associates in Process Improvement, 138
attributes, 106, 107
author guidelines, 390
Authors.jblearning.com, 390

B

bachelor of science in nursing (BSN), 182
balanced scorecard, 293, 295*f*, 354

Benedict, Deonne Brown, 12
Blue Cross Blue Shield of Michigan
        Foundation Student Award, 213
Boyer, Ernest, 6, 63
Brady, Stephanie, 166–167, 416*t*
bricoleur, concept of, 68, 69*t*, 71
budget tools, 297–298
    sample template, 319–320
Burke-Bebee, Susan, 417*t*
Business Source Premier, 120*f*

C

Canadian International Developmental
        Agency, 288*t*
care delivery innovation, 74
CARES tool, 146
caring science, 101
Carper, Barbara A., 101–102
cause and effect diagram. *See* fishbone diagram
Center for Nonprofit Management (CNM)
    organizational assessment tool, 288*t*
Centers for Disease Control and Prevention
        (CDC), 354
certified diabetes educators (CDEs), 70, 74–75
certified nurse-midwife (CNM), 39
certified registered nurse anesthetist
        (CRNA), 39
change management, 214
change theories, 162
    examples of, 163*t*
check sheet, 290, 291*f*
Chi square test, 266*t*
Chism, Lisa, 419–422
CINAHL®, 120*f*
Clark, Roy Peter, 249
client
    acceptance, 338–339
    needs, 335
clinical inquiry, 67, 352
clinical knowledge, 71
clinical nurse specialist (CNS), 39, 47
clinical nursing doctoral preparation,
        36–38

Clinical Practice Model (CPM)
        Framework™, 157, 158*f*
clinical question, 256–257
clinical significance, 266
close-out phase, 339
Cochrane Collaboration/Cochrane Nursing
        Care Network, 120*f*
collaboration
    components in the DNP project, 154–160
    with content experts, 209
    defined, 153
    interprofessional, 154, 156–157
    intraprofessional, 155–156
    successful scholarly project using, 163–167
comma usage, 268
Commission on Collegiate Nursing
        Education (CCNE), 27, 400–402
communication
    monitoring and, 336
    tools, 299–301
communication plan, 300
    sample of, 325
compassion, 332
competency assessment for practicum design,
        227–229, 228*t*, 308–313, 403
concept analysis, 106–108
concept mapping, 289, 314
conceptual framework
    defined, 133
    and theoretical framework, 258–259
conflict management skills, 180
*Consensus Model for APRN Regulation:
        Licensure, Accreditation,
        Certification & Education*
        (report), 39
Consolidated Standards of Reporting Trials
        (CONSORT), 253
construct, use of term, 97
Context-Input-Process-Product model
        (CIPP), 354
*Core Competencies for Interprofessional
        Collaborative Practice* (report), 164
Corker, Michele, 219–220
cost–benefit analysis, 297–298

cost-effectiveness implications, of project, 266

costs, direct and indirect, 260–261, 297

Council for Higher Education Accreditation (CHEA), 27

Crossing the Quality Chasm: A New Health System for the 21st Century (IOM, report), 4, 16, 36, 137, 156

Cumulative Index to Nursing and Allied Health Literature (CINAHL) database, 93, 119, 120*f*

D

data analysis, 366–368

data codebook, 364

data collection
 intervention and, 263–265
 methods, 357–362
 phase, 362–364
 resources for, 362

data entry, 365–366

data management, 364–365

data security, 364

database, defined, 119

declaration of originality, 129

Defining Scholarship for the Discipline of Nursing, AACN, 64

deliverables, 376–377
 determining, 240–242
 project, 333

Deming, W. Edwards, 368

depersonalization, 180

design choice, for DNP project, 348–356

diabetes educators, 70, 74–75

diagnosis phase, of nursing process, 191, 192*t*

direct costs, 260, 297

discovery scholarship, 65, 69*t*

dissemination of project findings
 from evidence-based practice and research to improving health outcomes, 368–369, 375–395, 414, 418

dissemination science. *See* implementation science research

dissertation, defined, 172

diversity, in DNP projects, 356–357

DMAIC (define, measure, analyze, improve, and control)
 process, 296
 strategy, 139

doctor of nursing (ND), 21, 62
 programs, 17–18, 18*f*

doctor of nursing practice (DNP)
 accreditation of DNP programs, 27
 Actualized DNP Model, 71, 72*f*, 414
 becoming expert in (story telling), 31–32
 DNP Inc., 403–404, 418
 "DNP Project," 5, 23–24, 51, 78, 406, 410
 "DNP Project Team," 52
 Essentials, 8–9, 37–38*t*, 39, 73–75, 73*t*, 74*f*, 152–153
 on evidence-based practice (EBP), 62
 exemplars, 415–417*t*
 and PhD, comparing, 40–42, 64, 67, 155–156
 phenomena of interest, examples of, 94*t*
 practice hours, 53–54
 Practice Outcomes Survey, 404–405*t*, 418, 419*t*
 program enrollments, 43*f*, 52, 407–409*t*
 scholar, 4–6
 scholarly project, 6–7, 51, 74*f*, 117–147, 172–173
 Task Force, 20, 49–54, 155, 403, 418
 Tool Kit and a Frequently Asked Questions reference, 20

doctor of nursing practice (DNP) degree, 38
 challenges and opportunities in moving forward with, 22–24
 evaluation of, 399, 401*f*
 evolution of, 16–21
 journey to, 15–32
 national initiatives from AACN and NONPF, 18–21
 opportunities for future, 28–29
 pathways to, 24
 viewpoints relating to, 21–22

doctor of nursing practice (DNP) education
current trends in, 43
essentials of, 39
interprofessional teams and, 153
reports affecting, 44–54
structure, 399–410
doctor of nursing practice (DNP) graduate, 29, 50
impact in practice, 418–422
doctor of nursing practice (DNP) project.
See also practicum; project implementation; proposal, components of
alternative approaches to traditional committee structure, 181–183
approaches, 349–351*t*
assessment tool for, 288–289
change theory, 162–163
choosing faculty mentor and team members, 174–176
collaborating with content experts, 209
components of collaboration in, 154–160
conducting literature search and writing literature review, 118–123, 120*f*, 122*t*
crediting the project team, 184
current views of, 77–78
data analysis, 366–368
data collection, 357–364
data entry, 365–366
data management, 364–365
design choice for, 348–356
development of, 118–136
dissemination of findings, 368–369, 375–395
and dissertation/thesis, differences between, 172–174
diversity in, 356–357
evaluation of, 397–423
evidence-based practice (EBP), 349–351*t*, 355
examples of, 137*f,* 352
formats for, 77
gathering resources for, 152–153

goals, achievement of, 131–132, 165–166, 398–399
healthcare delivery innovation, 143–144
healthcare policy analysis, 144–145
identifying the setting, for practicum, 225–226
implementation, 213–220
coordinating with organizations, 215–216
flowchart, 215*f*
forming the team, 217–218
intervention, 162
preparing the infrastructure, 216–217
project structure, 215
science, 135–136
training the team, 218–219
institutional review board (IRB) approval, 209–212
key stakeholders, 130–131
needs assessment, 125–128
nursing research, 139–141
organizational assessments, 123–124, 162
phase of project development process, 191–192
phenomenon of interest, identification, 92–95
pilot study, 141–142
plan, 192–208, 293, 315–318
policy analysis/evaluation for, 355–356
potential impact of, 76–77
problem statement, 128–130
program development and evaluation, 145–146, 349–351*t*, 354
purpose of, 7, 72–76
quality improvement, 134–135, 137–139
roles and expectations of team members, 176–177
sample outcome evaluation plans, 358–360*t*
scholarship beyond, 78–79
scope of, 132–133, 302
setting the stage for, 244
submitting grant proposal, 212–213
SWOT analysis, 124–125, 125*f*
team meeting, components of, 179

team productivity, enhancement of, 178–181

theory and framework, 133–134

timeline for, 177–178, 302, 304*f*

topic assessment format, 82

types of information needed to completion of, 160–161

doctor of nursing science (DNSc), 61–62

doctoral education, in nursing, 26

doctorate of nursing practice (DrNP), 62

doctorates, types of, 21

Donabedian model, 133–134, 258, 399, 400*f*

E

Eames, Charles, 348

EC as PIE, acronym of, 78

effectiveness, 37*t*, 137

efficiency, 38*t*, 138

80-20 rule, 131

Einstein, Albert, 364

electronic health records (EHRs), 161, 357, 361

elevator speech, 332

Elsevier CPM Framework™, 157–158

emancipatory knowing, 105–106

Emerald Fulltext, 120*f*

Emerson, Ralph Waldo, 13

emotional competence

behavior, 331

defined, 234

empirical knowledge, 102, 103

employment commitments, of DNP graduates, 410, 411*t*

engagement, 66, 69*t*

equitableness, 38*t*, 138

Essentials of Doctoral Education for Advanced Nursing Practice, The (document), 7, 20, 25, 37–38*t*, 40*f*, 49, 55, 173, 402*f*

esthetic knowledge, 102, 103

ethical knowledge, 102, 104–105

evaluation

of DNP project, 397–423

phase, 192*t*

plan, 265, 339

program development and, 145–146, 349–351*t*, 354, 356, 360*t*

tools, 302

of writing skills, 248–251

Evernote, 305*t*, 306

evidence-based practice (EBP), 62, 349–351*t*, 355, 359*t*

employing, 37*t*

healthcare delivery through, 412, 413*t*

Excel, 365

executive summary, 392

experimental design, 260

expert nursing practice, 91

Explain Everything, 305*t*, 307

explanation, of the phenomenon, 129

explication, 65, 69*t*

exploration phase, of knowledge development, 65, 69*t*

Exploring the Cost and Clinical Outcomes of Integrating the Registered Nurse, Certified Diabetes Educator in the Patient-Centered Medical Home (DNP project), 70

F

FADE model, 138

failure mode effects analysis (FMEA), 353

feasibility study. *See* pilot study

feedback, 336

Fetters, Lisa, 415*t*

figures, use of, 286

fishbone diagram, 290–291

flowchart, 294, 296*f*

force field analysis, 298–299

formative and summative evaluations, 26–27

forming stage, 217

free management library tool, 288*t*

Freeman, Bonnie, 146

Future of Nursing: Leading Change, Advancing Health, The (IOM, report), 4, 28, 36, 43, 46, 61, 90

G

grand theories, 98
grant proposal, submitting, 212–213
Grimaldi, Diane, 392–394
guerilla theorizing, concept of, 68, 69*t*

H

health, concept of, 98
health behavior theories, 101
health policy analysis projects, 355–356
Health Professions Education: A Bridge to Quality (IOM, report), 16, 36, 157
Health Resources and Services Administration (HRSA), 134
health services research. *See* implementation science research
healthcare delivery, 410–412, 413*t*
  assessment, by DNP graduate, 410–412
  challenges of, 42
  developing approaches to improvement of, 136
  integration of technologies into, 47
healthcare delivery innovation
  focus, 143
  methods, 143
  other considerations, 143–144
healthcare improvement, IOM recommendations on, 36–38, 137–138
healthcare issues, addressing, 4
healthcare policy analysis
  focus, 144
  methods, 144
  other considerations, 145
healthcare professionals, competencies for, 16, 36, 37–38*t*, 164
healthcare quality, defined, 137
Heer, R., 239
Henderson, Virginia, 67
hidden work of nursing, 91
histogram, 292
human becoming theory, 101
human caring theory, 259

I

impact factor (IF), 383
implementation process, 192*t*, 330–332. *See also* project implementation
implementation science research, 135–136
improvement, model for, 138–139
improvisation, concept of, 68, 69*t*
impulse control, 332
indication of central focus, 129
indirect costs, 260–261, 297
informatics, utilizing, 37–38*t*
information technology tools, 304–305
  to assisting DNP project process, 306–307
  to enhancing DNP project process, 305*t*
  functions and operating systems, 306*t*
innovation
  creation of, 191–192
  healthcare delivery, 143–144
Institute for Healthcare Improvement (IHI), 138
Institute of Medicine (IOM), 15
  aiming for healthcare improvement, 36–38
  Crossing the Quality Chasm: A New Health System for the 21st Century, 4, 16, 36, 137, 156
  DNP degree evolution, 16–21
  To Err Is Human: Building a Safer Health System, 16
  Future of Nursing: Leading Change, Advancing Health, The, 4, 28, 36, 43, 46, 61, 90
  Health Professions Education: A Bridge to Quality, 16, 36, 157
institutional review board (IRB) approval, 128, 141, 209–212
integration scholarship, 65–66, 69*t*
interdisciplinary, concept of, 154
interdisciplinary teams, work in, 37–38*t*
interpersonal relations theory, in nursing, 101
interprofessional
  clinical models, 157–160
  collaboration, 154, 156–157
  concept of, 154
  and leadership resources, 168*t*

interprofessionality, defined, 154
interrater reliability, 263
intervention
    and data collection, 263–265
    implementing, in DNP project, 162
intraprofessional collaboration, 155–156
intrarater reliability, 263
introduction, importance of, 255
iPad, use of, 307
Ishikawa diagram. *See* fishbone diagram
issues log, 301
iThenticate, 391

J

Jensen, Elizabeth, 55–56
Johnson, Maria, 306–307
Journal of Advanced Nursing, 61
journal submissions, 382
    author guidelines, 390
    editor's considerations, 384–385
    executive summary, 392
    finding out percentage of articles chosen
        for publication, 388
    matching the article to the appropriate
        journal and following specific
        guidelines, 388
    online manuscript submission, 391
    other considerations, 391
    plagiarism programs, 391
    points to understand when choosing
        appropriate journal for
        publication, 383–384
    process involved for selecting article for
        publication, 387
    recommendations for new authors
        and rejected manuscripts,
        385–386
    reviewer turnaround time, 387–388
    sending email to editor for status update,
        after 8 weeks, 388
    tips for, 382–394
    views on influx of DNP projects to a
        journal, 389–390

K

key performance indicators (KPIs), 293
key stakeholders, identification of, 130–131,
        334, 335, 338–339
Keynote, 305*t*, 307
knowing, fundamental patterns of, in
        nursing, 101–106, 102*f*, 106*f*
knowledge generation, scholarship and, 62,
        63–64, 66, 69*t*, 76
Kuebler, Kim, 417*t*

L

LACE, acronym, 29
lead-in statement, concept of, 129
leadership
    characteristics of, 331–332
    competencies, 163
    skills, 178
lean methodology, 294–295, 353
learning objectives model, 239*t*
Lenz, Betty, 19
librarians, consultation with, 120
literature review, 118–119, 121, 122*t*,
        257–258
    vs. annotated bibliography, 269
literature search, 119, 120*f*, 121
Logic model, 354
logical argument, 257

M

Magnan, Morris, 420–421
manuscript submissions. *See also* journal
        submissions
    requirements, 382
Marshall, Katherine A., 110–112
McConachie, Angela, 80–81
medication error rate, reducing, 132
MEDLINE, 120*f*
meeting agenda/minutes, 300
    example of, 326
mentoring, 231–234, 237–238
methodology, for project design, 260–261

Michigan Organization of Diabetes
Educators (MODE), 75
Microsoft Excel, 365
middle-range theories, 98
milestones, project, 300
mind mapping, 289–290
mindfulness, 332
meditation, 166–167
"model for improvement" framework,
138–139
modifiers, 268
monitoring
process, 335–336
and troubleshooting, 338
moral knowledge, 102
motivation, 336
multiple mentoring model, 233

N

National Center for Healthcare Leadership
(NCHL), 163
NCHL Health Leadership Competency
Model™, 164f
National Institute of Nursing Research
(NINR), 140
National League for Nursing (NLN), 25
National League for Nursing Accrediting
Commission (NLNAC), 27
National Organization of Nurse Practitioner
Faculties (NONPF), 403
Practice Doctorate Task Force, 18–19
national registries, 357, 362
needs assessment, conducting, 125–128
Nightingale, Florence, 67, 366
nonexperimental design, 260
norming stage, of team development,
217–218
North American Menopause Society
(NAMS), 421
nouns/pronouns, use of, 269
Nurse Author Editor (newsletter), 383
nurse practitioners (NPs), 12, 39, 47, 403

nursing informatics, 161
nursing phenomenon, 92
nursing practice, 411t
complex nature of, 89–90
expertise of, 90–91
history of scholarship and, 61–62
nursing process, 190f
nursing research
defined, 139
expertise, 141
institutional review board (IRB)
review, 141
research design, 140–141
research focus, 140
research method, 140
research question, 140
time and resources, 141
nursing theory
foundational tenets, 108–109
levels of abstraction in, 97–98
phenomenon of interest and, 97–100
practice scholarship and, 67–72
NVivo, 367

O

objectives of the project, 133
O'Brien, Denise, 383–389, 415t
Oermann, Marilyn H., 383–389
online manuscript submission, 391
operationalization phase, of project
implementation, 335
optimization, 66, 69t
organizational assessments, 123–124, 162
tools, 288t
Outcome and Assessment Information
Set (OASIS) Start of Care
document, 111
outcomes
DNP-prepared nurse impact on patients
and populations, 134, 399, 412,
414–418, 419t
overcoming, concept of, 107

P

p value test, 266*t*
Pace, Diane, 421
Pareto's principle, 131, 334
participants, choosing, 261–262
passionate optimism, 332
patient-centered care, 37*t*, 138
patient-centered diabetes project, 73
patient-centered medical home (PCMH)
    strategies, 75, 185
"patterns gone wild," 105
patterns of knowing, 101–106, 102*f*, 106*f*
Paull, Judy, 416*t*
Pearson's product-moment correlation, 266*t*
perception, 103
performing stage, 218
perianesthesia nursing, 212
personal humility, 332
personal knowledge, 102, 103–104
personnel recruitment, 335
phenomenon
    assessment worksheet, 109*t*
    concept analysis, 106–108
    defined, 92
    foundational tenets of nursing knowledge,
        108–109
    identification, 92–93, 96*f*
    of interest, for DNP project, 92–95
    looking through different lens, 100–109
    theoretical framework, 100–101
    using nursing theory to exploring,
        97–100
    ways of knowing, 101–106
Physician Health Organization (PHO), 74
PICO (Population, Intervention,
        Comparison, and Outcomes)
        approach, 140, 256
pilot study
    defined, 141–142
    expertise, 142
    focus, 142
    institutional review board (IRB)
        review, 142

    methods and design, 142
    time and resources, 142
plagiarism, 250, 271
    programs, 391
Plan-Do-Study-Act (PDSA) model, 139,
        220, 260, 353
planning, project
    disseminating, 299–301
    identifying the setting, 193–208
    management support, 333–334
    mission, 334
    operationalizing, 335–339
    schedule, 334–335
    template for, 293, 315–318
planning phase, 192*t*
Planning Pro, 307
podium presentations and posters, 379–381
Polarity Thinking™, 159*t*
policy analysis/evaluation, 355–356. *See also*
        healthcare policy analysis
portfolios, 381
Position Statement on the Practice Doctorate in
        Nursing, AACN, 44, 49
poster presentations, 380–381
PowerPoint presentation, 378–379
practice doctorate (DNP)
    defining, 36–40
    in nursing, 15, 17, 18–19, 21, 400
    and research doctorates (PhD/DNS),
        40–42, 50, 64, 67, 155–156
practice-focused doctoral programs, 25
    benefits of, 39
    graduates of, 50
    purpose of, 36
practice inquiry, 20
practice scholarship, 6, 76, 77
    and nursing theory, 67–72
practice theories, 98
practicum
    choosing a mentor, 231–234, 237–238
    closure of, 244
    competency assessment for, 227–229,
        228*t*, 308–313

practicum (*continued*)
    deliverables, determining, 240–242
    developing objectives for, 238–240
    evaluation, 244
    format for tracking the hours, 243*t*
    hours, in practice setting, 230–231
    implementation of, 243
    potential setting of DNP project for, 225–226
    presenting the plan, 242–243
    purpose, 224–225
    setting the stage for DNP project, 244
    site agreements, 230, 244
primary sources, 121
problem, defined, 128
problem statement, 255–256, 291*f*
    development of, 128–130
process
    flowchart, 294, 296*f*
    healthcare delivery by DNP, 134, 399, 410–412, 413*t*
process improvement tools, 294–297
professional writing, 248–251
program development and evaluation, 349–351*t*, 354, 356, 360*t*
    addressing healthcare needs, 145
    focus, 145
    methods, 145
    other considerations, 146
project, DNP. *See* doctor of nursing practice (DNP) project
project abstracts, 379
project aim/purpose, 256
project budget, 297
project charter
    sample of, 321–324
    tool, 299–300
project design
    analysis, 265–266
    APA format, 270–271
    appendices, 267–268
    citing references, 267
    intervention and data collection, 263–265
    methodology, 260–261
    participants, 261–262

    setting, 262
    significance/implications, 266–267
    tools, 262–263
    writing tips, 268–271
project goals, determination of, 131–132
project implementation
    balancing priorities, 330*f*
    barriers and issues, 336–337
    client acceptance, 338–339
    client's needs, 335
    close-out phase, 339
    communication, 336
    components of implementation success, 332
    factors involving in, 333–339
    feedback, 336
    key factors to improving performance during, 337–338
    mission, 334
    monitoring process, 335–336
    operationalization phase, 335
    personnel recruitment, 335
    planning, 333–339
    process, 330–332
    schedule, 334–335
    technical skills, 335
    top management support, 333–334
    troubleshooting, 338
    using leadership skills, 331–332
project management, 214
    tools, 292–294, 295, 296. *See also* communication, tools
project meeting agenda and minutes, 300
    example of, 326
project milestones, 300
project schedule, 301, 303*t*, 334–335
project scope, 132–133, 302
project status report, 300–301
    example of, 327
project time worksheet, 301, 302*t*
project timeline, 177–178, 302, 304*f*
proposal, components of. *See also* writing a proposal; project design
    abstract, 254–255
    clinical question, 256–257

conceptual and theoretical framework,
    258–259
introduction, 255
literature review, 257–258
problem statement, 255–256
purpose of project, 256
title, 253–254
proposal template, 274–286
public presentations, 377–381
podium presentations and posters,
    379–381
PowerPoint pointers, 378–379
*Publication Manual of the American
    Psychological Association* (APA),
    250, 382
PubMed, 119, 120*f*
purpose of project, 256

Q

qualitative inquiry, 353
quality, defined, 137
quality improvement (QI)
applying, 37–38*t*
approaches, 349–351*t*, 352, 353,
    358–359*t*
competence in, 353
data collection methods in, 357
defined, 134
focus, 138
methods, 138–139
opportunities, 356
organization's structure, process, and
    outcome of care, 134–135. *See also*
    Donabedian model
other considerations, 139
projects, in health care, 137, 210
stages of, 296
quasi-experimental approach, 352–353
questioning, 180

R

RAND Corporation, 15, 22, 44, 418
Ray, Kristel, 416*t*

references
citing, 267
types, 284
reflect and learn tool, 288*t*
reflection in action, 106
registered nurses (NPs), 17
registries, 357
and surveys, 362
reliability of the instrument, 262–263
research
defined, 139
design, 140–141
focus, 140
method, 140
question, 140
research doctorates (PhD/DNS) and practice
    doctorate (DNP), 40–42, 50, 64,
    67, 155–156
reverse mentoring, 233
rigor
concept of, 25
of DNP project, 77–78
risk assessment
matrix, 298*t*
tools, 298–299
root cause analysis (RCA), 353
rough draft, 252

S

SafeAssign, 391
safety, 37*t*, 137
scatter plot, 292, 293*f*
schedule, project, 301, 303*t*, 334–335
scheduling tools, 301–302, 303*t*, 304*f*
scholar, defined, 7
scholarship
defined, 60–61
evolution, 62–65
history of, and nursing practice, 61–62
knowledge generation and, 62, 63–64,
    66, 69–70*t*, 76
in practice, 59–83
practice scholarship and nursing theory,
    67–72

scholarship (*continued*)
    process of completing scholarly project,
        80–81
    recommendations, 79–81
    types of, 65–67, 69–70*t*
Scholarship Reconsidered: Priorities of the
        Professoriate (book), 63
"scope creep," 336
self-assessment tool
    competency assessment for practicum
        design, 289, 308–313, 403
self-awareness, 331–332
self-plagiarism, 251
semicolon/period usage, 268
Sheehan, Ann, 416*t*
Shewhart cycle model, 139
Sigma Theta Tau library, 24
Sirianni, Sue, 415*t*
situation-specific theory, 98–99
Six Sigma, 139, 260, 296, 353
skills
    conflict management, 180
    leadership, 178, 331–332
    technical, 335
    writing, 248–251
SMART acronym, 240
Soldier Readiness Process (SRP), 219
stakeholders, 130–131, 334, 337,
        338–339
Standards for Quality Improvement
        Reporting Excellence (SQUIRE)
        guidelines, 253
Statistical Analysis System (SAS), 365
Statistical Package for the Social Sciences
        (SPSS), 365
Stein, Jeanne, 30–32
storming stage, 217
Strengthening the Reporting of
        Observational studies in
        Epidemiology (STROBE)
        guidelines, 253
strengths, weaknesses, opportunities,
        and threats (SWOT) analysis,
        124–125, 125*f*

structure, of DNP education, 134–135,
        399–410
surveys and registries, 362
sustainability, 267
SWOT analysis, 124–125
    model, 125*f*

T

t statistic test, 266*t*
table of contents, template of, 276
Taylor, Elizabeth Johnston, 420
teaching, 70*t*
team leader, 65
10-10 rule, 380
theoretical framework, 134, 259
theory, research, and practice
    relationship between, 64*f*, 99*f*
thesis, defined, 172
threat, removing/reducing
        the perceived, 180
timeline, project, 177–178, 302, 304*f*
timely care, 37*t*, 138
title, choosing, 253–254
To Err Is Human: Building a Safer Health
        System (IOM, report), 16
toolbox, utilization of, 288–306
    assessment tools, 288–289
    budget tools, 297–298
    communication tools, 299–301
    connecting relationships and organizing
        thoughts, 289–290
    defining the problem, 290–292
    evaluation tools, 302
    information technology tools, 304–306
    process improvement tools, 294–297
    project management tools, 292–294,
        295, 296
    risk assessment tools, 298–299
    scheduling tools, 301–302, 303*t*, 304*f*
Tor, Carl G., 365
Tracy, Mary Fran, 383–390
tricky words, use of, 269
troubleshooting, and monitoring, 338

U

University of Arizona College of Nursing, 17
University of Washington, 20, 402
U.S. Department of Education (USDE), 27

V

Vanderbilt University School of Nursing
    (VUSN), 17, 26
verbal defense, 377
vulvodynia, care for, 56

W

ways of knowing, in nursing theory, 101–106
Wesorick, Bonnie, 157, 160
White Paper, 334, 337
who, framework of, 155

Willmarth-Stec, Melissa, 304
women with vulvodynia, improving
    the care for, 56
Worgess, Christina, 339–341
work breakdown structure, 302, 304*f*
writing a proposal, 248, 251
    approaching the first draft, 252
    developing the outline, 252
    tips, 268–271
    writing resources, 253
writing cinematically, concept of, 249
Writing for Publication in Nursing, 383
writing skills, evaluation of, 248–251
written manuscripts, 382

Z

Zajac, Lisa, 234–237